Tongue Diagnosis

Visible Responses to Pathology

Includes Tongue Diagnosis for all the Channels of Acupuncture

includes tongue diagnosis for all the
channels of acupuncture

TONGUE DIAGNOSIS

VISIBLE RESPONSES TO PATHOLOGY

ANN CECIL-STERMAN

DIAGRAMS AND ILLUSTRATIONS BY CODY DODO

Classical Wellness Press

www.anncecilsterman.com

First edition

Disclaimer and Note: The information presented in this book relates to the subject of what is known in the Eastern Medical Community as "Traditional Chinese Medicine" and "Classical Chinese Medicine" and is intended solely for use by Licensed Acupuncturists and students under the supervised study of acupuncture through an accredited educational institution. Under no circumstances is the information in this work to be used or acted upon by an unlicensed, untrained, or unsupervised individual. The Author and Publisher do not advocate or endorse self-diagnosis, self-medication, or treatment by unlicensed individuals under any circumstances. Chinese Medicine is a regulated profession and subject to the jurisdiction of the individual states as well as local and national professional and accrediting organizations. Individuals are strongly encouraged to perform their own due diligence and seek guidance and referrals from these organizations or other licensed professionals.

The teachings in this book are based on the oral tradition transmitted through the gracious generosity of my teacher, Daoist Master, Dr. Jeffrey Yuen. I have made interpretations, extrapolations, connections, additions, deductions, inferences, orderings, and, as in all my books, constructed piece-by-piece all the protocols contained in this book. This book contains many fine points developed through many years of clinical practice. May this book serve all those who practice and receive the precious gift of Chinese Medicine. Any mistakes are mine. A.C.S.

Cover design, book design, graphic design, and diagrams by Cody Dodo

ISBN: 978-0-9837720-2-6

By the Same Author

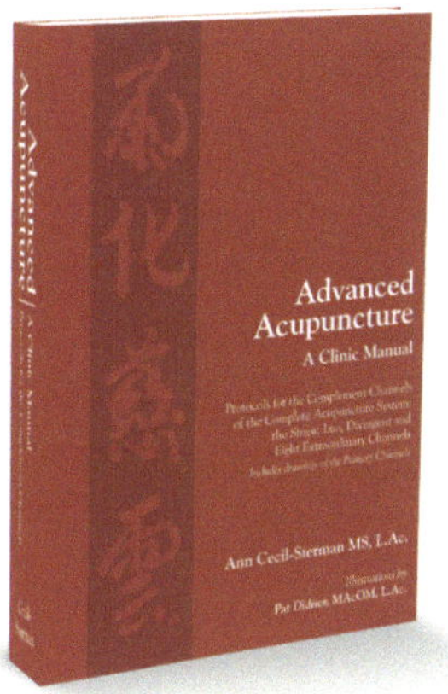

Advanced Acupuncture, A Clinic Manual

Protocols for the Complement Channels of the Complete Acupuncture System: the Sinew, Luo, Divergent and Eight Extraordinary Channels.

Classical Wellness Press, 2012, 2018 (2nd Ed)

Currently a required or recommended text in many acupuncture schools.

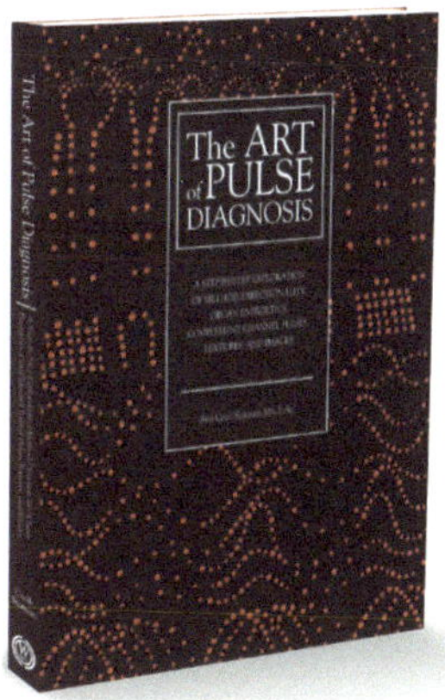

The Art of Pulse Diagnosis

A Step-by-Step Exploration of Method, Directionality, Organ Energetics, Complement Channel Pulses, Textures and Images.

Classical Wellness Press, 2015

Illustrations of the Complete Acupuncture System: the Sinew, Luo, Divergent, Eight Extraordinary and Primary Channels

Classical Wellness Press, 2014

(This is a companion volume to *Advanced Acupuncture, A Clinic Manual.*)

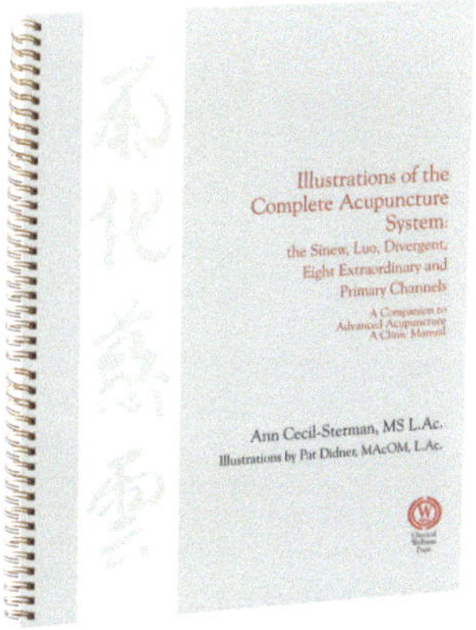

And introducing...

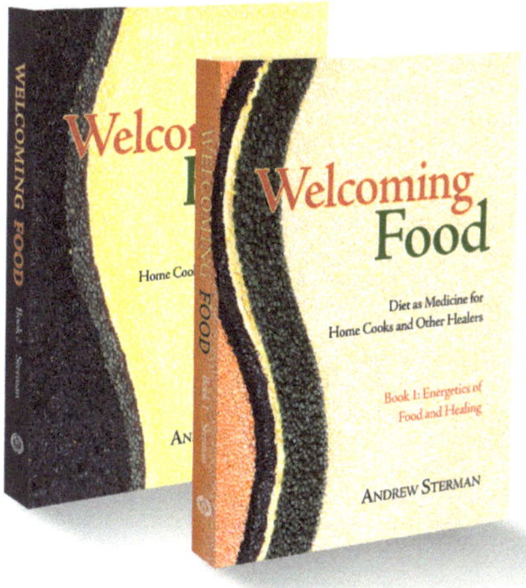

Welcoming Food: Diet as Medicine for Home Cooks and Other Healers

2 volumes

by Andrew Sterman

Classical Wellness Press, 2020

For Ravi

this tongue is
conversation
demonstrating
tasting

(don't think about it
so much!)

the tasting
and not the speaking

meaning
seeing feeling

touching
then sending

(not looking
so hard for it!)

rendering
being the feeling
talking
to seeing

placing meaning

open

glancing feeling

(touching seeing!)

—**Martha Oatis**

§

Contents

Foreword

In your hands you hold a remarkable book. Please don't be fooled by familiar thoughts—this isn't just another work on tongue diagnosis. In reality it's so much more.

When I received the manuscript from Ann, it came with a handwritten note stating that her aim in writing the book was "to eschew the idea that tongue appearances need to be memorized in order for tongue diagnosis to be learned." I was immediately captivated by the vision set out in these words.

I first met Ann during her teaching cycle of Advanced Acupuncture in Barcelona, in the Spring of 2014. There, amidst the bustling throng of downtown Barcelona—a stone's throw from Gaudi's Basílica de la Sagrada Família—something very special was happening. A medicine that had been meticulously so preserved—refined through cultivation, and incubated through the millennia—was being revealed by a softly spoken lady with razor sharp precision.

The resonance was strong, deep and, in today's troubled times, immensely relevant.

For those seeking a Classically trained teacher who is both faithful to the ancient traditions and highly innovative in adapting it for modern times, you're in the right place. Ann seamlessly blends classical scholarship with effective clinical practice. As all clinicians know, any high brow philosophy or irrelevant, obscure practice will not stand in the crucible of the clinic. There, having been counselled and prescribed to, all that matters to the patient is whether they feel better.

Everything in this work is faithful to the lineage of the author's esteemed teacher, but its real power is that it's also faithful to Ann's lived experience. It speaks directly to the times in which she lives and the people that she serves.

So to the subject of the work, Tongue diagnosis. Early in the text, Ann illustrates the application of this astonishing medicine through several case histories. She then follows with this passage: "The tongue is a marvellous window into the way the body responds to pathology. As a diagnostic tool we can use it to understand the multitude of responses the body can make. The tongue shows us where the body feels it can and cannot reach to enact those responses."

In the Classical traditions of Chinese medicine, pulse taking is the gold standard that any physician worth their salt needs to become proficient in. The layers and nuances of the animating presence of spirit on the physiology of the body—and its struggles with pathology—are all revealed to a still and receptive clinician. Ann has often remarked that you should be able to accurately and appropriately administer treatment to anyone after carefully listening to their pulse. When studying pulse taking with her, she takes you on an amazing tour of the landscape of the pulses—often taking a long time to deeply listen to all the layers, and noting the information that is yielded. Indeed her perception of pulses is so attuned that she creates paintings of them—capturing the images that they evoke in her imagination.

Here, in this remarkable text, the author conveys the precision and real life accuracy of a well honed pulse practice when applied to tongue diagnosis. No appearance of the tongue or symptom is left unaccounted for. Ann shows the reader how to deduce the clinical condition of anyone—even by a remote consultation—and prepare an appropriate treatment strategy by carefully examining what the tongue reveals. In some ways this is more accessible and swifter to learn than the pulses. It also has the advantage of being applicable to all patients regardless of location.

One might not imagine that the tongue could yield so much information. When I studied this subject I found it very dry, often contradictory and confusing. I rarely saw, nor could match, the tongue findings with the clinical presentation of the patient. I had a sense that there was something missing, but couldn't quiet discover what it was. It would be many years of seeking before the mysteries of this discipline were revealed to me.

When I first encountered the teachings of Dr Yuen, he revealed a very simple, dynamic and incredibly useful model for seeing the relationship of Qi as it pertained to the various terrains of the body. The model clearly reflected the functioning of physiology, and perhaps just as crucially for a clinician, the pathway of progress of pathology. This was the missing piece, the game changer. It was a model that enabled clear, real time clinical thinking. It enabled accurate selection of the appropriate channel system. And it was a way to track the effect of one's intervention immediately, as well as over the ensuing days, weeks, months and even years.

When you understand this model and keep it in mind when studying and practicing this medicine, you'll be able to stay rooted in the Classics, whilst innovating a specific treatment strategy to match the patient's presentation and guide their healing process.

The author has accomplished an incredible feat in conveying the spirit and the essence of this practice. The reader doesn't need to go around memorising a vast deal of tongue appearances. Within these pages, the art of tongue diagnosis is communicated with great clarity and precision, both nuanced and clinically relevant. I urge the reader to explore these pages with openness, and to marvel at how each person's history is clearly reflected on the tongue. This information, when skilfully relayed to the patient, will have a deep impact on them. They will feel seen and heard—invaluable in itself for establishing rapport and trust—and thus, the efficacy of the clinical encounter will be established before any treatment is formulated or administered.

Dr. Hung D. Tran, MBBS
London, April 2021

Author's Note

During the COVID-19 period, I performed remote treatments from my home. At first, I was quite worried about not having access to the precious and foolproof tool of pulse diagnosis. Tongue diagnosis became, temporarily, the principal diagnostic method, and not only did it stand up to the challenge, I found a new enthusiasm for the method emerge.

This book arises from decades of clinical practice and observation. As Chinese medicine unfolds for us, we begin to realize that if you understand the principles of the medicine you can practice with any tools that are in front of you. In all my studies with Dr Yuen, the underlying focus has always been awareness of one's chosen lens—look at everything but see through the lens that offers the most clarity. In countless tongue presentations, I remember Dr Yuen applying this principle with great virtuosity—integrating classical principles and channel theory along with the quite postclassical practice of tongue diagnosis. When the tongue is viewed within a wide array of parameters, a challenging and exciting arena opens. We have the opportunity, as modern practitioners, to methodically synchronize familiar modern tongue practices with the crystalline lens of classical Chinese medicine theory and practice. This book is intended to be a comprehensive guide to this process, and to function as a companion both in the clinic and to my book *The Art of Pulse Diagnosis: A Step-by-Step Exploration.*

In the clinic, I rely very much on pulses to show the location and nature of pathology and to tell me what I should do with it. I love listening to their depth, width, length, tempo, texture, and organ interrelationships—contemplating what it all means in the patient's physiological, emotional, and mental states. Then I look at the tongue for additional information about the degree to which Heat is responding to pathology, and the status of fluids. The tongue is wonderfully useful for this purpose. Often, I'll take a photo and give the patient a detailed tour of the conversation between Heat and fluids reflected on their tongue. When they actually see evidence of the pulse findings, compliance with gently communicated dietary and lifestyle suggestions increases.

If you are with the patient, I strongly recommend taking pulses first and crafting a diagnosis before looking at the tongue. Ask questions and look at the tongue later, considering the tongue an offering of additional information regarding the body's response to the pathology you found in the pulses. The Ten Questions and tongue diagnosis are each Ming Dynasty additions to acupuncture and therefore secondary in importance to pulses.

While this book is suitable for all acupuncturists with any kind of training and there are no specific prerequisites for its understanding, I have made references to the Complement Channels—the Sinew, Luo, Divergent and Eight Extraordinary Channels—all of which appear in the Han Dynasty (206 BCE—220 CE) Classical texts. (My book *Advanced Acupuncture, A Clinic Manual* contains my suggested protocols for the clinical practice of these channels.) Even though tongue diagnosis originated in the Yuan Dynasty (1279–1368 CE) and flourished in the Ming (1368–1644 CE), it would be remiss to discuss the tongue without some reference to these channels, since they are so celebrated in the classical texts that are the foundation and origin of acupuncture. The Complement Channels are those that preserve humanity; when the body is unable to release a pathogenic factor because of weakness, lack of Fluids, or other reasons, these channels create pathways that move pathology away from the organs, preserving life itself.

By the time of the tongue diagnosis texts, most of the Complement Channels had gone into disuse. The concept of latency—the body's ingenious and complex ways of hiding pathology—was also largely forgotten, and with it, the view that Cold and its vehicle, Wind, are the origin of all diseases. Diagnosis via the tongue alone, with its primary Ming Dynasty focus on Heat may leave us wanting for a completely comprehensive reading, but thankfully it reliably tells us volumes about the way the body is responding to pathology.

Lastly, in this book there are many photographs. It is expressly not intended to be a catalog of photos. I urge you not to memorize any tongue herein. The photos merely serve to illustrate the mechanisms, and the book should be able to stand without the photos. If the mechanisms are understood, diagnosis of any tongue is possible even with its inevitably unique, apparent, and seemingly puzzling contradictions. Chinese Medicine is an art as much as it is a magnificent and profound medicine. I'm so glad that we're here together to experience and practice it.

With best wishes for your practice,

Ann

New York, 2021

Abbreviations

At the first appearance of Chinese words, I've observed the convention of hyphenating their pinyin spelling with their English translation. Wei Qi means Wei-Defensive Qi, Ying Qi means Ying-Nutritive Qi, Yuan Qi means Yuan-Constitutional Qi, Jing means Jing-Essence, Thin Fluids means Jin-Thin Fluids, and Thick Fluids means Ye-Thick Fluids. When words such as Heat and Cold are capitalized, it signifies a complexity in the word that exceeds its basic meaning in English. Heat implies a response generated by the body that is viewed later as inflammation as it becomes trapped by its complicator, Damp. Cold, when capitalized, captures the notion that Cold is constrictive and destructive and creates complications such as stagnation and tightness.

Left and Right

The words "left" and "right" always refer to the patient's left and right. As you look at a photograph, the right side of the photograph shows the left side of the patient's tongue. The left side of the photograph shows the right side of the patient's tongue.

Glossary

Bean: a unit of pressure in pulse taking

Bi Syndrome: pain caused by Wind (instability in the channel).

Cold: the contraction, tightness and slowing of functions caused by cold foods and drinks, climatic cold, or from the depletion of Yang Qi.

Cun, guan, and chi, translate to "measurement, gateway, template": the three locations on the wrist occupied by the fingers during pulse taking.

Dai Mai, translates as "the Belt Channel": the channel that runs around the belt line, responsible for releasing what has been held onto for a long time, or holding onto things that cannot be released.

Dampness: stagnated or accumulated Fluids, creating swellings, phlegm, and congestion. Dampness is often present as compensation for dehydration or other deficiencies.

Diaphragm: the very large muscle that separates the abdomen from the chest, shaped like a giant mushroom and spanning the entire lower ribcage. It moves with the breath but tightens under various stresses.

Heat: the inflammation that arises from the consumption of irritating foods (fried, spicy foods, allergens, GMOs), or from the naturally generated response to pathology, including internal cold.

Jiao, translates to "Burner" or "Heater": any one of three regions of the torso. These are divided at the belt and at the diaphragm. Broadly speaking they are the chest, the middle abdomen, and the area below the waist. The area above the diaphragm is the Upper Jiao. The area between the diaphragm and Dai Mai is the Middle Jiao. The area below Dai Mai is the Lower Jiao.

Jing-Essence: the deepest level of Yin, Yin at the constitutional level.

Latency: the act or state of having hidden away pathology somewhere in the body so that they cannot access the organs. The Divergent and Luo Channels achieve this for the body.

Mediumship: any fluid: thin fluids (Jin), thick fluids (Ye), blood, or essence (Jing)

Pathology: any challenge to the immune system, to Wei-Defensive Qi.

Qi: the animating life force related to breath, warmth, and spirit.

Wei-Defensive Qi: the Qi that flows in the exterior anatomy, gut and smooth muscle, defending the body against entry of pathogens. It also flows to energize muscles for responses to challenges. It is a subset of Yang Qi.

Wind: Instability in the flow of Qi or/and Blood. External Wind is contracted by exposure. Internal Wind is caused by deficiencies in mediumship (substance).

Yang: moving, warming energy

Yin: substance; anything that can be weighed. However, the term Yin nearly always applies to some kind of fluid. Yin can mean the collective fluids, but can also refer to the mediumship of the Kidneys. Usage depends entirely on context.

Ying-Nutritive Qi: the collective of Qi that builds us through gathering and transforming nourishment from the outside world, and flows in Blood and Fluids.

Yuan-Constitutional Qi: constitutional vitality that flows in the deepest level of the body: in the reproductive system, bone, bone marrow, spine, brain, and Eight Extraordinary Channels.

I
Tongue Diagnosis and Visible Responses

Tongue diagnosis examines responses to pathology and the compensations that result from those responses. Understanding the responses enables the practitioner to deduce the nature of the pathology.

Case 1

My patient, Lina's husband Chad, sent me an urgent text. They had been chatting and enjoying lunch together when the phone rang. The caller was Jay, a close friend and regular visitor to their apartment. Chad answered, "Hi Jay! Yeah, that was fun yesterday, we had a great time. Can I call you back? Lina and I are having lunch." When Chad returned to the table, Lina said to him, "I know that I should know who Jay is, but I really can't place him. Can you remind me who he is?" Chad thought she was kidding, but then saw that she was serious.

Chad wanted to take her to the emergency room but Lina insisted that he send me a text first. I asked for a photo of her tongue. It was deep red, shiny with no coat except for a diagonal area of the tongue behind a line starting a third of the way back on its right side, extending to the rear of the tongue. The majority of the tongue was so peeled that it appeared to be missing the top two millimeters of flesh. The features were gone as though polished off. No evidence of taste buds or texture were evident in the peeled region. I asked was it shaking. Yes. Were there one-sided neurological signs? No. Was there a problem with vision? Yes, the lower right portion of the visual field in both eyes had black and white zigzagging patterns. Internal Wind, I thought, with an underlying Yin deficiency. I had them pinch and pull upward very hard on GB-21 (the top of the shoulder) and to immediately eat something Yin (a mushroom, some leftover rice, some soup, a banana, anything Yin). They had some carrots and Chad quickly steamed them. After the pulling on GB-21, the vision issues subsided then disappeared, and after eating the carrots, some almond milk, and a banana, her memory fully returned. Throughout the day, Chad—fascinated by the notion that a diagnosis could be made by looking at the tongue—asked to see Lina's tongue. Later he told me that over the course of that day, the coat gradually "grew back" on the tongue, like a curtain being drawn diagonally across a window. The tongue became covered as it normally would be and the return of the coat correlated exactly with the rate of her return to normal. With a change in diet to include much more wet food, she has not experienced it again.

Chad was witnessing the tongue's display of the body's response to pathology. The extreme Yin deficiency had called for an emergency response from the body to accumulate Yin to stem the escape of Kidney Yang. The body was drawing Yin from the Lungs and the digestive tract down to the Kidneys to anchor Yin back there. The event was relayed in chronological order for all to see.

The tongue is a marvelous window into the way the body responds to pathology. As a diagnostic tool we can use it to understand the multitude of responses the body can make. The tongue shows us where the body feels it can and cannot reach to enact those responses.

Case 2

A patient arrived with a very deep and very wide midline crack extending from the middle toward both tip and rear of the tongue. The crack was filled with a coagulated gray-colored phlegm. His main issue was insomnia. He couldn't quiet his mind sufficiently to be able to enter a restful state. He was certain from his searches on the Internet that his underlying issue was Dampness—an accumulation of Phlegm. He'd been to several acupuncturists demanding that they treat him for Dampness, but the insomnia persisted. I told him that I didn't agree with his diagnosis of himself. The wide midline crack indicated a profound Yin deficiency to which his body was responding by accumulating as much pathological Dampness as possible. The clue that Damp was the response to the Yin deficiency was the "gluing together" of the tongue on either side of the crack, with the body reaching for any and all resources it could obtain to build back Yin. The treatment, therefore, was to nourish Yin and regulate Dampness. It would take quite a while for the tongue to repair itself completely, but the crack did become noticeably shorter and narrower quite rapidly and sleep was dramatically improved within the month.

Case 3

A young man came in carrying an iced coffee; he was bent double and wearing a diaper so that he could venture away from home with a severe illness diagnosed in Western medicine as Crohn's disease. Upon questioning, the usual suspects implicated in this type of illness were in play: garlic, onion, hot spices, coffee, chocolate, gluten, and sugar. Removal of these culprits was not going to be sufficient to get him through to health, because the tongue showed a distinct band of tension at the level of the diaphragm. The body was responding to the possibility that the extreme Heat might affect the Heart. The Heat, therefore, could not vent upward due to this tension and was being forced downward, where it played havoc in the Lower Jiao. The daily diet—frying and sweating the gut—added to the turmoil, and the organs themselves were becoming eroded. Apart from the immediate cessation of all the causative factors in the diet, the treatment required the releasing of the chest first, then the clearing of Heat. The utterly amazed patient was free of debilitating symptoms within ninety days.

2

A Brief History of Tongue Diagnosis

Examination of the Tongue in the Classical Period

The history of tongue diagnosis is surprising; what many don't realize is that it's a late addition to acupuncture practice. If you're a clinician practicing medicine according to the Han Dynasty texts (206 BCE—220 CE), it's strangely liberating to think that the early clinicians were not really thinking about the tongue much at all. I say "liberating" because sometimes you can look at a tongue and marvel at how much of the information you just found in the pulses is not showing on the tongue. There are good reasons for this.

Tongue diagnosis developed to replace abdominal palpation during a period when touching the patient was taboo. The Song Dynasty (960–1279 CE) was a time of puritanism: abdominal palpation[1] and pulse taking were not widely practiced. Patients pointed to the locations of their complaints on ivory dolls, and court physicians diagnosed by feeling the vibrations in strings tied to patients' wrists. Imagine, even as a practiced clinician, trying to do that. Something had to change. Puritanism ultimately called for something to look at, rather than touch. If the abdomen was not to be palpated, then perhaps the beginning of the alimentary canal, the tongue, should be able to provide information about the digestive system. The tongue would surely reflect the abdomen.[2] It was in this cultural environment that tongue examination developed to become an actual system of diagnosis.

In the Ming Dynasty, two other major events occurred: the great plague (also known as "the Black Death") swept through Europe and China, and the printing press arrived. The West would like to think Europeans invented it, but no, it was yet more Chinese brilliance: Bi Sheng (990–1051 CE) brought us movable-type printing a full four hundred years before Johannes Gutenberg's innovations. As the technology became widespread, printers joyfully disseminated fashionable material of the time. In the field of medicine, the topic *du jour* happened to be tongue diagnosis, so there happens to be a comparative plethora of material about the tongue dating from that early printing period. The very first tongue diagnosis text was the 1341 book, *The Golden Mirror Records*. The Heat of the plague projected a changing, technicolor show on the tongue, making these materials all the more fascinating, especially with the advent of multicolor printing in the early Ming Dynasty.

The broad coinciding of these three events—puritanism, plague and press—led to the innovation of using the tongue as a diagnostic tool.

---

[1] Abdominal diagnosis and palpation were practiced extensively until the end of the Tang Dynasty (618–907CE).

[2] Later emerged a significant focus on the Spleen, whose Primary Channel emerges from the chest at LU-1 and then spreads throughout the root of the tongue. The tongue can be seen as an extension of the flesh which is controlled by the Spleen.

But what was the status of the tongue before that—in the period spanning the Han and Tang Dynasties? How was it viewed clinically, when acupuncture was at the pinnacle of its development—when all the channels of acupuncture were in use, when pulse diagnosis was sophisticated, and when practitioners, in command of the entire network of over sixty acupuncture channels, were confident and successful in treating everything?

In the classical texts, there is no mention of the tongue being examined and analyzed to derive a diagnosis. This is because, in order for the tongue to be a diagnostic tool, there would need to be a diagnostic *system* applied to the tongue. This system would cover all the aspects of the tongue—varieties of coatings, distributions of moisture, lists of movements, colors, and textures—along with a translation of these into assessments of Wei, Ying, and Yuan Qi and all the various media.

But when the tongue is cited in the classical texts, it's listed only as a sign—a sign of prognosis perhaps worth noting, but not at all a diagnostic system. For example, chapter 32 of the *Su Wen*, a chapter on internal Heat, says: *When the Lung has a Heat disease, at first the patient shivers, there is receding Qi and the finest body hair rises. The patient has an aversion to Wind and Cold. The upper surface of the tongue is yellow. The body is hot*. Chapters 4 and 31 of the *Su Wen* say that diseases of the Spleen will show at the base of the underside of the tongue (where the Spleen Channel ends). Elsewhere in the *Su Wen*, in chapters 16, 17, 41, 47, 52 and 63, it's noted that the tongue might be misshapen or curled, or that speech is affected because so is the tongue, especially when the disease is advanced. Chapters 31 and 33 describe dryness of the tongue as a symptom. Chapter 48 of the *Su Wen* says that if the tongue can be moved, there is hope for recovery. A little later, Zhang Zhong Jing (c. 150–219 CE) referred to the tongue coat with the radical for fetus. He says that upon the invasion of the body by an external pathogenic factor (EPF), the coat becomes impregnated by that EPF and shows the Yang stages of penetration of that EPF.

In the *Nan Jing*, the four diagnostic tools are discussed, but when it refers to looking (in chapter 13), it is referring to the complexion, not the tongue. The *Nan Jing* mentions that Cold and Heat will cause the lips and tongue to become dry. It also mentions that when the Liver Channel is diseased, the testicles and tongue will be retracted.

The tongue is mentioned twenty-one times in Hua To's (c. 140–208 CE) book, *The Central Treasury Classic*. He, too, writes that the general appearance of the tongue can signify the severity of disease, that a curled tongue indicates impending death (Scroll 3, chapters 48 and 49). He lists several signs that, if concurrent with a black tongue, deem a disease terminal. Scroll 1, chapter 26 says that the tongue may become stiff enough to affect speech, and includes rigidity of the tongue in a long list of symptoms of Spleen pathology (quoting Bian Que, born c. fifth century BCE, in the last instance). Scroll 1, chapter 25, mentions the relationship of the Heart, Small Intestine and tongue. Scroll 2, chapter 41 mentions heat toxin sores.

In the *Jia Yi Jing* (scrolls 7 and 8) Huang Fu Mi (215–282 CE) lists either a degenerating tongue or a curled tongue midway through several long lists of signs and symptoms. Each of these lists relates to a different type of illness, including rebellious Qi, Tai Yang, Shao Yang, Shao Yin, and Jue Yin presentations.

Chao Yuan Fang's (550–630 CE) book, *The Origin of Symptoms of Diseases* discusses signs and symptoms that appear with certain simple presentations of the tongue. Scroll 28 relates the following to the tongue: oral and tongue sores, rigidity, dryness, scorching, swelling, and heaviness. It also describes systemic Heat rising to the Heart and Spleen, affecting their connection to the tongue and mouth. If the tongue is dry, the teeth are also checked for dryness and yellowing. In scroll 10, he says the colors of the sublingual veins demonstrate Heat in the Heart and Spleen. Scroll 5 says that Qi stagnation is often accompanied by a white slipperiness on the tongue. He also mentions that during febrile diseases, if the root of the tongue is shriveled or withered, one should not needle.

In his book, *Prescriptions Worth a Thousand Ducats*, Tang Dynasty giant Sun Si Miao (581–682 CE) postulated that the tongue may contribute to diagnosis, mentioning the Qi of the tongue in its flaccid or rigid state, that a hyperactive tongue can accompany epilepsy, and that a fetus will die if the mother's tongue is blue or green.

Throughout the classical texts there is no mention of a system of diagnosis that involves the tongue. But the tongue does offer a marvelous reflection of the body's responses to its challenges. It's a thesis on the body's responses to pathology.

The Beginning of Tongue Diagnosis and the Advent of Focus on Heat as Pathology

During the Song Dynasty, there were invasions of nomadic Mongolian tribes from the north. A series of rapid, sweeping epidemics, including the Black Death, spread along the Silk Road, both east into China and west into Europe, killing almost half their populations. Flares of the epidemic would erupt, as epidemics do, killing swaths of the population, then disappear. During this time, most medical and religious practitioners died.[3]

Until the Black Death, China had experienced diseases that were routinely treatable—chiefly acute diseases—not pestilence. The sheer intensity of the plague and its high mortality rate led the remaining people to feel that the *old medicine* was ineffective, eliciting a shift in attitude toward disease. Heat, once known to be crucially important as a generated response to pathology, was now seen as a chief evil, the new primary pathogenic factor. The resulting Wen Bing school, of the late Ming Dynasty, eventually prevailed. Its popularization by the new printing press led to the emergence of more written information on the tongue and on Wen Bing theory perhaps than any other tradition.

In modern Chinese Medicine (known as TCM), which is heavily influenced by Wen Bing theory, Heat is still seen as a principal pathology. Today, therefore, tongue diagnosis has its focus on the observation of Heat and the movement of Heat through the body. In this book we'll examine how practitioners can benefit from the tongue's revelations about Heat.

[3] In defense, China turned inward; contact with the outside world ceased. This shift is reflected in Japanese acupuncture even today, as developments that occurred later in China do not appear in Japanese practice. Examples of Chinese Song Dynasty practices preserved to this day by Japanese practitioners are abdominal palpation, the Earth School, and the School of Nourishing Yin.

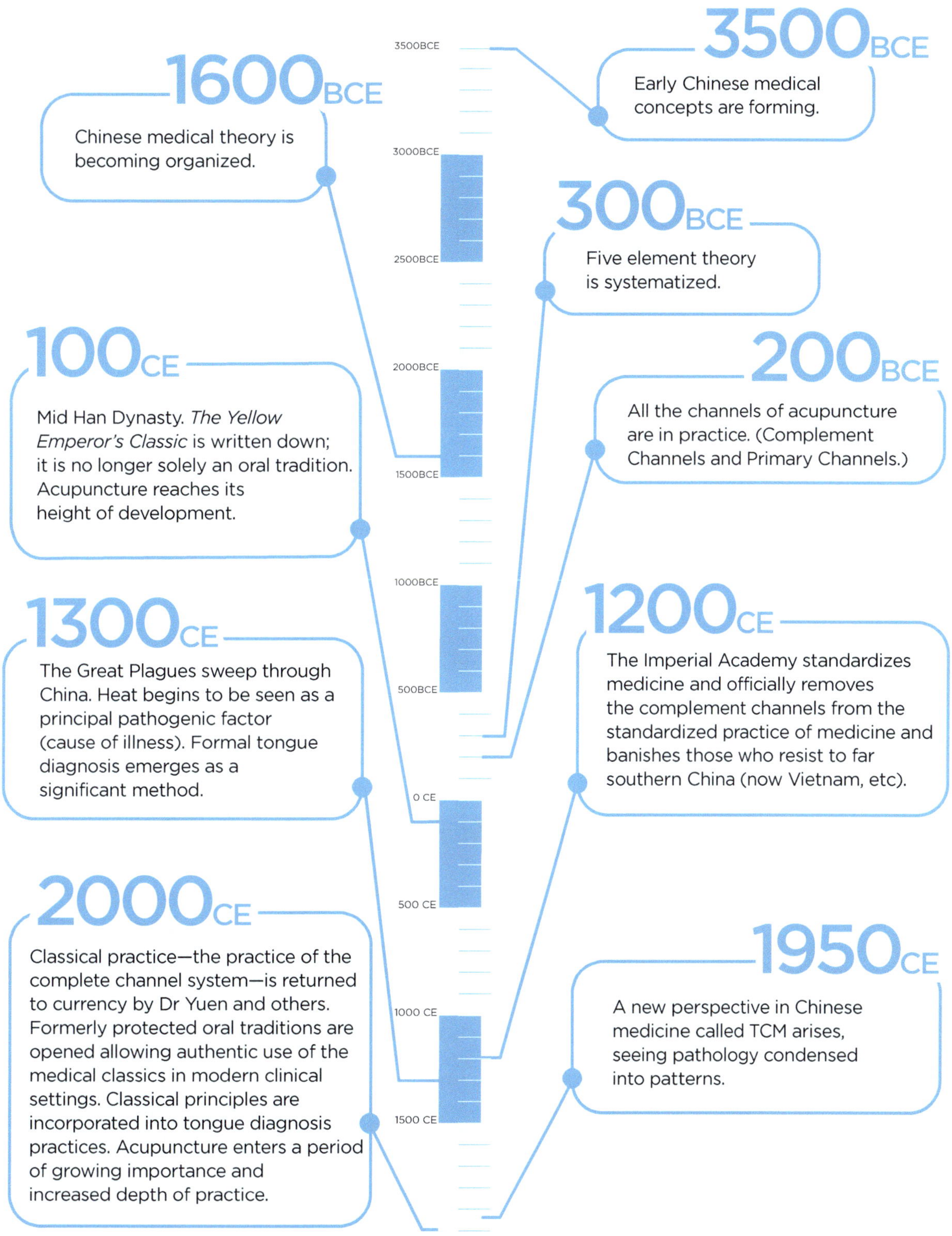
3500BCE
Early Chinese medical concepts are forming.
1600BCE
Chinese medical theory is becoming organized.
300BCE
Five element theory is systematized.
200BCE
All the channels of acupuncture are in practice. (Complement Channels and Primary Channels.)
100CE
Mid Han Dynasty. *The Yellow Emperor's Classic* is written down; it is no longer solely an oral tradition. Acupuncture reaches its height of development.
1200CE
The Imperial Academy standardizes medicine and officially removes the complement channels from the standardized practice of medicine and banishes those who resist to far southern China (now Vietnam, etc).
1300CE
The Great Plagues sweep through China. Heat begins to be seen as a principal pathogenic factor (cause of illness). Formal tongue diagnosis emerges as a significant method.
1950CE
A new perspective in Chinese medicine called TCM arises, seeing pathology condensed into patterns.
2000CE
Classical practice—the practice of the complete channel system—is returned to currency by Dr Yuen and others. Formerly protected oral traditions are opened allowing authentic use of the medical classics in modern clinical settings. Classical principles are incorporated into tongue diagnosis practices. Acupuncture enters a period of growing importance and increased depth of practice.
3500BCE
3000BCE
2500BCE
2000BCE
1500BCE
1000BCE
500BCE
0 CE
500 CE
1000 CE
1500 CE

3
Cold in Tongue Diagnosis

Tongue diagnosis focuses on Heat, but the primary pathogen in classical medicine is Cold (or Wind-Cold). How do we reconcile the two?

The principles of Chinese Medicine—the roots of our practice—are explained in the classical texts of the Han Dynasty—the *Nei Jing*, the *Nan Jing*, and the *Shang Han Lun*. There we learn that Wind-Cold is the origin of all diseases (in Western terms, Wind-Cold is the common cold, a routine viral infection, and even a pandemic viral infection). Seventy percent of the *Shang Han Lun* (second century CE) is devoted to treatment of the initial invasion of Cold, the Tai Yang stage. The text shows that Heat arises as the body's response to Cold. The body wants to expel it, or burn it up. This is in clear contrast to the understandable bias of the Ming, where the progress of unforgiving, scorching epidemics was so rapid that Heat—in Western terms, bacterial infection—came to be seen as the origin of disease, rather than the response. In the COVID-19 period, we experienced the same kind of scenario: people did not report sneezing, stiff back of neck, runny nose; they reported internal Damp-Heat signs instead. The virus (Wind-Cold) was strong enough to bypass the Tai Yang stage and people witnessed and identified the Shao Yang and Yang Ming response to COVID-19 as the actual pathology, rather than complications impeding the patients' responses.

The adoption of the tongue as a diagnostic tool in the Ming Dynasty challenges us to hold the foundational theory of the classical texts firmly, while incorporating something that is very useful from tongue diagnosis—that is, tracking the effects of Heat in the interior.

It's now time to do this—to fuse these two parameters together; time to ask: in what way is the necessarily generated Heat going out of control or how has it become trapped by blockages or Dampness? What mediumship (fluids) is it consuming? And how is the body trying to compensate for the erosion of Yin that occurs as a result of trapped or rampant Heat? This is the blessing of the art of tongue diagnosis, the fusion of theory and a reframing from the perspective of the roots of Chinese Medicine.

External Cold and the Tongue

The notion that Wind-Cold is the origin of disease is a constant in the foundational theory of the channels also. Sinew Channel theory begins with Cold entering the Tai Yang (Bladder) Sinew at the Wind gates at the back of the head and neck. Wei-Defensive Qi is a product of Kidney Yang and Stomach Fluids. It is the Qi of immunity carried in the Sinew Channels that responds immediately to Wind-Cold, in a series of perfectly orchestrated actions.

First, the Tai Yang Sinew tightens to confront the Cold. The body enters a defensive stance: the posterior neck contracts, the shoulders rise, the head moves down and forward. Constrictive in nature, Cold concentrates in the center of the face, causing the nose to run. Then, a bolstering surge of Yang is brought up from the Kidneys to create more Wei-Defensive Qi to respond to and break up the Cold. Wei Qi is thereby fortified, able to instigate sneezing and sweating; the Cold is expelled. If this happens quickly, as it is designed to, there may be no sign of the entire process in the tongue. The pulse, however, will change dramatically during the process, as the Wei-Defensive level of the pulse becomes very tight, between one and six beans of pressure, and resumes its relaxed state once clear.

Though the body's responses are organized and wise, illness will progress if the body cannot ward off the pathogen due to insufficient resources: there are not enough fluids or Yang Qi to mobilize those fluids. If there are inadequate fluids to finance a sneeze and the accompanying micro-sweat that releases the exterior, or if there is not enough Yang to generate a sneeze in the first place, the Cold together with the Wei Qi that is chasing it begin to move inward. The body responds perfectly and powerfully again, now generating a fever to burn up the pathogen, compounding the Heat. The pathogen must not be allowed into the interior. The pulses become rapid at the superficial level since the battle is still located at the exterior. The body's perfect (Heat) response shows as the perimeter of the tongue becomes red. If the fever is allowed to run and do its job while the patient rests and hydrates, the Cold is overcome, the pathogen doesn't reach the interior, and the patient benefits from a new, improved level of health and outlook, since Wind (Cold's vehicle) brings positive change.[4]

If the fever is not high enough, or if the fever is suppressed through medication, the pathogen is not resolved and remains unchecked. It then can move to the interior, through the zones, into Shao Yang, Yang Ming, Tai Yin, Shao Yin, and Jue Yin, in one order or another. Heat from the Wei Qi accumulated around the pathogen creates havoc as it goes. The pulses become rapid at the Ying, and later the Yuan, level as the disease consumes Fluids, Blood, Yin, flesh, and eventually Jing-Essence, developing into any manner of disease along the way. The tongue goes through its rainbow of reds and purples as the disease worsens.

At every stage, if resources are available, there is an opportunity for the Complement Channels (especially the Luo and Divergent Channels) to assume responsibility for the pathogen and put it into latency (into hiding). While the pathogen is in latency, the patient appears symptom-free. If the channels fail in their quest to hide the pathogen away, the pathogen continues on its inward course. Signs emerge in the tongue to indicate the pathogen is no longer in latency

4 The survivors of the Ming Dynasty plagues failed to understand that epidemics will never be fully treatable because they are like a terribly miraculous force that we cannot understand; they come, do their work, and disappear in their own time. It's no coincidence that in Europe, after the Black Plague came the Renaissance, a wholesale shift in human consciousness, and that after the 1918 flu came the dramatic shift of the end of World War I and then the Roaring Twenties. Viruses (Wind-Cold)—barely living fragments of DNA—work directly at the level of evolution. To think that we can stop viruses is to think that life must not change; the virus—even the common cold virus—is constantly mutating: an agent of change in the world.

and is consuming resources with its accompanying Heat. Ultimately, the Heat breaches the giant membrane, the peritoneum, then enters the organs and becomes fatal. This process is endlessly fascinating as it leads us through the genius theory of the Complement Channels—the Sinew, Luo, Divergent, and Eight Extraordinary Channels.

Pestilent Qi Response and the Tongue

Invasion of pestilent Qi—highly infectious diseases, including the bubonic plague—differs from the regular appearance of invasion of Wind-Cold in three aspects. First, it is so hostile that the Tai Yang and Shao Yang defenses are overcome; pestilent Qi appears to enter the body at Yang Ming, becoming internal seemingly on contact. Second, the body's response is heightened to match the extreme nature of the pathogen. Using its mighty Yang Qi, the body creates much more Heat (Wei Qi) to battle *Yersinia pestis* (the bacterium of the plague), for example, than it would less potent pathogens. Third, the pathogen's passage through the zones and the Complement Channels, though theoretically standard, is so rapid that it quickly reaches the organs—the most interior treasures. Death approaches rapidly. Throughout this process the tongue moves through gradations of redness: bright red, dark red, crimson, deep crimson, purple, and deep purple. The pulse progresses from rapid to extremely rapid.

Those who survived the dramatic, valiant response to pestilent Qi faced decimation of their Yang Qi; their tongues were left pale. Since the central tenet of the Ming Dynasty was that Heat is likely the principal cause of illness, and since tongue diagnosis is a Ming Dynasty invention, the tongue diagnosis tradition focuses on viewing the tongue in terms of Heat damage. A pale tongue was understood to be the result of Heat having consumed Yang Qi, leaving Cold in its wake. In times of pestilence, this view of the tongue may be accurate but it is not always true for other conditions. Unfortunately, the notion that Cold was a prime pathogen was largely disregarded during the Ming.

Internal Cold and the Tongue

This book focuses on the tongue's reliable demonstration of the body's purposeful generation of Heat in response to complex pathology, and on the damage Heat leaves in its wake.

But damage done by incoming Cold is also important, however; sometimes Cold signs are signs of actual Cold—full Cold, you might say, rather than empty Cold (Cold from Yang deficiency). If the tongue is pale, and inquiry reveals that the patient is engaged in Cold-related habits, the pathogen is likely Cold. Cold constricts and creates stagnation of Qi, which in turn stagnates Blood, leaving the tongue pale, pale purple, blue, or difficult to extend. Heat would have difficulty arising since Cold also depletes and can stifle Yang, but if it were able to break through and create a fever, it would be a natural response—an attempt to break up that Cold.

During the last few decades, a new breed of Cold-origin diseases has emerged. These imbalances occur in long-term vegans, strict vegetarians, raw foodists, iced water drinkers, and other refrigerator frequenters.[5] These are in addition to the already established group of Cold imbalances in skiers, outdoor and refrigeration workers, and people who go barefoot on ceramic-tiled floors or other cold places. All this is fast-tracked internal Cold, gravely damaging Yang Qi, leaving the tongue various shades of pale. When Yang Qi is depleted, so too is its warming function. There may be insufficient Yang Qi to make enough Wei-Defensive Qi to generate a response (including fever) to the interior Cold. The Wei level pulses will be absent. The Ying and Yuan level pulses will likely be weak, slow, and tight in some combination. Ask questions related to lifestyle and diet and take pulses to determine the cause of a pale tongue.

[5] Strict vegetarians can avoid Cold by ensuring their food is cooked and served warm or hot and by ensuring their protein intake is regular and adequate.

4
Orientation

The Four Layers of Assessment

Historically, four layers of inquiry are considered during the assessment of a patient:

1. **Looking** gives an impression of the illness. Looking can give clues. Tongue diagnosis is a Ming Dynasty addition to this category.
2. **Listening** and Smelling reveal the expression of an illness. Sounds in the chest, breathing sounds, the tone of the voice, and smells, and noises from the digestive tract show how the body is conveying the illness outward.
3. **Asking Questions** helps determine what information is not being shared and what information gained so far may need more evaluation. Asking questions can confirm observations about the tongue. The Ten Questions are a Ming Dynasty addition to the medicine, and include questions related to diet, menstrual history, and emotional history, which can be important in corroborating findings in the tongue.
4. **Palpating** reveals that which is latent (hidden) and enables the practitioner to determine what the body might be repressing. Palpating includes the art of pulse taking. This is the most accurate, and therefore is the chief of the four routes of inquiry.

Note that the tongue is a natural instrument of expression and therefore does not reveal what is being hidden, although we will see that it is possible to deduce what is being repressed in many cases.

This "four layer" style of inquiry forms a complete set. "Looking" gives an impression of the illness, but certain basic ideas must be factored in before a diagnosis is possible.

- Most tongues have a thick coat in the morning. This might not be an indication of Damp, but simply be a reflection of the generation of Yin, a key function of sleep. So an 8:30a.m. patient who presents with a thick coat might not have a Damp condition at all.
- Also in the morning, in some, tongues are commonly red on the sides and the tip. This is not necessarily an indicator of Heat, but may be an indicator of Yang being mobilized to the surface of the body, since Yang Qi, and its subset, Wei Qi, are most active in the morning. So an early morning patient who presents with a tongue with a red tip and red sides might have had a hard workout in the gym that morning or may have rushed to the appointment. That tongue may be representing temporary overheating or temporary overactivation of Yang Qi—it might not indicate pathology at all.

- Children have a natural exuberance of Yang, often causing the perimeter of their tongues to appear redder than the rest of the tongue. However, if that red perimeter or other areas of the tongue have indicators of pathology, the redness is of interest to the practitioner.

If you're unable to take pulses, it's important to ask questions about activity, habits, and foods eaten to get the fuller picture pulse taking would provide. It would have been clear from the pulses that the Heat was in fact from the earlier gym visit and is not systemic (since the pulses will not be rapid at the moderate or deep levels). In the earlier example, you may see that the Yin on the tongue was accumulated during sleep and is not pathological, since the pulses will be wide and deep rather than slippery. Still, tongue assessment is very useful, it just needs to be approached with clarity and awareness of the various possible explanations for its appearance.

The Tongue as a Complete Diagnostic Tool

If the tongue is to be a complete diagnostic tool, it must show the practitioner all three levels of Qi, since they are the basis of physiology: Wei-Defensive Qi (the Qi of the exterior), Ying-Nutritive Qi (the Qi of Blood and Fluids), and Yuan-Constitutional Qi (the deepest level of Qi).

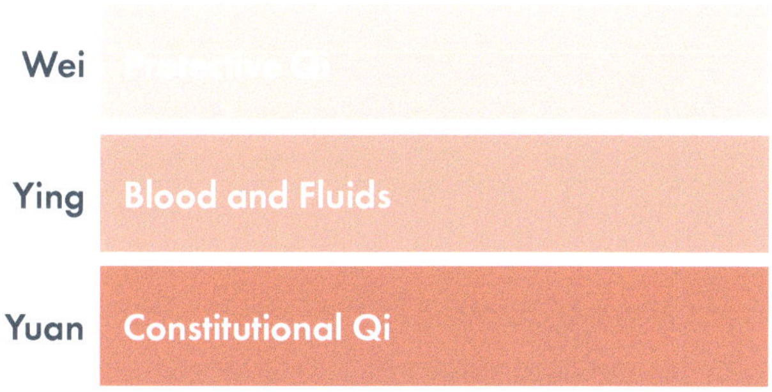

In the following chapters we will see that by casting an especially broad net of inquiry pertaining to the three levels of Qi, the tongue can yield information worthy of adding to our pulse findings:

The Three Levels of Qi

- The Tongue **Coat** reflects Wei-Defensive Qi.
- The Tongue **Body** reflects Ying-Nutritive Qi.
- The **Sublingual Veins** reflect Yuan-Constitutional Qi.

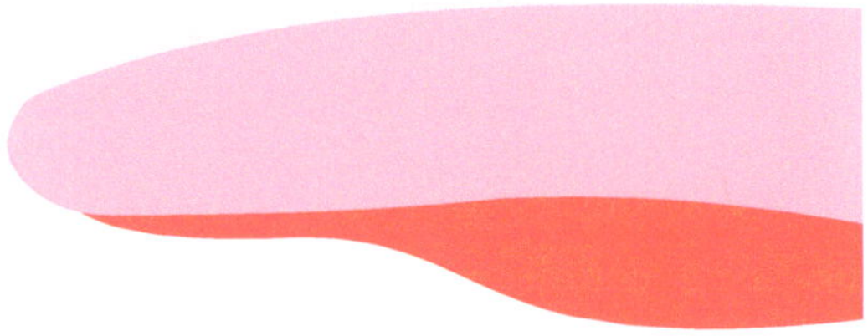

Each level of Qi is assessed. The practitioner examines:

- the **coat** and its moisture, texture, color, coverage
- the **body** and its movement, posture, orientation, moisture, length, thickness, size, shape, color, luminescence, spots, protrusions, accumulations, swellings, silhouette, profile, cracks, and erosions
- the **sublingual veins** and their color, shape, and integrity
- the **map** of the organs as reflected on the tongue. This, however, is very much secondary in importance to the above observations.

Channels Connecting Directly to the Tongue

Channels that connect to the tongue also inform the diagnosis:

- The **Spleen Primary Channel** goes to the root of the tongue. It controls the integrity of the flesh (tonicity) of the tongue and manages Blood going to the tongue.
- The **Kidney Primary Channel** goes to the root of the tongue where it spreads its Qi. This channel initiates movement of the tongue and relays information from the constitution to the tongue.
- The **Heart Luo Channel** goes to the tongue. This channel allows the tongue to express emotions and enables speech to project the truth of one's life purpose. It also allows the tongue to express emotions that may be in latency, freeing them through speech. (Note: The Heart Primary Channel goes to the throat and resonates through the eyes; it does not go to the tongue.)

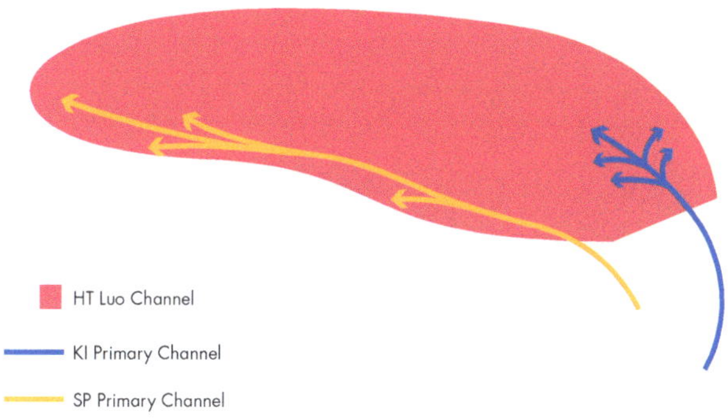

What Does This All Mean in Practice?

In practice, the appearance of the tongue is separated into three broad considerations:

- the appearance of the **coat**
- the appearance of the **body** of the tongue, and
- the appearance of the **sublingual** veins

Diagnoses are made by:

- gaining a **general impression** of the tongue
- observing the qualities of the **coat**
- observing the qualities of the tongue **body**
- observing the qualities of the **sublingual veins**
- observing the status of the **channels** as they attach to the tongue
- superimposing the **map** of the organs on the tongue and deducing where the response to pathology is focused

We will arrive at step-by-step diagnosis protocols at page 124.

5

The Tongue Coat Reveals Wei Qi Status
(The Immune System and Musculoskeletal Movement)

Analysis of the tongue coat reveals the status of Wei-Defensive Qi—the Qi of the immune system. Wei Qi guards the exterior and governs our ability to ward off disease through sneezing, sweating, coughing, vomiting, defecation and urination. Without strong Wei Qi, we are weak and vulnerable, unable to resolve illness, acute or chronic. Internally, Wei Qi controls the movement of smooth muscle—in the bronchi, heart, gut, bladder, blood vessels, and uterus. Wei Qi also governs the movement of the musculoskeletal system, allowing us to move away from harm.

Assessment of the following four factors of the tongue coat helps determine where pathology is influencing the formation or management of Wei Qi.

1. Moisture of the coat
2. Texture of the coat
3. Color of the coat
4. Coverage of the coat

Tongue Moisture

Observation of moisture on the tongue is perhaps the most important observation in tongue diagnosis and is far more important than the coat color. When I was in acupuncture school, during my favorite class, Clinical Case Review, where we presented our cases from the clinic, if a student mentioned the tongue but didn't report the status of tongue moisture, Dr. Yuen would ask for it without fail, reminding us that the moisture is of greatest importance. *Without adequate fluids, pathogens can be neither resisted nor evacuated.*

Wei Qi and the moisture on the tongue arise from Jin (Thin) Fluids. The Stomach produces two broad types of Fluids: Jin-Thin Fluids and Ye-Thick Fluids. Thin Fluids are further divided into two classes: pure and turbid.[6] (Turbid means denser, not to be confused with polluted.) Pure Jin-Thin Fluids go to the sensory orifices to irrigate the ears, eyes, nose, sinuses, throat, and mouth, including the tongue. Turbid Jin-Thin Fluids go to the Sinews to allow Wei Qi actions, including the production, and enabling of, sweat.

[6] The word turbid simply means denser and has no negative connotation unless the balance of pure and turbid is off, in which case there is "too much turbidity" or "a turbid coat."

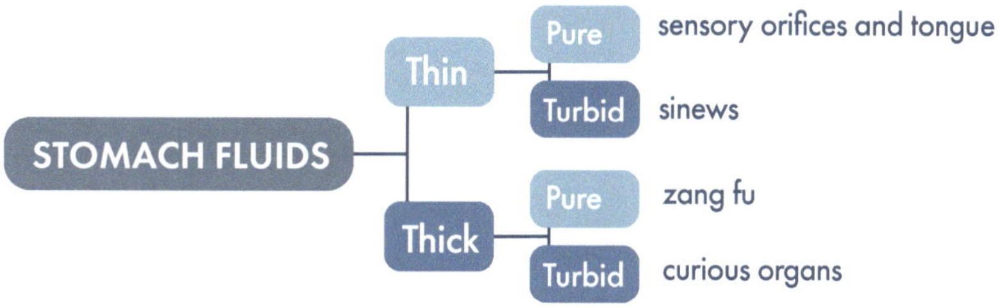

The coat reflects the general status of all Fluids, but the actual stuff of the coat itself is Jin-Thin Fluid. A normal tongue coat is moist: it has clear-looking, clean moisture, indicating that Pure Fluids are being produced. That means the immune system has the resources it needs to expel Wind-Cold (the pathogen and aftermath of the action of a pathogenic factor). It is able to create the micro-sweat or sneeze necessary to defend the exterior. Also, a tongue coat that is neither sticky nor turbid and without accumulations reflects a free moving gut. A free moving gut ensures freedom from stagnation and the Damp conditions that follow, including parasites and fermentation (yeast conditions), lassitude, brain fog, weight gain, phlegm accumulation, and generally weakened digestion.

Tongue coat moisture is also a mirror of Stomach Yin (including the mucosal lining) and hydration levels in the entire alimentary canal. A dry coat is a sign of insufficient hydration for the complete and efficient transformation of food and drinks. Transportation in the gut becomes unreliable; elimination may become irregular or incomplete.

If the tongue coat is absent, Wei Qi (the immune system) is extremely weak; the patient may be deeply vulnerable to external pathogens. If the body is unable to expel a pathogen, it must at least have sufficient fluids to put that pathogen into latency, to hide it away from the organs.

Aside from digestion and defense, fluids must be available to temper Heat and to prevent its progression. When Heat is unchecked or when uncontrolled Heat (inflammation) creates fire toxins (free radicals), terminal diseases may result.

Dehydration

Though a "normal" coat is quite thin, lightly white, and evenly distributed over the entire surface of the tongue, in our deeply dehydrated, overstimulated and underslept culture, it is a treat to see one. Your treatments will be undermined if the patient is engaged in dehydrating habits. Dehydration along with imbalance in the emotions are a root of all diseases.

When I first encounter a dehydrated patient, I find that they are usually doing one or more of the following: not eating enough soup, not drinking enough water, not eating enough saturated fat (they are often adhering to a low-fat diet), eating sugar, eating processed foods, going to bed late, drinking carbonated beverages, coffee, alcohol, too much tea, taking unnecessary supplements they can't handle anyway, or eating garlic, onion, hot spices, or chocolate. All these strip the body of its hydration. In the first encounter, while you don't want to alienate your patient, it may be a good idea to make sure they know that these things adversely affect not only the treatment, but also their immune system, by robbing it of its currency—systemic fluids.

Tongue Coat Texture

The texture of the tongue coat is determined by the Qi of the Spleen and Lungs, which is in turn dependent on the strength of Kidney Yang. The "steaming" action of the Spleen transforms the food and fluids the Stomach churns. The Spleen ascends its Qi, carrying that steam with it all the way to the beginning of the alimentary canal,[7] to the tongue. The Lungs then diffuse those fluids—at this stage known as Lung Yin—spreading them over the surface of the tongue.

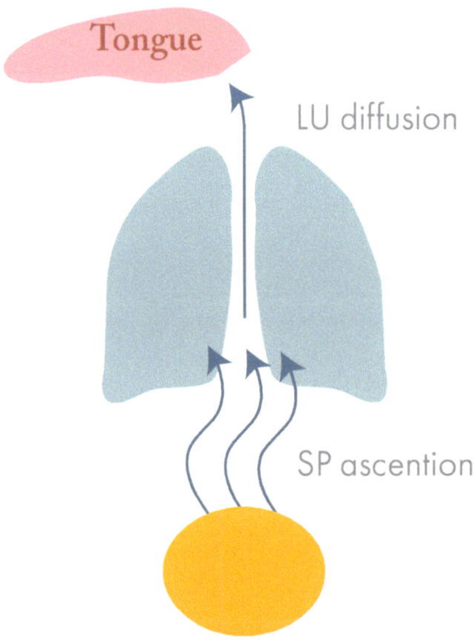

If this steaming mechanism is compromised, the tongue coat shows an uneven *texture*; the coat will not be smooth but will have some roughness as fluids are stagnating. Often you'll see tongue coats that look rough, sandy, grainy, pasty, fibrous, powdery, gluey, glassy, or perhaps gritty. All these coats show pathology involving fluids managed by any combination of the Kidneys, Spleen, and Lungs and indicate that Wei Qi is adversely affected. The Thin Fluids that finance Wei Qi are not being properly derived in the first place.

[7] The end of the Spleen Primary Channel terminates as it disperses at the tongue.

Tongue Coat Production Chain—Basic Observations

If the coat is too thin or too dry and concurrently Spleen Qi is weak, distributable fluids are not being generated in the Stomach. There is dehydration; the mucosal lining of the gut is inadequately hydrated. Or there may be stagnation (lack of movement of fluids) in the gut. Qi is not moving adequately or freely.

If the coat is too thick, there is too much turbidity; too much turbid fluid is coming up to the tongue. This means the Stomach and Spleen are not separating Fluids properly. The Spleen is not transforming Fluids (or food). Spleen Qi is deficient.

If the tongue coat is reduced or absent, Spleen Qi might not be ascending. Moisture cannot reach the tongue.[8]

If the tongue coat is not covering the entire surface—even if there are plenty of fluids available (the Stomach and Lung pulses are wide)—the Lungs are not able to diffuse fluids to the exterior; there are issues with systemic fluid distribution.

Kidney Yang is the driving force behind this entire process. If Spleen Qi (good digestion) is the cornerstone of health, Kidney Yang is the bedrock beneath that stone. The Spleen ascends Kidney Yang to the Stomach to begin the initial phase of digestion, rotting and ripening. If the Kidney Yang pulse (right chi position) is weak, digestion and therefore ascension of the coat will be compromised.

What Does All This Mean in Practice?

Your diagnostic process must find the weak link in the chain of production of Wei Qi and treat it.

In nearly all cases, underlying all these issues are errors in diet, mentioned earlier. Either the diet is not hydrating; or it is dehydrating by draining or clearing; or there are factors in the diet consuming fluids. The most common dehydrating causes are: coffee, sugar, garlic, onion, hot spices, liquor, dried foods, processed foods, and additives. For excellent information about food and about cooking for health, See Andrew Sterman's *Welcoming Food*, volumes 1 and 2.

[8] See chapters 3 and 4 of *The Art of Pulse Diagnosis* for information on detecting directionality (the communication between organs) in the pulses.

Tongue Coat Moisture and Texture Diagnosis

If the tongue coat is:

- dry, fluids are damaged or not being ascended. Since fluids are the domain of the Lungs, Spleen, and Kidneys, ask questions related to these organs and find the location of stagnation or weakness to determine what is preventing the creation of the tongue coat. One of the above organs is weak, or there is an error in their communication. Or Stomach Fluids are deficient in the first place.

- dry and thin, there is stagnation of Fluids in the Middle Jiao. If the coat is white, there may be stagnation in the Upper Jiao also.

- dry with difficulty speaking, Kidney Yang cannot ascend sufficiently to assist in diffusing Qi at the root of the tongue. The Kidney Channel normally enables the initiation of tongue movement.

- dry at the front of the tongue, Wind has dried the coat.

- thick and dry, the body has become tired trying to move pathology out. Qi has become deficient, taxing the Stomach and damaging or stagnating fluids. This causes the body to try to hold on to fluids. This is not Dampness. Tonify Stomach Qi, move Qi, and most importantly nourish Stomach Yin.

- dry, with thick white coat, Heat has consumed Fluids, and Dampness has responded to that Heat, smothering it. Find where the Damp-Heat is trapped. Clear Heat before you transform the Dampness. If you clear Damp first, the Heat will run rampant, causing disease.

- greasy, dryness in the Middle Jiao (deficient fluids) has weakened the Spleen and created Heat. Dampness has responded and combined with the Heat to create a greasy coat. Heat pushes the Dampness up to the surface, reflecting the Hot-Phlegm that is developing.

- thick, yellow and greasy, there is Summer Heat (the inability to sweat sufficiently to relieve Heat).

- thin, greasy and white, there is oppression in the Upper Jiao (often chest oppression with nausea).

- thin but too moist, there is not enough Qi to push pathology out. The body has accumulated the fluids to deal with a pathogen but cannot complete the task because Qi is deficient.

- very moist, there is Dampness.

- moist, dark, and gray, Damp in the Lower Jiao is damaging the Essence. The Kidneys are taxed. The gray color reflects Kidney involvement.

- very thick, the coat can become thick as the body tries to move Yin to expel an external pathogenic factor.

- very thick and discolored, there is Phlegm or swellings. Interestingly, people with Phlegm often don't have a thick coat because the Phlegm itself can block moisture from being expressed. In these cases, the tongue body will swell. To confirm that there is Phlegm, or advanced Dampness, ask questions about heaviness, lethargy, and poor focus and look for slippery pulses. Ask about bowel movements and ensure elimination. If there's a sense that signs and symptoms are worsening, the Phlegm is continuing to accumulate.

- very thick and yellow, there may be too much Stomach Fire. The Spleen can ascend that Heat to the Lungs, which (under the influence of the Heat) diffuse Fluids too rapidly. Fluid can then accumulate in the Lungs, leading to a thicker coat. The Stomach Fire causes the coat to turn yellow.

- sticky with strands of mucus on the tongue as the mouth is opened, the body is in purging mode. There are loose stools or diarrhea.

- powdery, there may be a Spleen Qi deficiency. The Spleen is unable to hold onto the coat.

- white and powdery on the rear of the tongue, Heat has consumed Kidney Yin.

- very shiny, Wei Qi is being lost. There is a pathological emission of Qi. Or too much Wei Qi is meeting a pathogenic factor and has become blocked at the exterior. Heat is actually pushing Qi out of the body. The concentration of Yang in the exterior creates a kind of illumination. This concentration of Heat consumes Yin. There is then insufficient Yin to dissipate Heat, resulting in a physiological circuitous situation. Strengthen Wei Qi by nourishing Yin.

The Difference Between Slippery Moisture and Greasy Moisture on the Tongue

Not that you would, but if you were to scrape the tongue and find thin, watery liquid dripping off the tongue, you would call that slippery moisture, indicating turbidity in the Stomach.[9] But if you were to scrape the tongue and find the coat thick, greasy, or clotted, you would call that greasy moisture, indicating a Spleen imbalance. Differentiate between the Stomach and Spleen in treatment. Dampness can be a positive response of the Stomach (to Heat), or it can indicate a deficiency of Spleen Qi as it fails to transform and transport. Differentiate by assessing pulses; remember, the Stomach sits higher in the guan position than the Spleen.

[9] The patient should not scrape their tongue on the day of treatment.

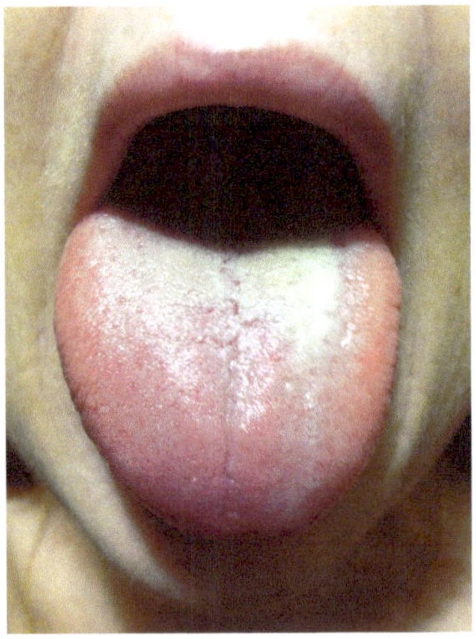

Gluey coat

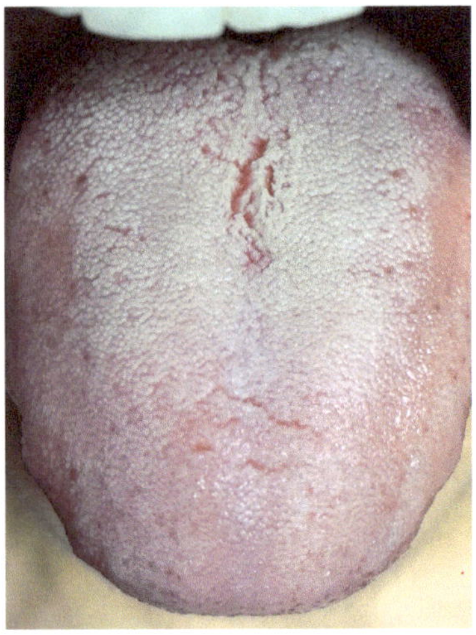

Rough coat

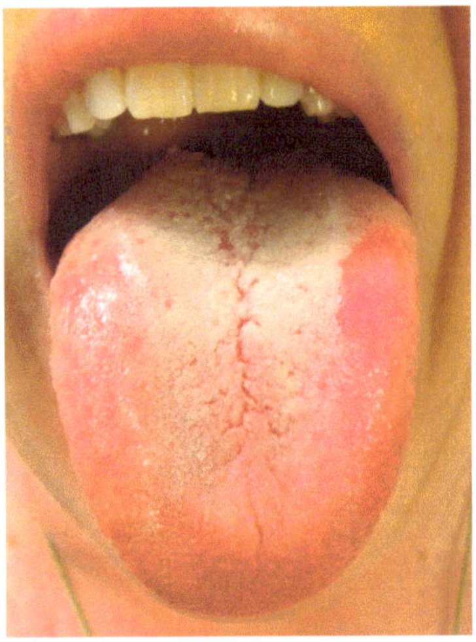

Pasty coat

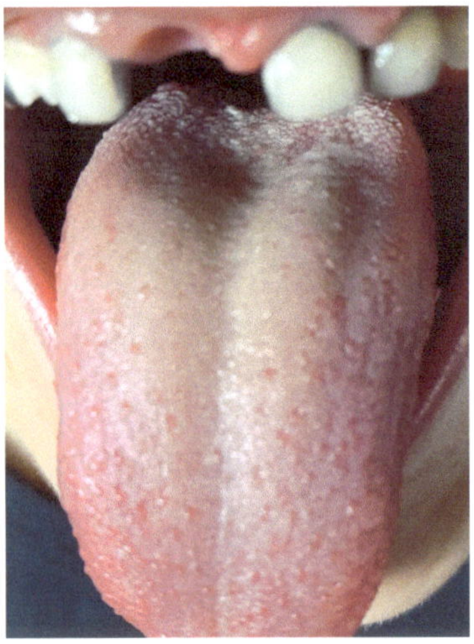

Powdery coat

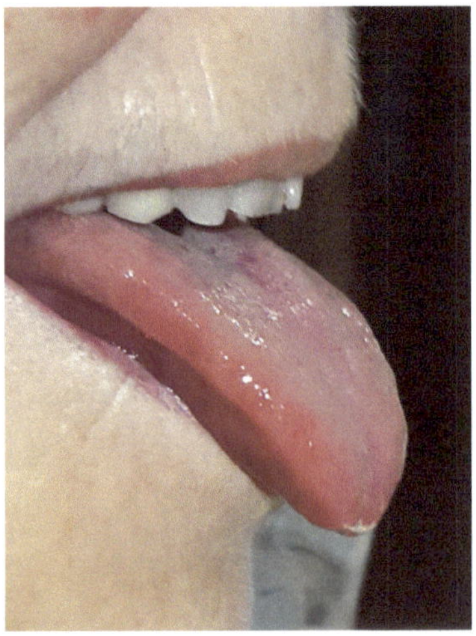

Glassy coat

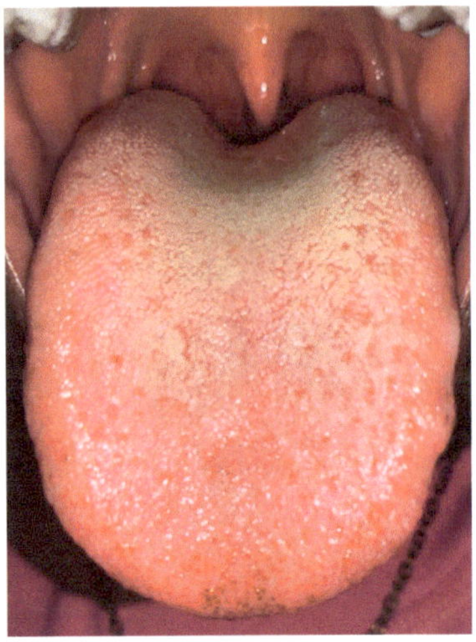

Grainy coat

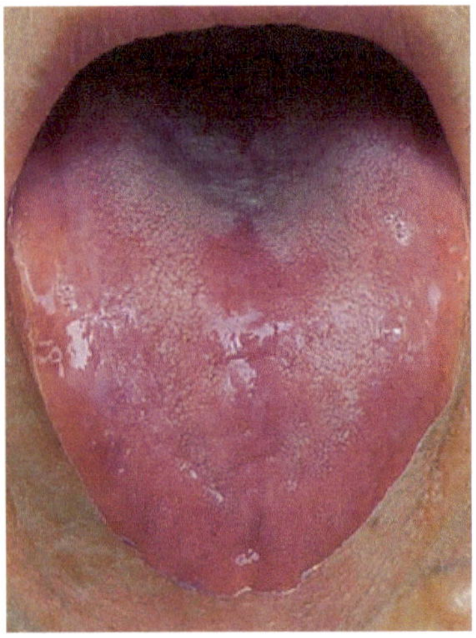

Wet coat

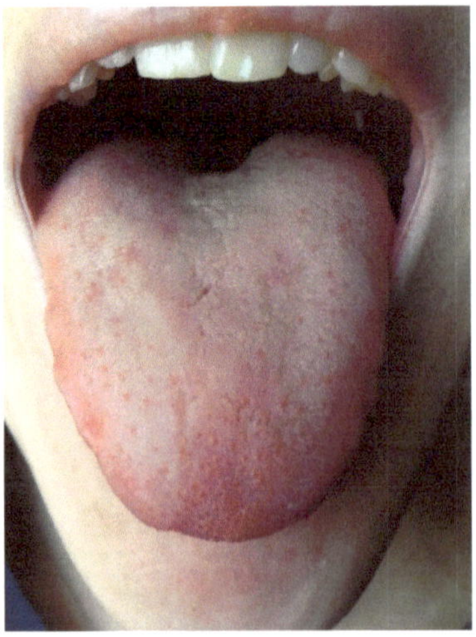

Dry coat

Tongue Coat Color

Additional comments on color are included in the previous section.

The tongue coat is expected to be thin and white. The white color reflects:

- the Lung's effusion of fluids to the exterior.
- the efficient functioning of the gut in terms of transformation and transportation, especially the potency of the transformative Qi of the Stomach. If there is excess turbidity in the Stomach, the coat may be discolored (and thickened). The lack of clarity of the coat's color indicates digestive strength is insufficient to fully separate Fluids.

Tongue Coat Color Diagnosis

If the tongue coat:

- is thicker than normal and white, there may be an external pathogenic factor, Wind-Cold. Wei Qi is responding to Wind-Cold, in its early stage, by moving to expel it. This movement of Wei Qi closely involves the Lungs' movement of fluids to expel the pathogen, hence the thicker white coat. Release the Tai Yang Jing-Well points to release the pathogen from the exterior.
- is very slightly yellow, the body is responding to the pathogen with Heat. The tip and the sides of the tongue may be red as Wei Qi, which is very warming, activates to scatter the Cold. The Heat is seen as a response to a Wind-Cold invasion as it tries to burn up or transform the pathogen. As it does so, it begins to turn the white coat yellow.
- is greasy and white, the condition is in Shao Yang. The pathogenic factor is lingering due to Dampness. The body is unable to expel it but hasn't given up yet. The tongue body may be slightly pale due to the underlying Qi deficiency. The patient may have Bi Syndrome since Qi is partially stagnant.
- is yellow, the condition has penetrated to the interior and Heat is in Yang Ming. There is Heat in the digestive tract. Ask about nausea and coughing.
- is golden brown, long-term Heat is now affecting the bowels.
- is brown, the Heat has been there a long time and is advancing.
- is black or gray, the Heat has been there so long it has scorched the interior or it has moved to the Kidneys (Lower Jiao). This happened because there were insufficient fluids in the Lungs to create sweat, or insufficient fluids in the Stomach to initiate vomiting

to rid the pathogenic factor. The Kidneys are profoundly taxed while responding to this assault—trying to provide more Yang to move the pathogen to the exterior. The extended Kidney involvement gives the coat a gray hue.

- is black and moist, Heat has damaged the Kidneys causing Cold-Phlegm to accumulate.
- is quite black, the patient is in a critical condition. There is injury to both Yin and Yang at the Yuan level. Remember, all conditions can be turned around if that is the patient's path.
- has a bluish/purplish hue, the longitudinal Luo is having difficulty containing a pathogenic factor. It may be trying to express an internal pathogenic factor to the exterior. Look for spider veins on the Luo Channels, bleed Luo points and then the related spider veins.

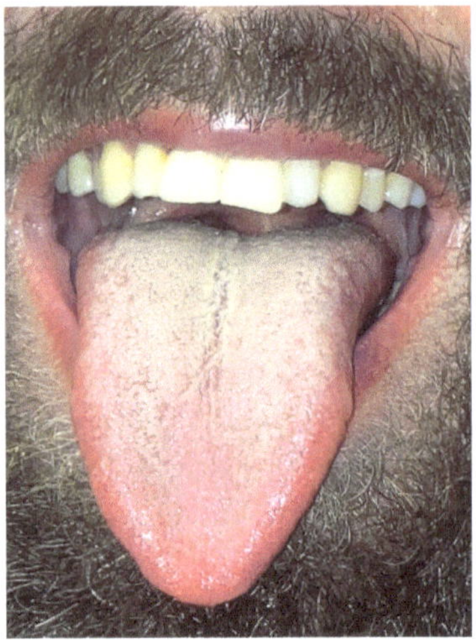
Very slightly yellow

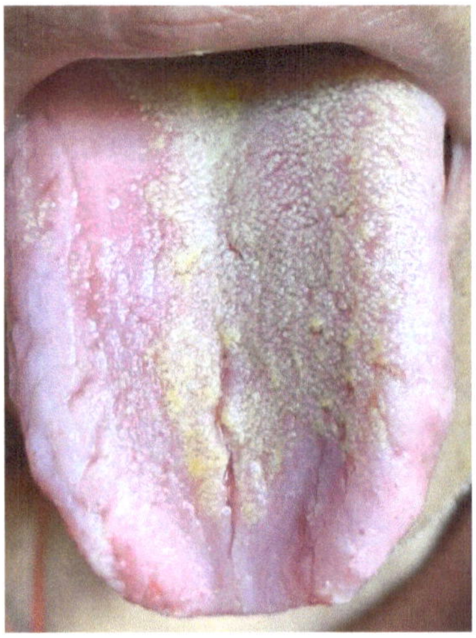
Yellow

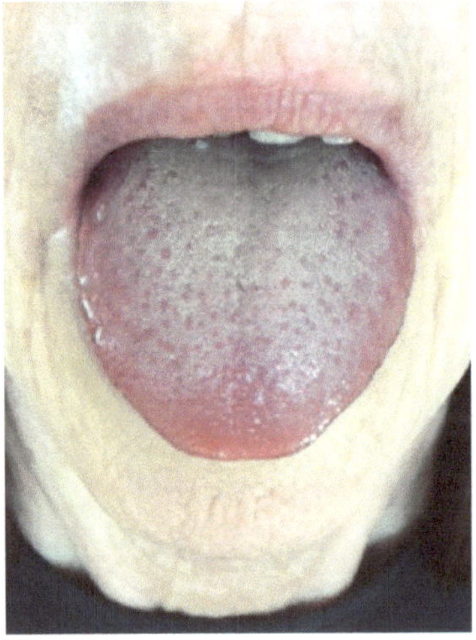
Dirty gray

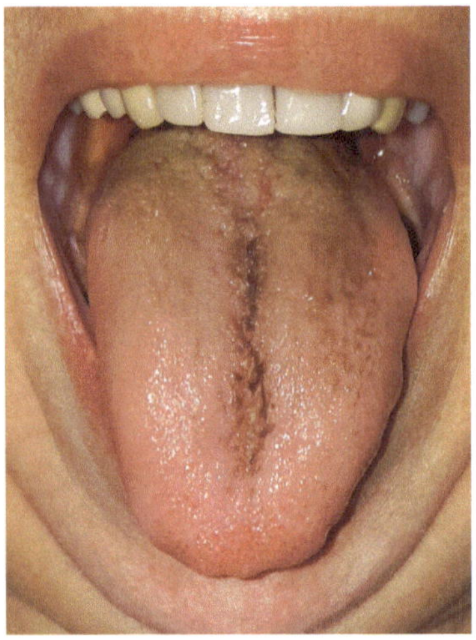
Dark brown

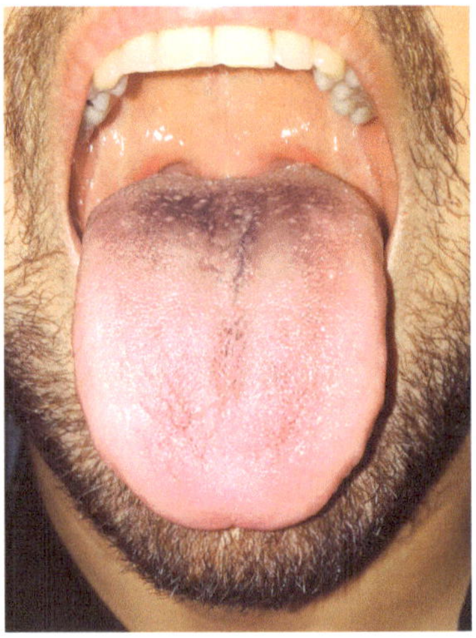
Black

Tongue Coat Coverage

The tongue coat:

- is normally thicker in the early morning.

- is normally thicker after menstruation because the body is trying to generate more Blood and in so doing must generate more Fluids.

- can easily change with food and herbs. To see the full and deeper picture beyond the influence of the patient's recent meals, rely on detailed pulse taking.

- interestingly, shows the waxing or waning of Stomach fluids during the course of a lifetime: in babies, the tongue coat develops slowly, beginning at the back of the tongue and slowly spreading to the tip. As people get older, the Yin slowly disappears like a curtain, beginning at the tip of the tongue and slowly extending all the way to the back of the tongue.

Tongue Coat Coverage Diagnosis

If the coat is:

- patchy, the body is trying to accumulate Yin. As the body gathers Yin, you may see pockets or patches of coat. The body is trying to respond to the lack of Yin. This is not to be confused with the Lungs failing to disperse fluids over the tongue. The appearance of a "patchy" tongue is different because it has a feeling of having been there but having been lost. The patchy tongue is accompanied by pulses showing deficient Yin in the left chi position at the deep level.

- trying to glue together cracks all over the tongue, there is a deficiency of Yin together with stasis of Yin. As Heat damages Yin, whatever coat there is evaporates. The body attempts to gather Yin and hold on to it out of desperation to repair the loss, while Yin continues to be eroded or Heat-damaged.

- peeling off, there may be a Yin deficiency; the body is not able to retain Yin by banking and consolidation. The coat starts to peel off. Heat damages all Fluids. Treat full and empty Heat and pay attention to Kidney and Heart communication since the consolidating action is dependent on the Heart being able to communicate downward to the Kidneys.

- absent long term, if there is no coat for an extended period, there is deficient Yin. This can include deficiency due to loss of Fluids causing dehydration. If there is no coat at the back of the tongue, the deficiency of Yin is due to loss of Yin, or aging. Wei Qi is weak if there is no coat.

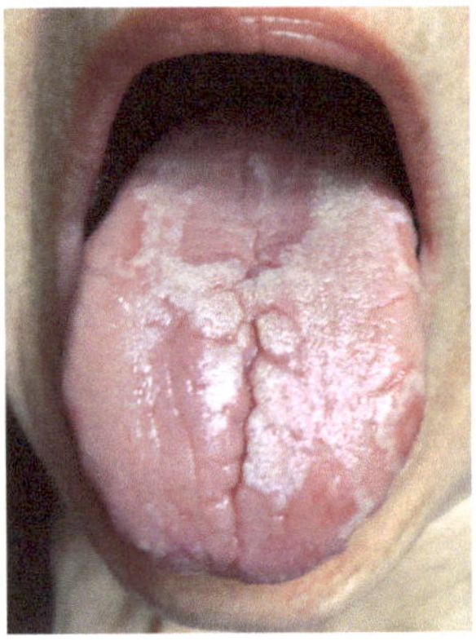

Patchy coat.

Yin deficiency causes the tongue to attempt to build back Yin.

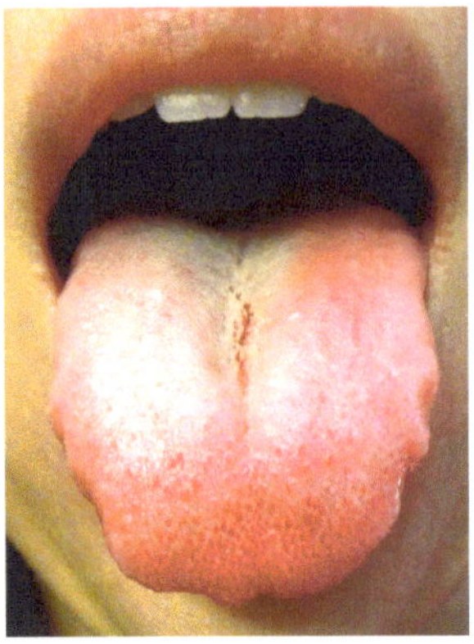

Glueing together.

The tongue coat attempts to patch up the tongue crack, since pathological Dampness is accumulated as compensation for Stomach Yin deficiency.

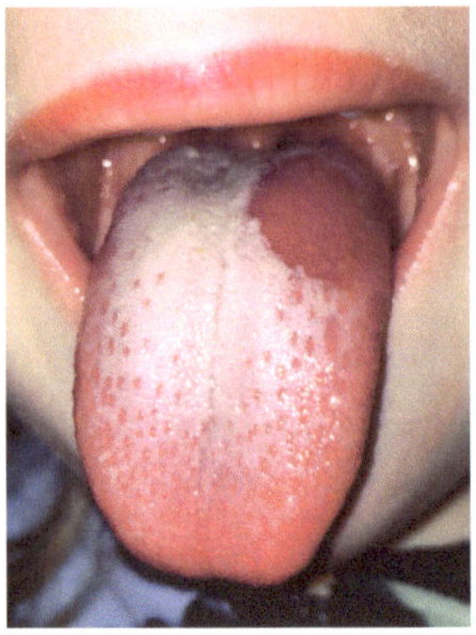

Peeling off.

Processed food and sugar has decimated Kidney Yin in this young child, causing the coat to peel.

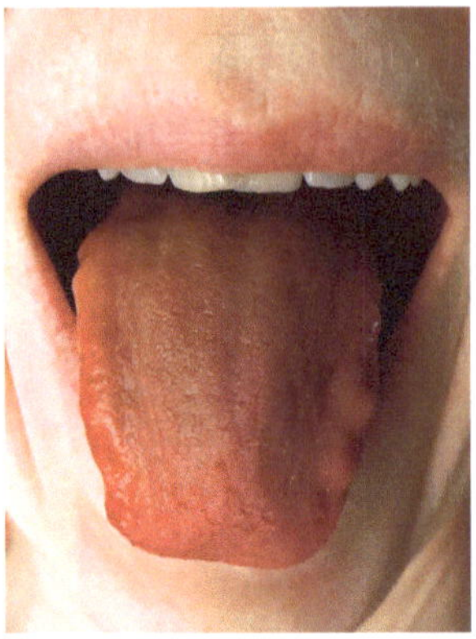

Missing coat.

This patient has chronic insomnia, a very late-night habit, and deep anxiety, all of which have created a cycle of diminishing Yin.

The Tongue Coat, Wei Qi, and Pulse Diagnosis

If there is no coat, or the coat is not well formed according to the criteria above, Wei Qi is compromised. But deficient Wei Qi is always a branch of an underlying pathology. Treatment must focus on the root of the pathology, the weak link in the chain of Wei Qi manufacture. The tongue is showing you the result of the pathology that has weakened Wei Qi, not the root cause. To find the cause, if you can, take the pulses. To identify where Wei Qi production is weak, consider the following list of factors to find where the root cause lies. Of course, you'll have your own way of treating these things, but in case it's useful, I've included quick treatment suggestions I often use to address the weakness. The responses can be astonishing in their immediacy and effectiveness. These changes leave you freer to continue within the hour, moving to a next phase of treatment.

If the tongue coat appears to reflect pathology, the following may be in play:

1. Kidney Yang is deficient.
2. Spleen Qi is not ascending.
3. There is Systemic dehydration.
4. Stomach and Spleen are failing to transform fluids.
5. Heat is damaging fluids and the fluid mechanism.
6. Lung Qi is not dispersing fluids.
7. There is Liver Qi constraint.

These pathologies are explained below in more detail.

1. Kidney Yang is deficient. Wei Qi flows in the Sinews and is a subset of Kidney Yang; it's warming and moving. It provides Yang to the Spleen and Stomach for the transformation and transportation of food and fluids.

    Pathology: The absence of a good tongue coat may be showing you that there is a deficiency of Kidney Yang. Or Kidney Yang might not be supplying Yang to the digestive tract where the coat is manufactured. To find out if this is the case, perform the following diagnosis.

    Diagnosis and treatment: Listen to the deep level of the Kidney Yang pulse (the deep level of the right chi position). If it is weak or absent, tonify Kidney Yang, perhaps with moxa at KI-3. Check the pulse again.

2. Spleen Qi is not ascending. The coat is brought from the digestive tract to the tongue by the ascending action of the Spleen. But first, the Spleen must access Kidney Yang for its own strength then ascend more Kidney Yang to the Stomach, which is the origin of fluids.

    Pathology: The absence of a good tongue coat may be showing you that the Spleen is weak. If the Spleen is not able to access or ascend Kidney Yang, the Spleen might not have enough Qi to ascend fluids from the Stomach to coat the tongue. To find out if this is the case, perform the following diagnosis.

    Diagnosis and treatment: Press down on the Spleen pulse and release a tiny amount of pressure from the Lung pulse. You should feel the Qi moving upward from the Spleen toward the Lung pulse. If you don't feel that, ascend Spleen Qi, boosting its function of connecting Kidney Yang to itself. Use the only trajectory that does this: the third branch of the Kidney Primary Channel. It has two points: KI-2 and SP-8. Needle and moxa both points, imagining they are connected together. Moxa safely until the patient reports they can feel the two connected by an unmistakable line. Check the pulse again.

3. There is Systemic dehydration. Wei Qi is derived from Gu Qi, specifically the turbid aspect of Stomach Fluids.

    Pathology: The absence of a good tongue coat may be showing you that there is significant systemic dehydration. To find out if this is the case, perform the following diagnosis.

    Diagnosis and treatment: Note the width of the Spleen position at the moderate level. It should be nice and wide. If it's narrow or thin, nourish Stomach Fluids by tonifying ST-42 or/and CV-12. Check the pulse again.

If the tongue coat is not clean, thin, white, and evenly distributed, the following may be occurring.

4. **Stomach and Spleen are failing to transform fluids.** The color and texture of the coat indicates how efficiently the Spleen and Stomach are transforming and generating Fluids. If the coat doesn't look clean, the Spleen and Stomach are not transforming and transporting Fluids.

    Pathology: If the tongue coat is discolored or impure-looking, it may be showing you that the transforming capability of the digestive tract is weak. To find out if this is the case, perform the following diagnosis.

    Diagnosis and treatment: Listen to the strength of the moderate level of the Spleen position and listen to the deep level of the right Kidney position (Kidney Yang). Tonify Spleen Qi and ensure you have sufficient Kidney Yang. Simple moxa on SP-3 and KI-3 can work beautifully if these are missing.

5. **Heat is damaging Fluids and the fluid mechanism.** Wei Qi is damaged by Heat as Heat damages the Fluids that form Wei Qi. The texture of the coat indicates to what degree Heat is damaging Fluids and affecting fluid mechanisms.

    Pathology: If the coat looks scorched or dry and yellow, there may be Heat damaging the digestive tract and its transformation and transportation of Fluids.

    Diagnosis and treatment: Take pulses and locate the rapid pulse. Clear Heat from the Stomach, perhaps through ST-44, and then clear Heat related to the location you found in your pulse findings. Check the pulse again.

6. **Lung Qi is not dispersing Fluids.** The distribution of Wei Qi to the surface of the body is governed by the Lungs. The evenness of the tongue coat coverage is a reflection of how well the Lungs are able to distribute Fluids systemically.

    Pathology: If the coat is uneven, the tongue may be showing you that the Lungs are not dispersing their Qi to the exterior. To find out if this is the case, perform the following diagnosis.

    Diagnosis and treatment: If the Lungs are not diffusing Lung Qi, you will find that as you lift your finger very slowly from the moderate level of the Lung pulse all the way to the surface of the skin, the pulse will not follow your finger all the way; you will not feel it against your finger as you release pressure from the pulse. To get the Lungs to diffuse Wei Qi, needle LU-1 or LU-7 and pull the needle up to the surface with the intention of bringing Wei Qi to the surface. Check the pulse again.

7. **There is Liver Qi constraint.** The Liver is responsible for the smooth flow of Wei Qi, both to the exterior and in the smooth muscle.

   Pathology: If the coat appears uneven or has accumulations, it may be showing you that Wei Qi is constrained by the Liver. To find out if this is the case, perform the following diagnosis.

   Diagnosis and treatment: If the moderate level of the Liver pulse is tight or wiry, release the tightness by reducing LR-14 or LR-13 or BL-17 or 18. Stay very oblique, not perpendicular on any or all of these points.

The tongue coat is further discussed in chapter 9, The Tongue Map.

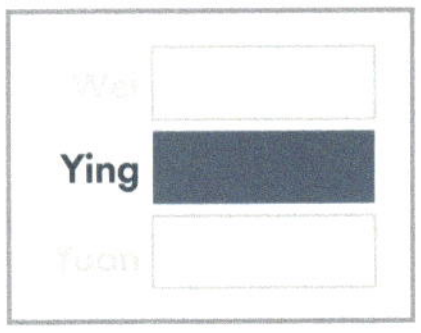

6

The Tongue Body Reveals Ying Qi Status
(Blood and Fluids)

The body of the tongue reflects Ying-Nutritive Qi (the Qi of Blood and Fluids). Analysis of the tongue body tells us about the effect of Heat on Blood and Fluids. It also tells of the effect that Heat is having on the organs that deal with Blood: the Heart, Liver, and Spleen.

Movement and Posture of the Tongue Body

Movement and posture of the tongue is governed by the channels that connect to the tongue: Kidney Primary Channel, Spleen Primary Channel, and Heart Luo Channel. [10]

Kidney Channel

The Kidney Primary Channel goes to the root of the tongue, where its Qi initiates tongue movement. If the tongue is dry and there is difficulty initiating tongue movement, Kidney Qi is inadequate.

Spleen Channel

Movement and posture of the tongue rely on Qi reaching it. The Spleen Primary Channel goes to the root of the tongue, and so the Spleen is responsible for its posture, general movement, swallowing, and chewing. If the tongue appears flaccid, droopy, flopping, or hanging, there is insufficient ascension of Spleen Qi.

Heart Luo Channel

The tongue is known classically as the sprout of the Heart. The connection between the Heart and its sprout is the Heart Luo, a conduit of Blood. Since Blood houses the emotions, the Heart Luo enables the tongue to express emotions. When the mind overrides the tongue in the expression of emotions, the tongue becomes stiff as Blood flow to the tongue slows. The tongue acquires shades of purple as a result. This in turn reflects emotional pathology: a state where the patient is seeking to find latency for unexpressed emotions. When the Blood is in free flow and the emotions are free, the tongue exhibits its natural bland red color, a color we now call pink.

Movement and Posture Analysis

Analysis of the movement of the tongue is an important part of diagnosis. The first part of the

[10] The Heart Primary Channel does not go to the tongue, though it does go to the throat and the eyes.

analysis of movement involves consideration of the three channels that attach to the tongue.

1. If there is difficulty in the initiation of movement—for example, if the patient cannot initiate movement because of paralysis, shock, trauma, stuttering, or damage—the Kidney Channel should be treated. If these are a chief complaint, key points would be KI-27 and CV-23, paired with individually appropriate distal Kidney Channel points.

2. If there is a lack of tonicity of the tongue, Spleen Qi is not sufficiently ascending to enable movement to be vital.

3. If the tongue is stiff and purple, the Heart Luo Channel is enabling the withholding of speech for emotional reasons.

Wind and the Tongue

When mediumship (Fluids, Blood, Yin or Jing) become deficient, the channels lack the stability they are provided by the mass of that medium. The instability manifests as twitches, tremors, shaking, moving pain, and ultimately stroke. The tongue reflects wind as tiny erratic movements, major unpredictable movement, stiffness, and deviation.

In addition to all the above, the following can be considered:

If the tongue is:

- stiff,
    - Liver Qi is stagnated. The smooth flow of Liver Qi enables free movement of the musculature, or
    - the Heart is not adequately moving Blood, or
    - the Lungs are not adequately moving Blood, or
    - Heat has depleted fluids in the tongue, causing stiffness, or
    - Heat has either consumed Stomach Fluids, or blocked the passage of Stomach Fluids to the tongue, or
    - Blood stasis is causing the tongue to stiffen.
- so stiff it is curled or retracted, one or more of the above conditions is advanced.
- stiff and has purple spots on it, there is Blood stagnation, due to either emotional trauma, or intellectual stagnation.
- pointing upward, examine the color of the tongue body.

- If it is red, Heat is rising.
- If it is pale, there are accumulations or swellings and the resulting constriction is causing the pathology to move upward.

- darts out and is long, Blood flow is pathologically increased. Perhaps there is bleeding or systemic Heat, or Wind, or exuberant Yang.
- flaccid, Spleen is not managing Blood and Fluids, Spleen Qi has collapsed, or there is a deficiency of Kidney Yang.
- shaking, there is imbalance in the Kidneys.[11] Since the Kidney Primary Channel connects to the tongue, shaking is often due to Kidney deficiency:
    - Either Kidney Yin is deficient, allowing Kidney Yang to escape and float upward, causing instability as it cannot come to rest, or
    - Kidney Yang is itself insufficient, unable to support the tongue.
- incessantly moving, wiggling, Kidney Yin is insufficient to anchor Yang and bring it to a state of rest.
- wiggling but with intermittent short periods of stiffness, a Yin deficiency has led to congestion of Liver Qi as the Liver tries to stagnate Yin in response to a Yin deficiency. Yin then fails to circulate effectively. Wind in turn arises due to the vacuity and compromised circulation, causing the tongue to shake. The stagnating Liver Qi causes tiny periods of stiffness within the shaking. Treat Kidney Yin deficiency, which is the root.
- shaking rapidly, systemic Heat can cause shaking as Heat rises. Locate the origin of the Heat, ideally by taking the pulses and finding where they are rapid. Exuberant heat results in Wind due to consumption of fluids.
- reluctant to move, hesitant, remember that the tongue will only receive Blood from the Heart if there is sufficient Blood engendered in the Liver. If Liver Blood is stagnant, it won't move to the Heart, so it's essential that the treatment move Blood. If the Heart does not receive sufficient Blood, it cannot manage the emotions.
- deviated, it must be determined whether it is misshapen or whether it appears deviated because of the way the tongue is moving.
    - The imbalance could be in the Spleen not controlling the shape of the tongue muscle.

[11] From the point of view of neurology, it's tempting to think of the Liver as being implicated in shaking. That possibility should be explored but it's important to note that the Liver Primary Channel does not reach the tongue. Therefore a shaking tongue indicates a Kidney Yin deficiency since that channel connects to the tongue and controls the initiation of movement.

- Constraint in the Liver can sometimes shift the tongue to the right. Constraint in the Gallbladder can sometimes pull the tongue to the left.
- The Divergent Channels may also be implicated as they fail to hold pathology in latency and struggle to contain pathology, shifting the pathology to the other side of the body.
- Wind can deviate the tongue.

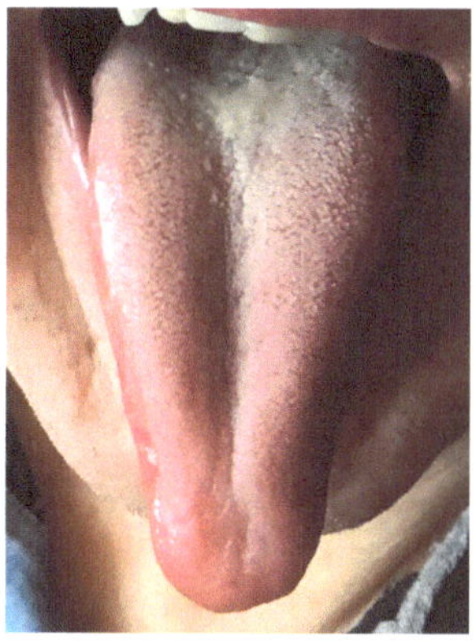
Stiff

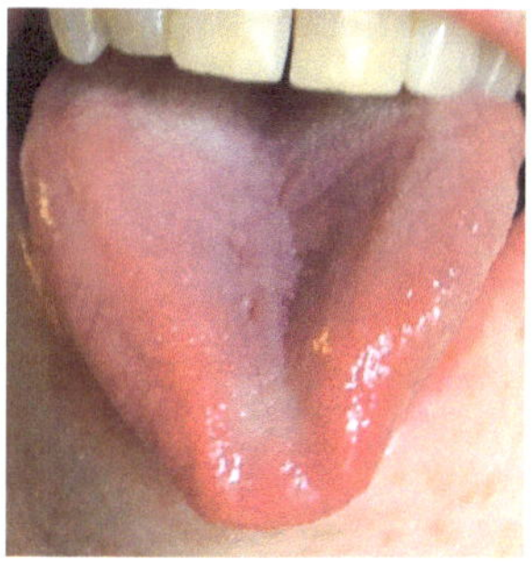
Stiff and curled or retracted

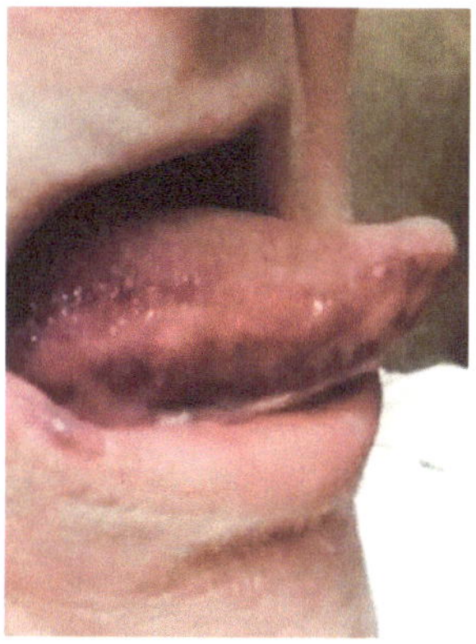
Pointing upward

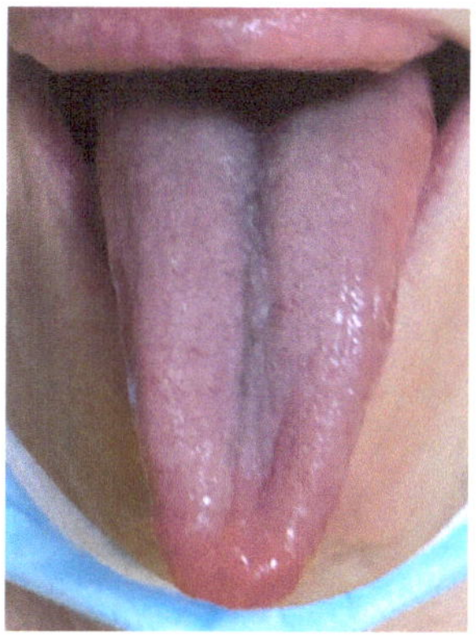
Long and darting

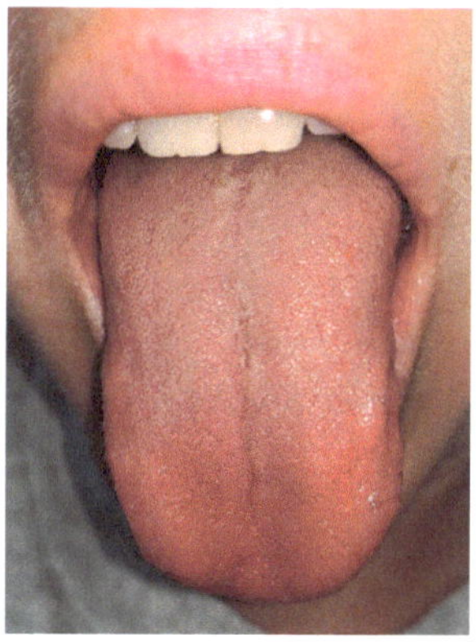
Flaccid

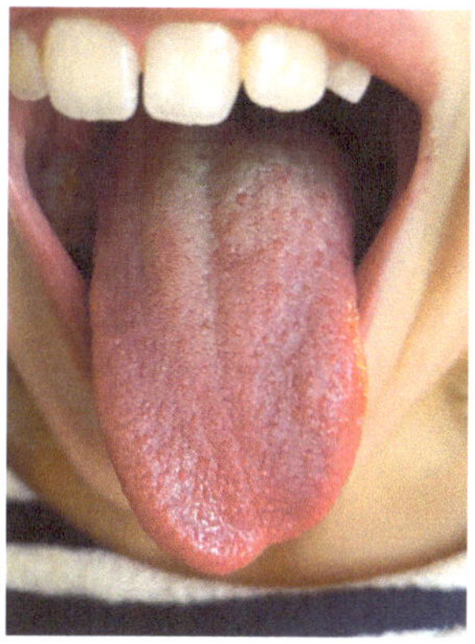
Deviated

Length of the Tongue Body

The length of the tongue body is determined by the amount of Kidney Yang available to assist in the action of extension.

The tongue appears **short** if the muscles can't extend due to a lack of Kidney Yang. There might also be insufficient Qi to lift the tongue. If so, tonify Yang.

Sometimes, you'll see there is no curve downward at the back of the tongue because it is retracted and compressed. This is a sign of Cold contracting and **retracting** the tongue.

Turbidity building in the Stomach as weak digestive function fails to separate the pure from the impure can also impede the movement of Stomach Fluids, and result in an apparent **shortening** of the tongue.

If the tongue appears **long**, there is too much Heat. The tongue can be particularly long in menopause when Heat rises from the Kidneys and at the same time the tongue tapers at the front because there is a Yin deficiency. The tongue can also redden as Yang escapes when there is insufficient Yin to anchor it. In these cases, the tongue will also be shiny.

If the tongue is **curled under**, there is insufficient Yin to maintain integrity (that is, to follow the movement of Yang) in the extension of the tongue. Disappointment can show in this way, also.

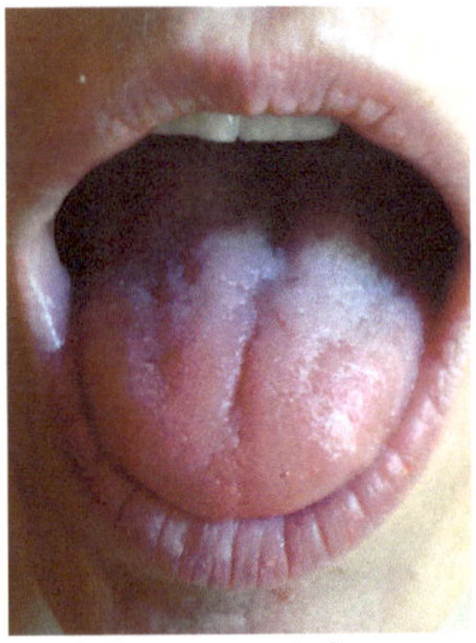

A short tongue indicates a Yang deficiency.

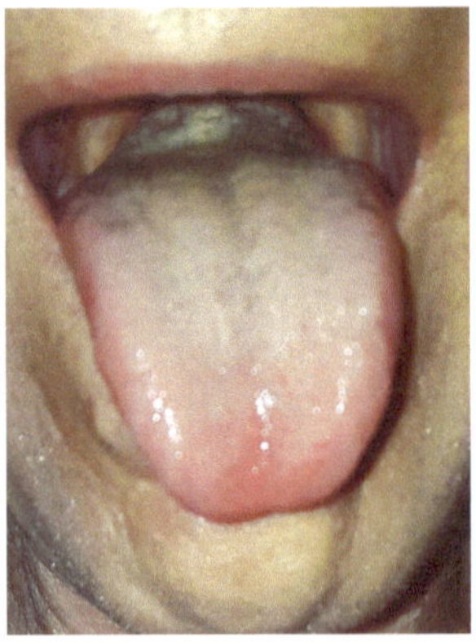

Cold retracts the tongue, preventing its natural downward curve at the rear.

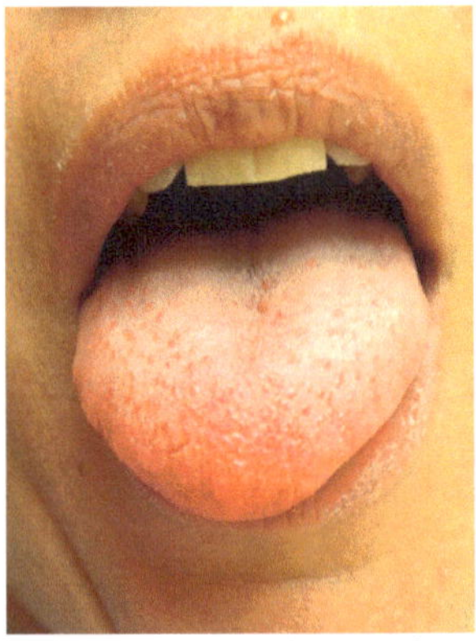

Weak digestion shortens the tongue.

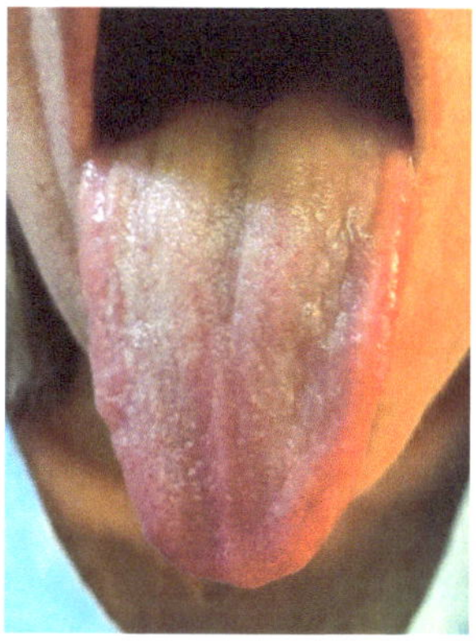

A long tongue indicates too much Heat.

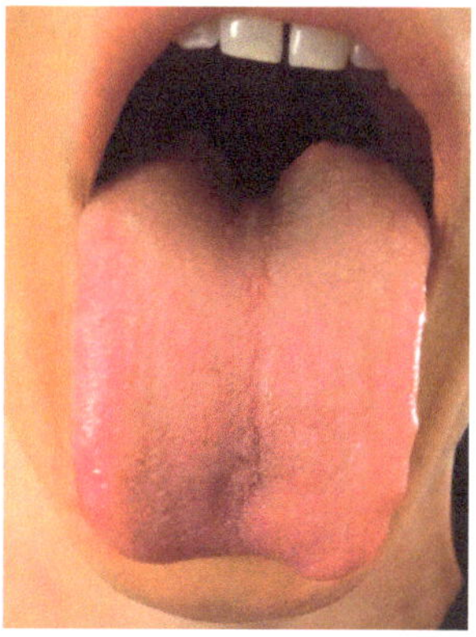

A tongue that curls under indicates a Yin insufficiency.

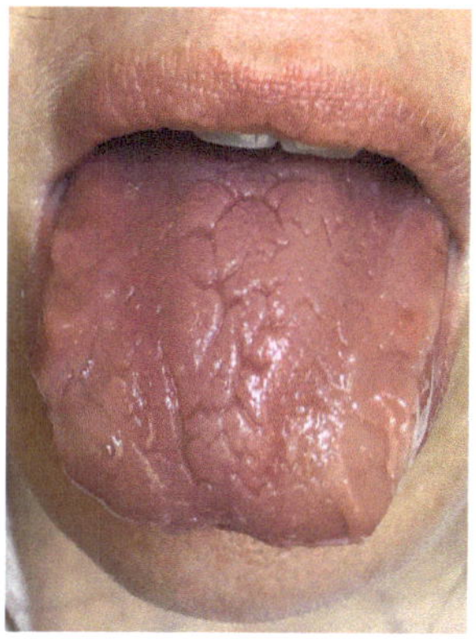

Curled under due to disappointment

Thickness and Moisture of the Tongue Body

The thickness of the tongue body is determined by the complement of mediumship (Fluids, Blood, Yin) and pathological mediumship, Dampness.

If the tongue body is:

- thin like a crepe and pale, there is a deficiency of Blood. Strengthen the Spleen in a way that enables it to generate more Blood. Many of these patients are not eating grains, the principle food of the Spleen and Stomach.[12] Just as a swollen tongue can indicate a digestive tract overwhelmed with refined carbohydrates, a very thin or crepe-like tongue can indicate a deficiency of grain. Although Blood building can be achieved with other foods, safe grains naturally bolster the Spleen and Stomach in all their roles, including Blood-building.

- thin and pale along the sides, there is a deficiency of Blood, usually at the Liver.

- large or fat, there is too much mediumship, usually Dampness. There are too many grains and other carbohydrates in the diet, nearly always refined, and usually sugar. If the tongue has been swollen for a long time, it will have toothmarks. Reduce refined carbohydrates and eliminate sugar, sticky foods, and processed foods.

- large all over, hitting all the teeth at sides and front, the tongue has been swollen for quite some time. It will likely be scalloped all the way around (front and sides). It could be discolored, bruised-looking, or dark. Reduce grains, especially the sticky grains (wheat, oats, rye, barley). Phlegmatic accumulations are being sent outward or upward. If being sent upward, the swelling will either be in the middle section of the tongue sides (the

[12] The non-glutinous grains are preferable here since the Spleen is weak. Watch for responses in the gut that may reveal an intolerance to gluten.

Middle Jiao) or the front of the tongue (the Upper Jiao as Phlegm is sent further upward). Mucus membranes of the gut have become saturated with fluid that was initially intended to get rid of a pathogenic factor but developed into phlegmatic congestion instead.

- thick and scalloped on the sides only, the Liver is tightening its hold on Blood so that it can return blood to the Kidneys. As the Liver tightens, it overpowers Spleen Qi, weakening it, leading to Spleen and Stomach signs and symptoms. This scenario is often seen during menses as the Liver tries to conserve blood.
- rough and has the texture of sandpaper, Stomach Fluids are drying up.
- appears dried or shriveled under the coat, Fluids, Blood, and/or Yin are deficient.

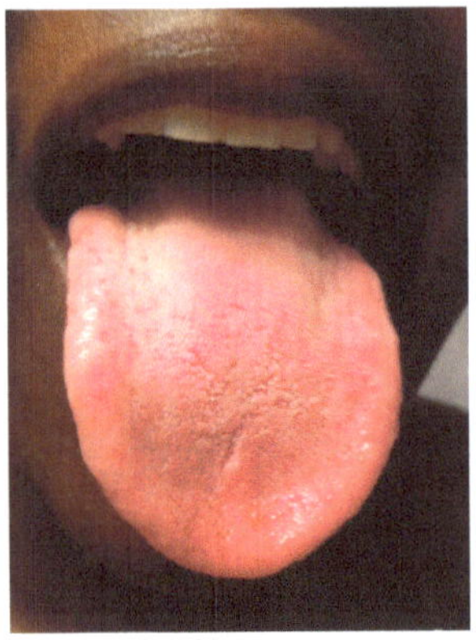
Thin like a crepe

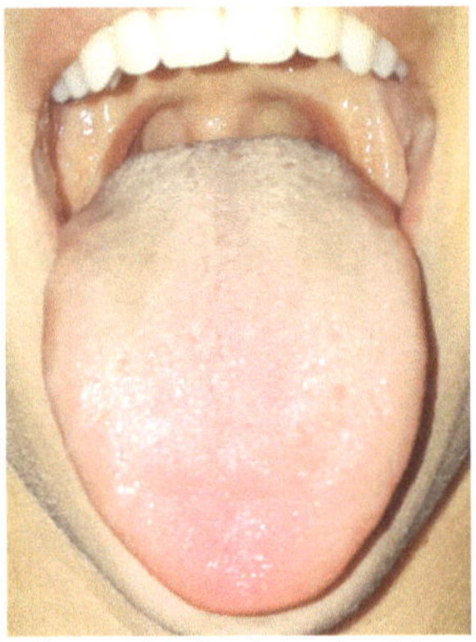
Thin and pale along the sides

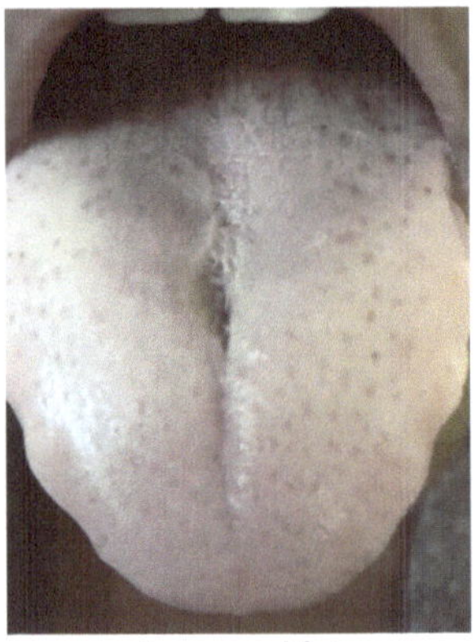
Large and fat

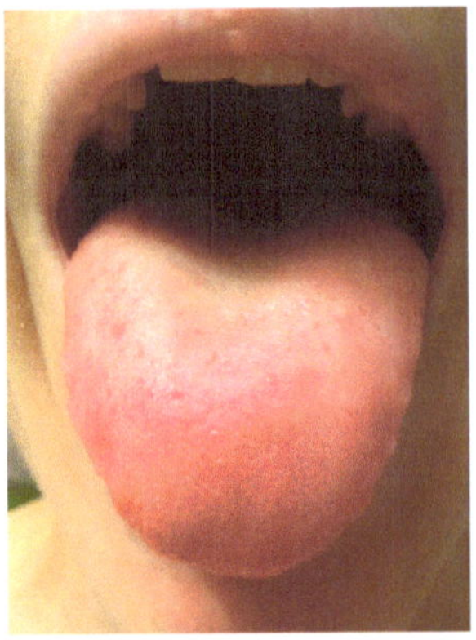
Large and hitting teeth sides and front

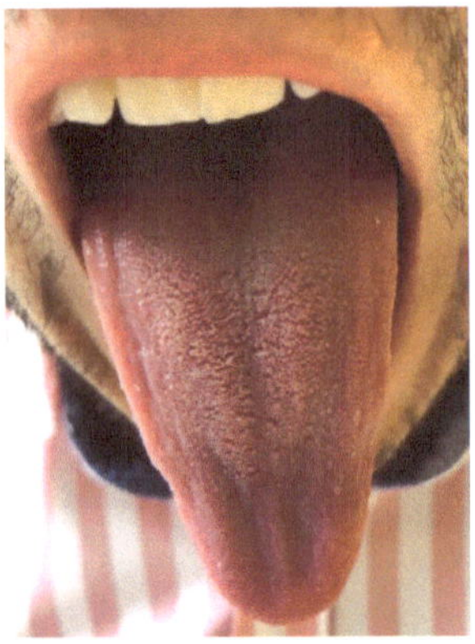
The texture of sandpaper

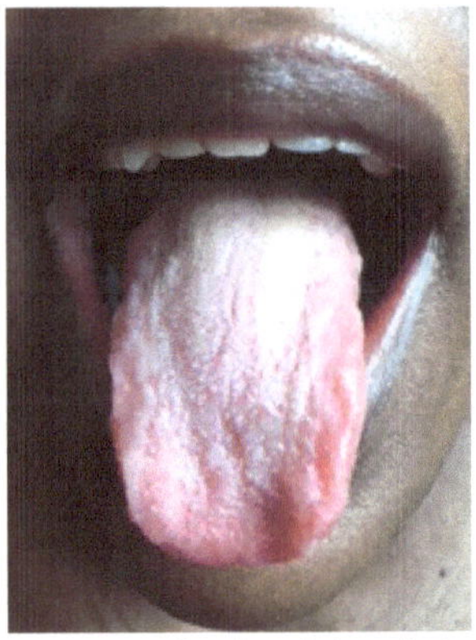
Appears dried and shriveled under the coat

Shape of the Tongue Body

The Spleen is key to the maintenance of the shape of the tongue body because its channel terminates at the root of the tongue, compounding its roles of control over the general musculature and the management of Blood.

Basic Tongue Shapes

A squared tongue shows that Wei-Defensive Qi is not adequately dispersed to the exterior.

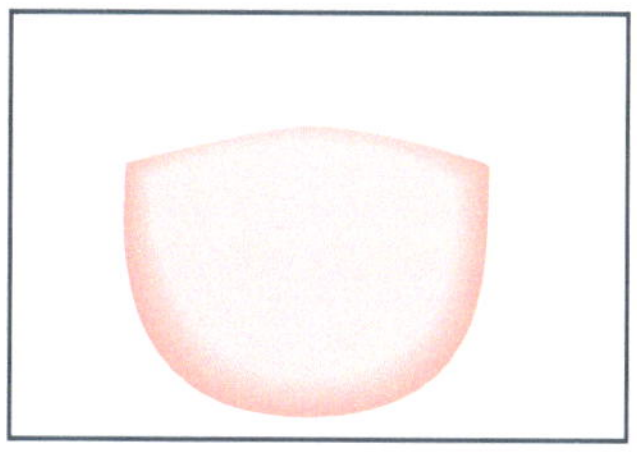

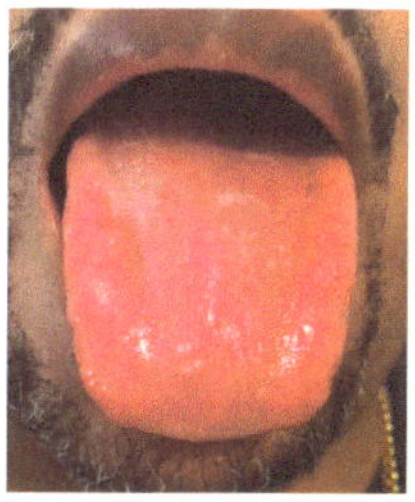

This patient suffered insomnia, as Wei Qi was unable to home to the chest at night.

A pointed tongue means that Liver Qi constraint is advancing, and forcing the tongue to a point.

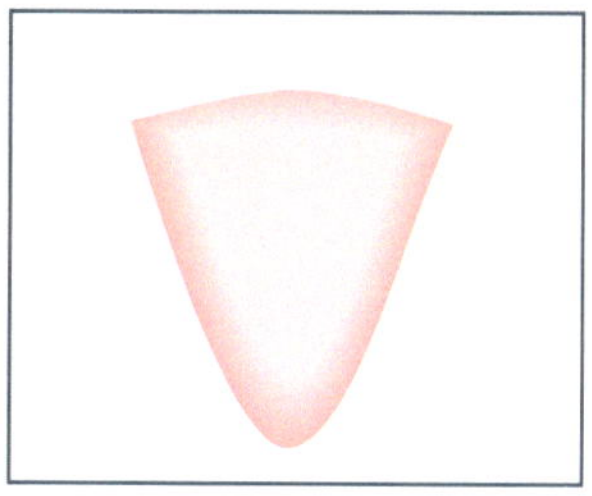

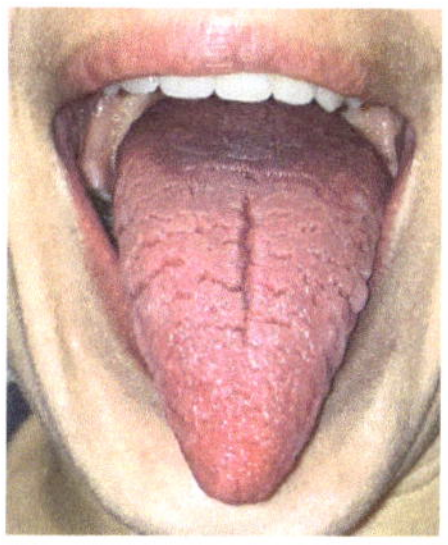

This young patient accumulated so much Heat that Blood has been consumed, cracking the tongue and causing constraint in the Liver as it struggles to store what Blood it can.

A swollen, rounded tongue indicates that systemic Dampness has accumulated in the Upper Jiao. The Middle Jiao is usually affected also.

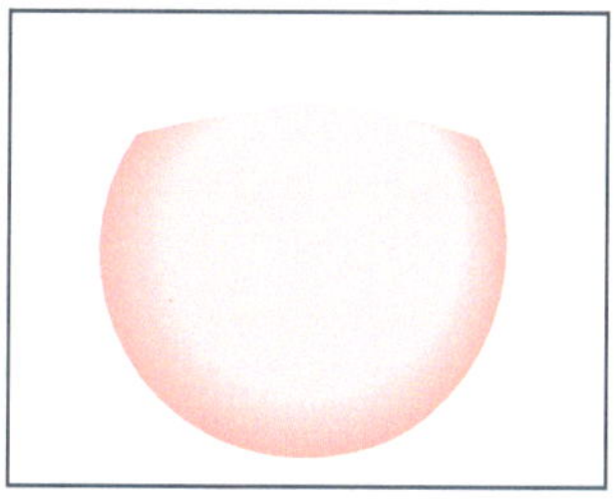

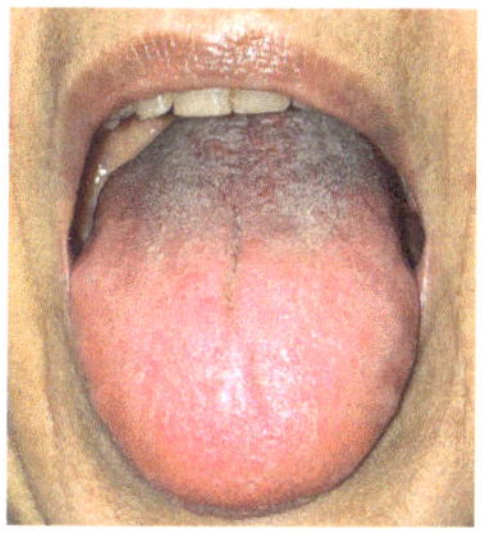

This patient has digestive weakness resulting in Dampness that is now affecting the Lungs.

A swollen, rounded tongue that is wider than the mouth indicates that the body is overwhelmed by systemic Dampness. If the pulses are slow, Dampness is the pathology.

If the pulses are rapid, Dampness is the response. Do not drain this latter Dampness.

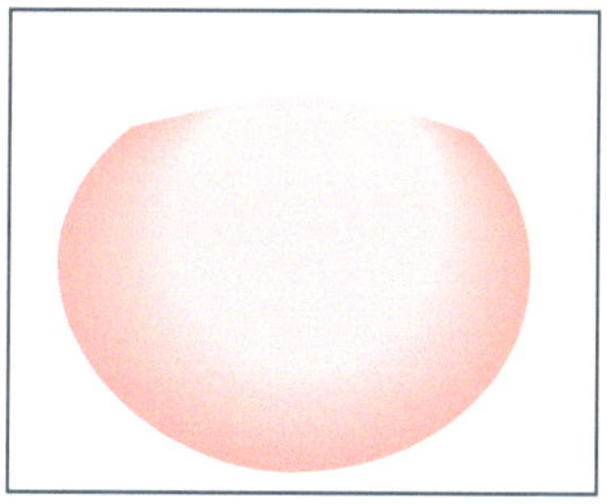

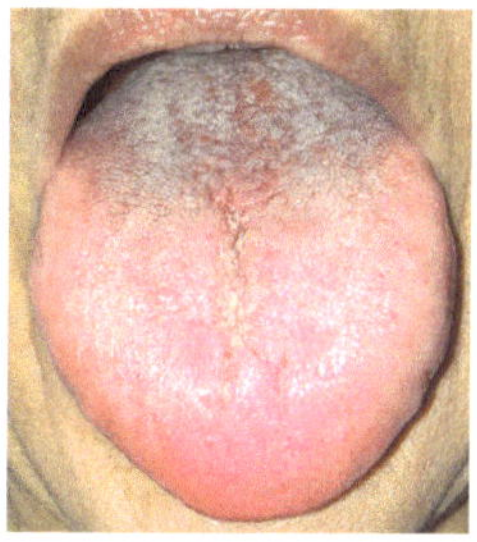

Systemic Damp is manifesting in gas and bloating, tiredness, constipation, and anxiety.

If the tongue is:

- swollen, the Spleen is not managing Blood and Fluids. Dampness is resulting.
- narrow, resulting in gaps between the extended tongue and sides of the mouth, there is a deficiency of Blood, usually at the Liver, or there is a Yin deficiency. There is insufficient mediumship to fill the tongue out.
- narrow across the rear, there is deficiency of Yin or Jing, or Cold is contracting the Lower Jiao.
- narrow across the front, there is a deficiency of Blood and Fluids nourishing the Upper Jiao, or the Pericardium is tightening to protect the Heart.
- narrow across the middle, there is a deficiency of mediumship (Blood or Fluids) in the Middle Jiao.
- thin and narrow, the Spleen is not managing Blood and Fluids or there is a depletion of mediumship (Blood or Fluids), Qi or Kidney Yang.
- pointed with tight sides, there is frustration with life, resulting in Liver constraint. This stagnation tightens the sides of the tongue, pushing the front of the tongue forward, demonstrating the extension of Heart constraint. The patient feels they are unable to do as they wish.
- scalloped, either Spleen or Liver is deficient. See box on page 40, *Differentiating Scalloping*.
- concave in shape, there is not enough Qi to allow the tongue to fully fill in and occupy its space. The Spleen may be failing to ascend Qi. Kidney Yang may be deficient.
- concave in the middle, the Spleen is not ascending because it can't gather Qi.
- concave in the rear, there is weakness in Kidneys or a deficiency of Jing.
- small, there is a deficiency of Yin.
- shriveled, Yin has been consumed to a serious degree.

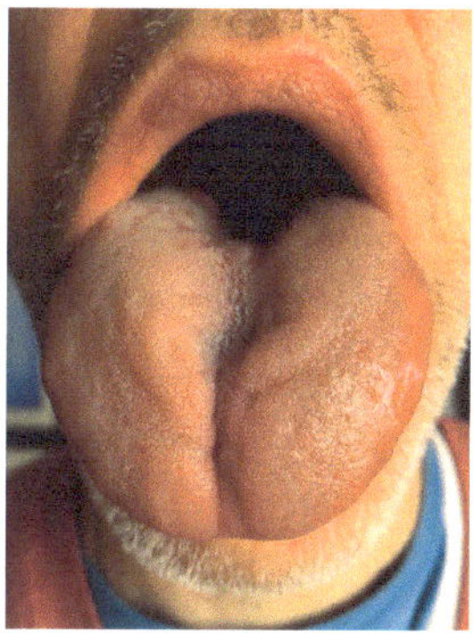

Swollen

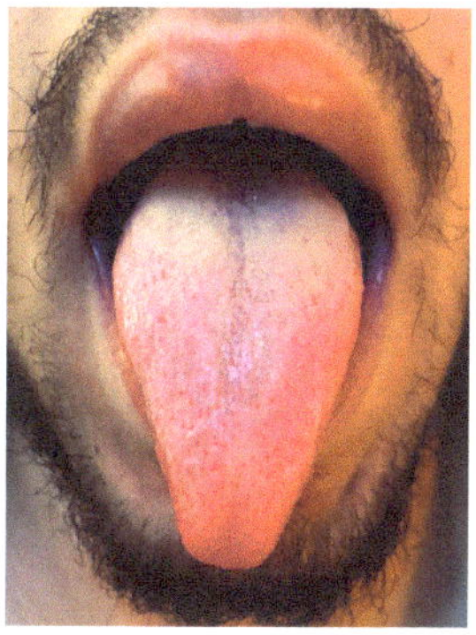

Narrow with gaps

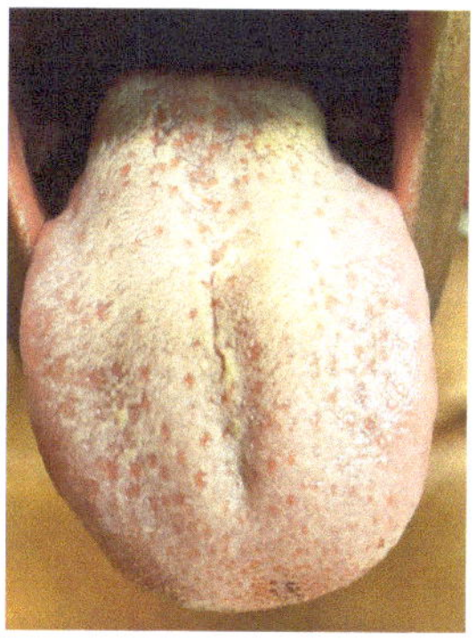

Narrow at the rear

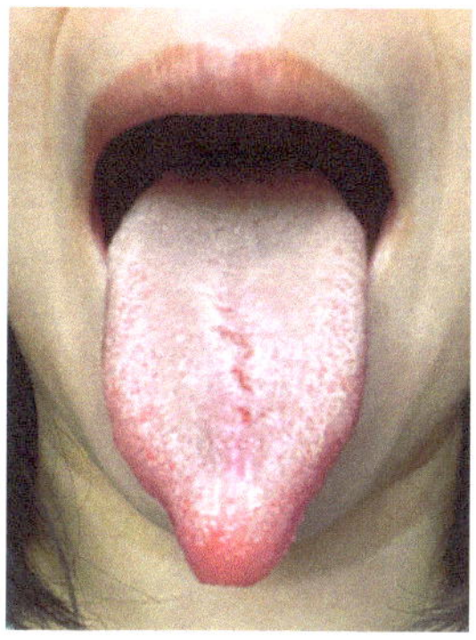

Narrow across the front

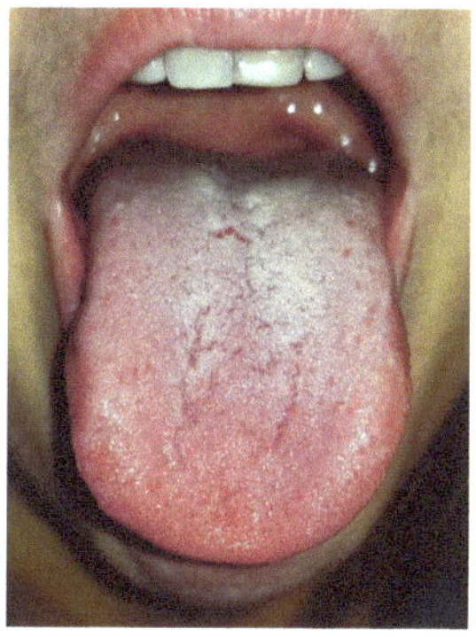

Narrow across the middle, affecting the rear

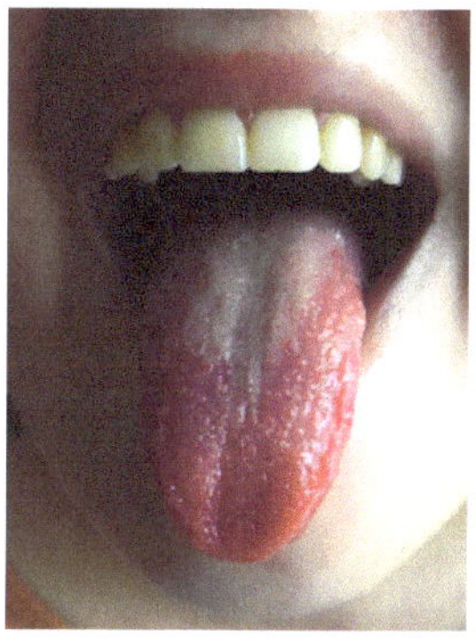

Thin and narrow

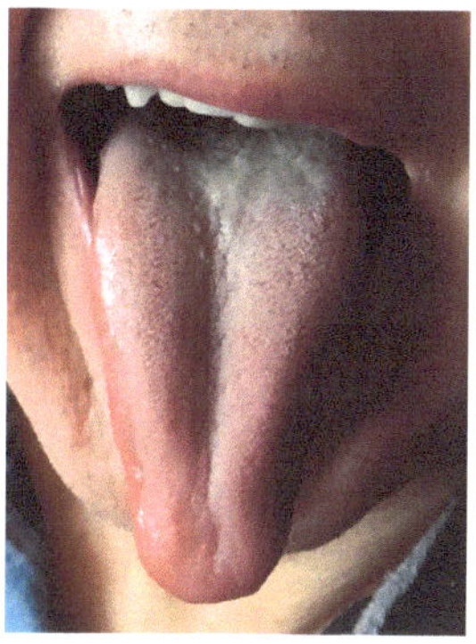

Pointed with tight sides

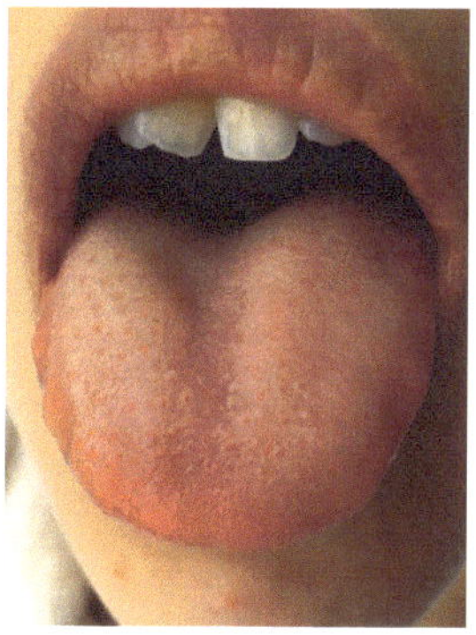

Scalloped

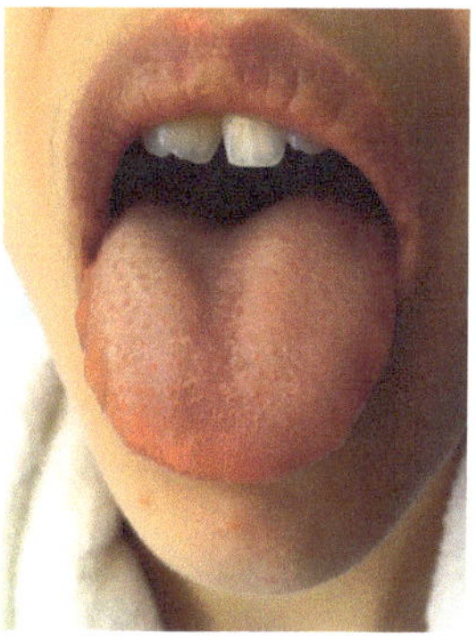

Concave

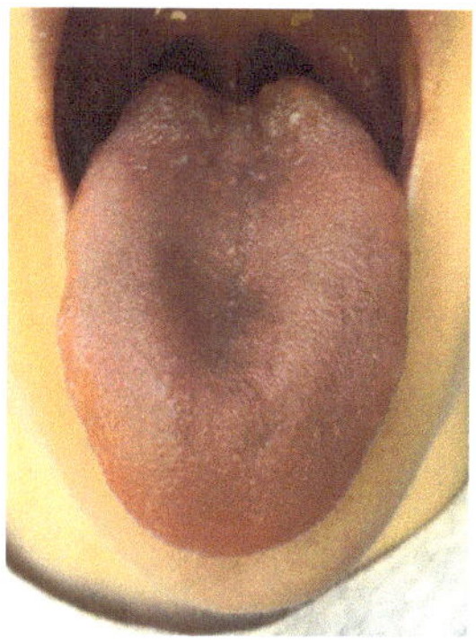

Concave in the middle

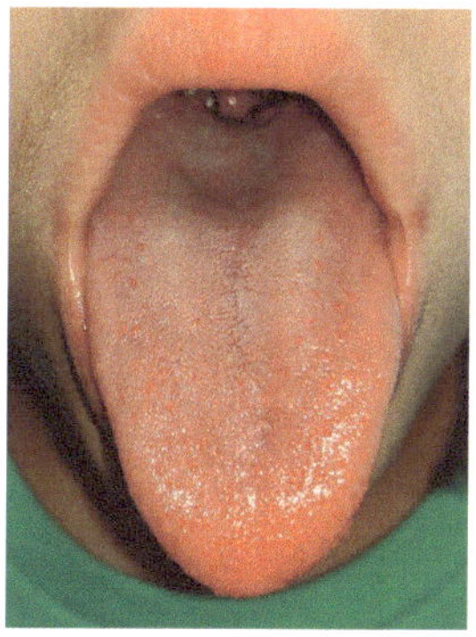

Concave in the rear

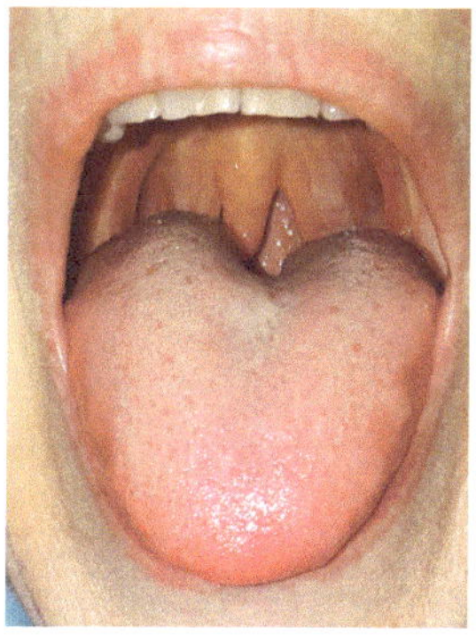

Concave in the rear II

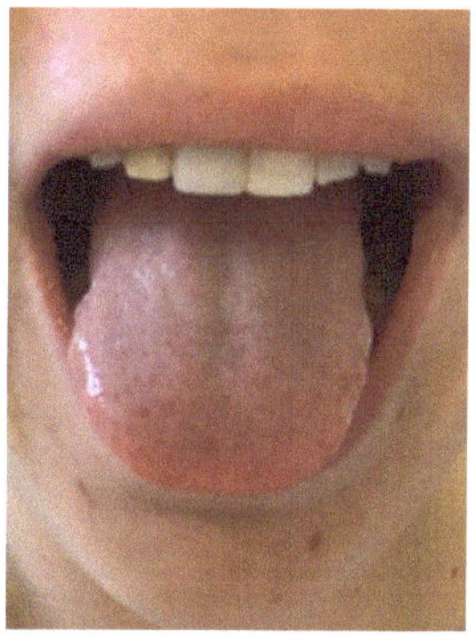

Small

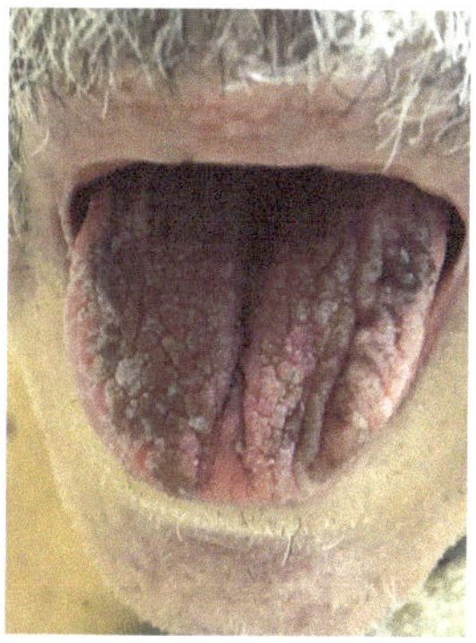

Shriveled

Differentiating Scalloping

Scalloping is a term given a swollen tongue that bears impressions of the teeth on its sides. There are two types of scalloping:

- Spleen Damp scalloping
- Liver Compensation scalloping

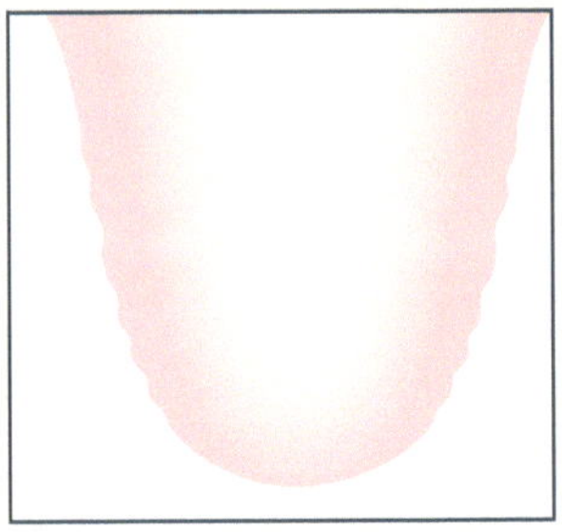

Spleen Damp scalloping occurs when the swelling in the middle of the tongue begins to affect the sides of the tongue. The tongue is swollen from the middle and the swelling extends to the sides of the tongue. This occurs when the digestive tract and the Spleen-Pancreas are weakened and unable to run digestion efficiently.

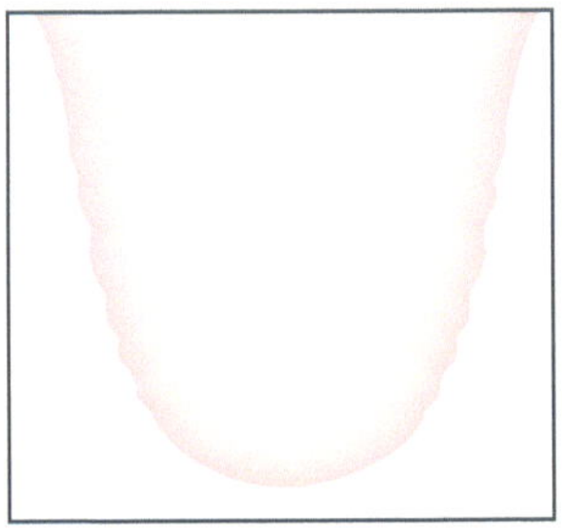

Liver compensation type scalloping is seen at the sides and is clearly not emanating from the center. The center could be slightly swollen or not swollen at all. There might also be no elevation of the center at all; it could even be concave. This constraint reflects the Liver having difficulty either storing Blood or moving Blood because Blood is insufficient. There might also be constraint as the Liver holds back the smooth flow of Qi to prevent deep penetration of a pathogenic factor.

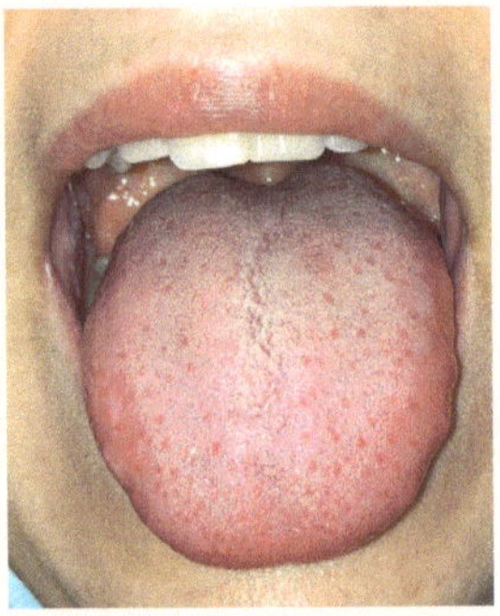

Spleen Scalloping

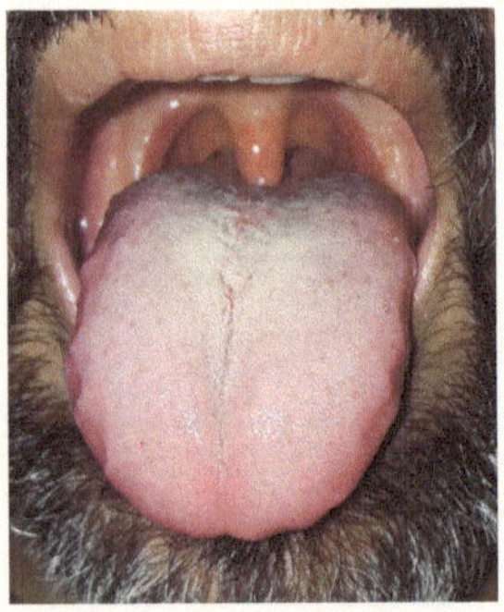

Liver Scalloping

The Three Jiaos

In a general sense, the tongue can be divided into thirds, each representing a Jiao (Burner, or center of Qi). These divisions are delineated by the diaphragm and Dai Mai.

Beyond breathing, the function of the diaphragm is to act as a barrier to stop further penetration of pathology from Upper Jiao to Middle or Lower Jiao, or to open the way to releasing pathology. Since the diaphragm is controlled by the Liver, constriction of this area denotes Liver Qi stagnation. The Liver also commands Wei Qi. Related signs and symptoms may appear in the musculoskeletal system or in smooth muscle.

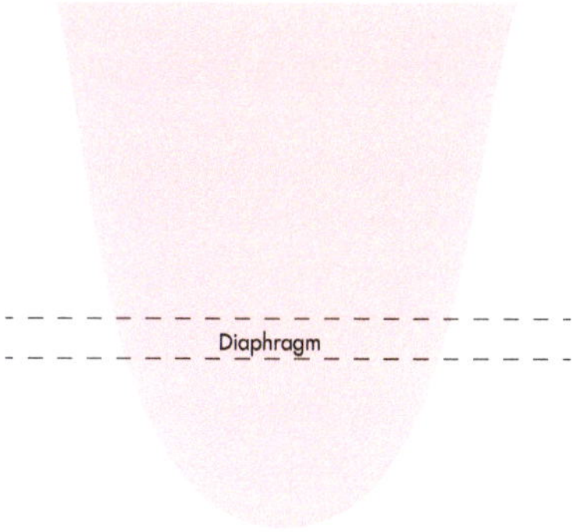

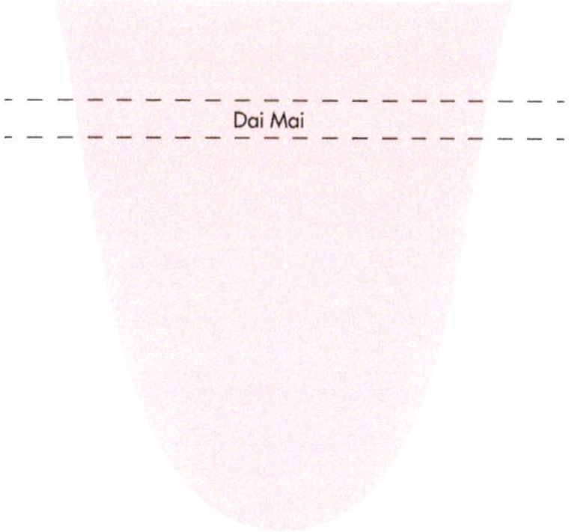

Dai Mai is the second barrier. It separates Middle and Lower Jiaos. The function of Dai Mai is to release pathology, or to hold on to pathology if there is insufficient mediumship to clear it effectively. Constraint in Dai Mai shows as the tongue appears indented, cinched, or subdivided across its line.

The diaphragm and Dai Mai separate the Jiaos. They rarely show in a healthy tongue. When they are constrained, they manifest as visible demarcations in the tongue.

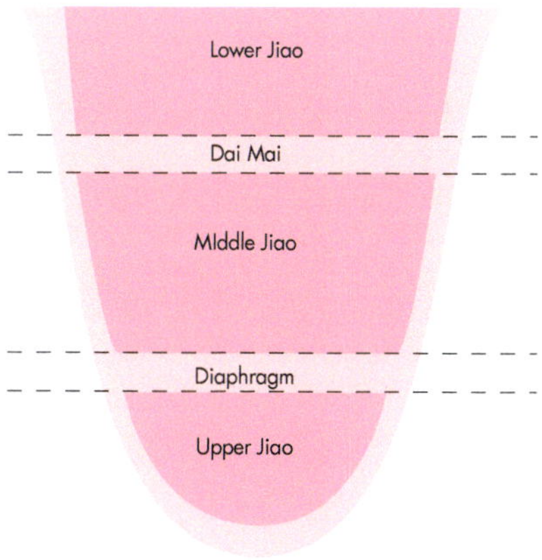

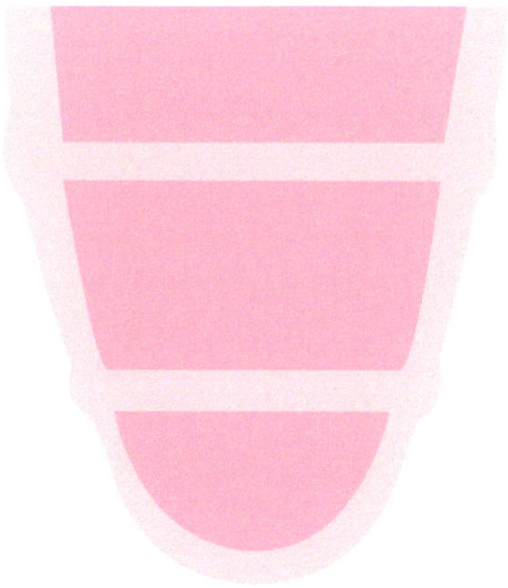

Constraint due to excess

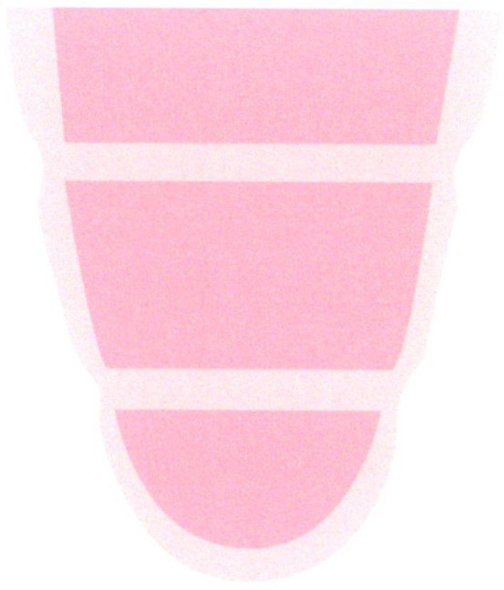

Constraint in response to deficiency

Swelling and the Tongue Silhouettes or Profiles

Swelling can affect the profile (side view) of the tongue. From the tongue profile, the practitioner can ascertain whether there are swellings confined to any of the three Jiaos (regions or burners) which are separated by the diaphragm and Dai Mai (the Belt Channel).

If the distal third of the tongue is swollen, there is an accumulation of Dampness in the Upper Jiao, most likely in the lymphatic system. You might choose to drain the Dampness through the Bladder.

If the middle third of the tongue is swollen, there is an accumulation of Dampness in the Middle Jiao. You might choose to transform the Dampness by treating the Spleen.

If the distal and middle thirds are both swollen, there is a failure to transform or refine food and fluids, resulting in food and fluid stagnation.

If the proximal (rear) third of the tongue is swollen, there is an accumulation of Dampness in the Lower Jiao. You might choose to disinhibit or drain the Dampness, unless the Dampness is compensating for Heat. (Treat the Heat before dealing with the Dampness.)

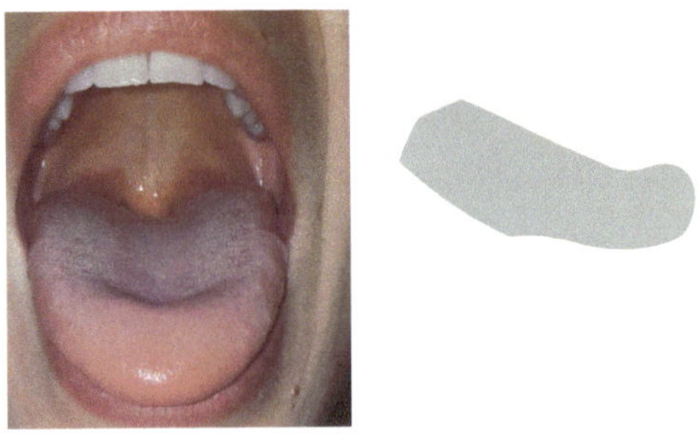

Swollen Upper Jiao

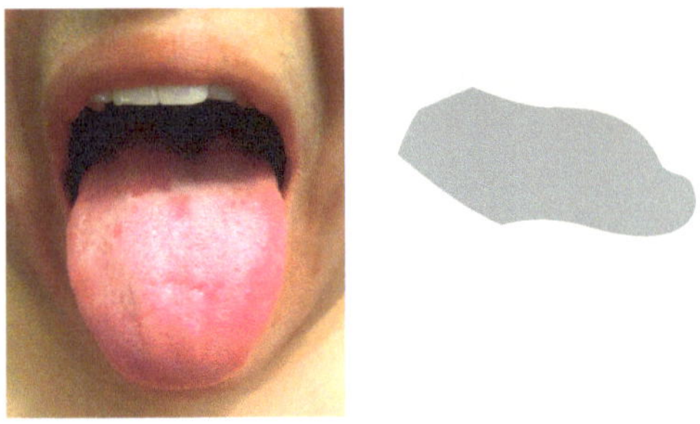

Swollen Middle Jiao

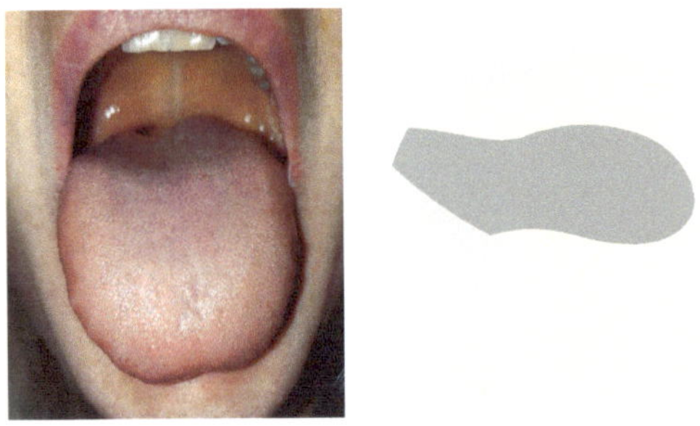

Swollen Upper and Middle Jiao

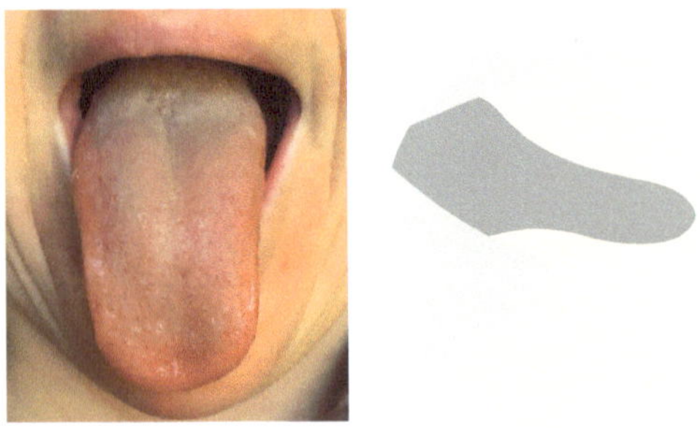

Swollen Lower Jiao

Dampness accumulated in the Upper Jiao can be clearly visible in profile:

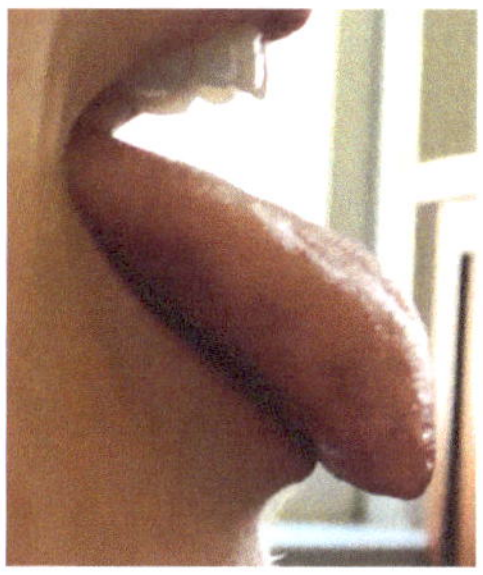

This patient is working through long-standing anxiety: lack of Heart-Kidney communication.

Note that these swellings can also mean the diaphragm is constrained, causing accumulations in the Upper Jiao as it is unable to communicate downward to the Lower Jiao. Also, the Middle Jiao is unable to communicate across the diaphragm to the Upper Jiao. This can result in deficiency conditions in the Upper Jiao such as palpitations, depression, chest oppression, and the like.

Dampness accumulated in the Middle Jiao can be clearly visible in profile:

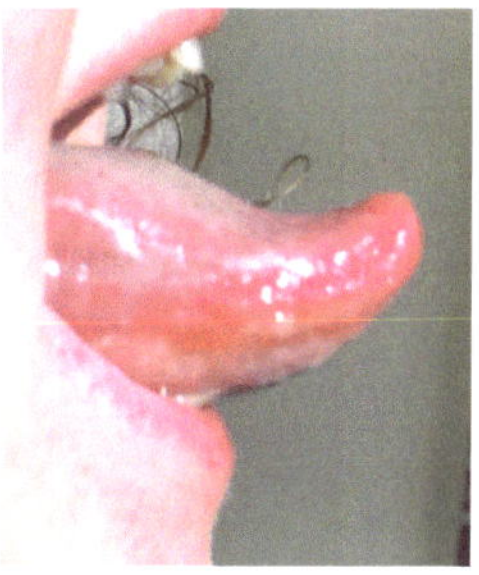

This patient has accumulated Dampness in the Middle Jiao and constraint in the diaphragm, each interfering with Heart-Kidney communication, leading to hypertension.

Dampness accumulated in the Lower Jiao can cause the rear of the tongue to swell upward toward the palate. Note that a blockage in Dai Mai can result in the loss of communication between Upper and Lower Jiaos, impeding communication between Heart and Kidneys, Lungs and Kidneys, and Lungs and Large Intestine. Also impeded is communication between Middle and Lower Jiaos resulting in impaired communication between Liver and Kidneys, and Kidneys and Spleen.

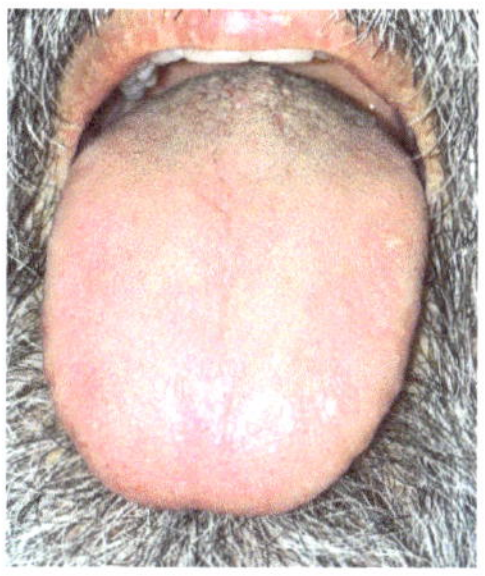

Sluggishness and congestion in the Lower Jiao compromises the distribution of Kidney Yang in a patient who presented with a low heart rate.

The profile can also show a collapse of Dai Mai.[13]

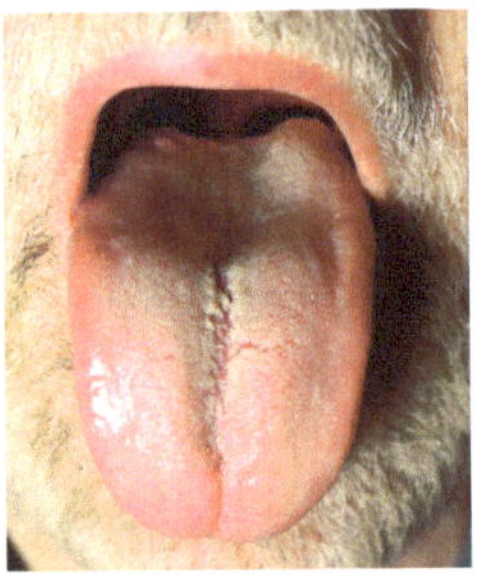

After taking a well-known drug prescribed for acne, this patient reported symptoms including irritable bowel diarrhea, requiring twenty bathroom visits a day. The photo clearly shows a collapsed Dai Mai.

Other Profile Types

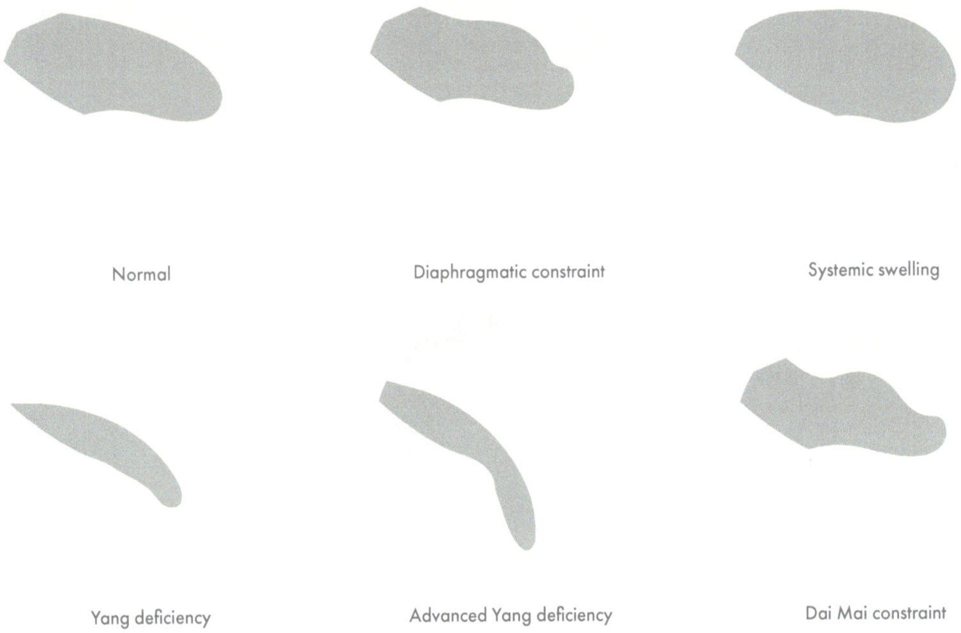

Origins of Dampness in Tongue Body Swellings

Swellings indicate Dampness. Dampness can be a response to Heat (inflammation), often located in the digestive tract. Gut inflammation arises when substances that create strong Wei Qi responses are introduced. These include garlic, onion, hot spices, liquor, coffee, chocolate, and for some people, gluten, milk, and cheese. If the tongue is dry and swollen, there is likely more Heat than Damp. This can mean that the body is overwhelmed by the offending foods or that the body cannot generate enough Dampness to extinguish their effects.

If the tongue is moist and swollen, there is likely more Damp than Heat. This can mean that the body is overwhelmed by damp foods (sugar, dairy, and gluten) or that the Damp response to inflaming foods is stagnating Fluids. Check whether Heat or Dampness predominates in the

[13] The profile of the Lower Jiao is deduced since a profile photograph is not possible.

pulses to identify the root pathology. The pulses may be clearly more slippery than rapid or vice versa. If you are not confident taking pulses, ask the patient their historical tendencies. Over the course of their life, have they tended to swell with "water weight", or do they tend to run hot?

Accumulations on the tongue body also result from improper elimination due to impairment of the Spleen's transportation function. This can be caused by allergies or intolerances in the gut, often to grains. While moderate amounts of grain are essential to the proper functioning of a healthy gut,[14] an overly sticky diet will adversely affect the gut.

Other causes of accumulations on the tongue include:

- failure to chew well
- processed food (food that came through a factory). Choose whole grains instead.
- genetically modified foods (GMOs). These contain rogue proteins unrecognizable to the Spleen. The immune system is activated in response, and inflammation can develop.
- eating too much, or eating too soon after a previous meal. If a person eats a meal before they have separated, absorbed and prepared to eliminate the previous meal, the gut will become progressively stagnated. Elimination is compromised, since it is not keeping up with incoming food, be it grain, protein, or lipid.
- too much cold and raw food
- too much spicy food irritating the mucus lining of the gut and negatively affecting the absorption of nutrients
- sugar
- vaccines, as they often contain nut, soy, wheat, pea, and egg by-products
- improper combining of foods[15] for the individual. Food combinations that the person does not have the capacity to digest, or for which their digestion is too slow, allow the food to ferment in the gut, causing autointoxication and eventually damage to the gut. The gut protests against the food combinations, but if each food were eaten alone it might be well digested.
- Grains and dairy don't get along well. Bagels and cream cheese, crackers and cheese, macaroni and cheese, pizza, etc., can ferment in the system.
- Grains and sugar don't get along. Peanut butter and jelly on bread, sugary doughnuts, pies, etc., may eventually cause a reaction because of the combination.

---

[14] Even nomadic peoples chewed on grasses (grains) as they moved. Grains did not suddenly appear with the advent of agriculture.

[15] See Andrew Sterman's writings on food for more discussion. These are listed in the Further Reading.

- Fruits are designed to be eaten alone and to exit the Stomach quickly. If eaten right after a meal of grains, fruit will digest slowly, creating fermentation (gas and bloating) and compromise transport.

Dampness: To Drain or Not to Drain

When Dampness is responding to Heat, do not try to clear the Dampness. Leave it there. The Dampness is the body's response to Heat (inflammation). Even more importantly, swellings in the tongue can be a sign of latency; the body is using pathological fluids (Dampness) to contain a pathogenic factor, averting a threat to the organs. In this way, Dampness is very often a response to Heat, quelling it and allowing it to become quiet. If any of the deep pulses are rapid, approach Dampness with great caution. Removing Dampness in these cases may result in auto-intoxication since the pathogen will have lost its container, becoming systemic as it unleashes fire toxins (free radicals). Fluids will be further damaged by the additional Heat being released into the system. The body may try to mount an eradication of this pathology but the lack of fluids may cause insufficient bowel movement, vomiting, or sweating for it to clear, leading to further autointoxication as the toxins are caught in the bowels. Clear Heat first if the deep pulses are rapid. If the tongue is pale, Qi has been consumed and there is inadequate Qi to elicit a clearing. To go forward, the Heat must be cleared first, then the Fluids nourished. It is essential to have enough fluids to flush the toxins out through sweat or defecation, otherwise the fire toxins will become systemic. (ST-44, LI-1, LI-2, and LI-11, all clear Heat. CV-12, ST-25 generate Fluids and move the bowels.) The Divergent Channels are invaluable in this type of scenario, which includes many cancers. (See *Advanced Acupuncture, A Clinic Manual.*)

Flares

When either or both diaphragm and Dai Mai are tight or blocked, Qi can accumulate in a particular Jiao. Unable to move up or down, the trapped Qi causes swelling toward the sides.

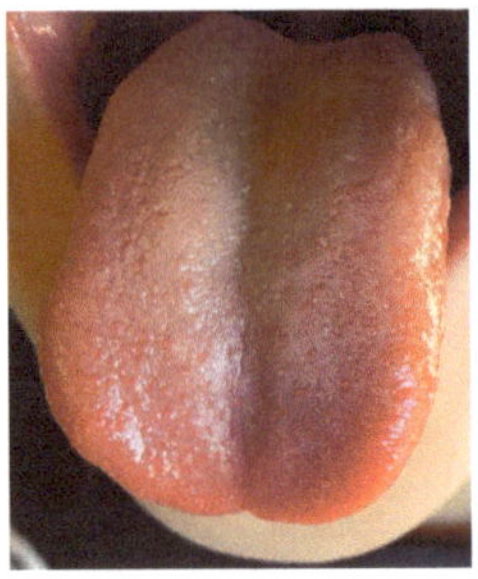

Flaring of the Upper Jiao in a deeply private child

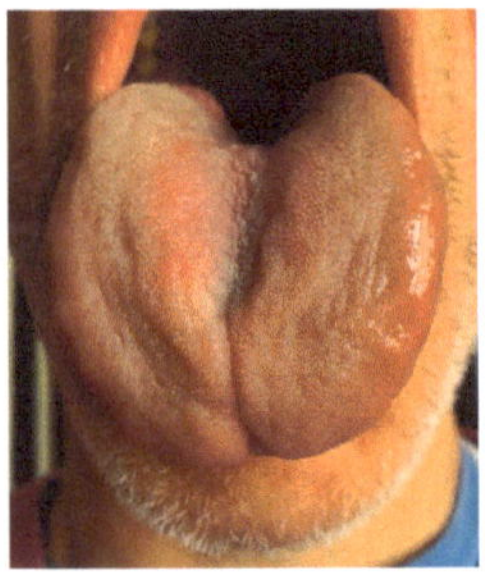

Flaring of the Middle Jiao in a patient who presented with deep chronic fatigue to the point of being unable to move, headaches, and repeated burst blood vessels in the eyes

General Color of the Tongue Body

The color of the tongue body is affected by:

- Heat and whether the Heat is moving or trapped
- the quantity of blood going to the tongue and the freedom of that flow
- the availability of the various Fluids and their free flow
- Cold
- stagnation in the channels that connect to the tongue, the Spleen Primary, Kidney Primary, and Heart Luo Channel

Some starting points for diagnosis are below:

1. A pink tongue body is normal.
2. A red tongue body is reflecting the presence of Heat.
3. A purple tongue body is reflecting either advanced Heat or blood stagnation due to Cold or Heat.
4. A blue tongue body is reflecting Cold due to the exhaustion of Yang Qi.
5. A blackened tongue body is showing deep illness due to advanced Heat.

Beyond those basic observations, fine-tune your diagnosis with the following:

If the tongue:

- is pink (translated from "pale red"), it is healthy.
- is pale, with tight and rapid pulses at the deep level and very weak Kidney pulses, there may be long-term stagnation. Long-term Heat that accumulates as a response to stagnation consumes Qi, resulting in Qi and Yang deficiencies. A pale and purple tongue results as there is not enough Qi to move Blood.
- is pale with slightly slow pulses, Yang Qi is not fully circulating.
- is pale with slightly slippery pulses, Spleen Qi has become weak, causing Dampness to accumulate. This has compromised the movement of Spleen Qi and with it, blood, to the tongue.
- is pale, with weak pulses in the guan position, there may be insufficient Stomach Fire (gastric acid), due to the inability of the Spleen to ascend Yang Qi to the Stomach, resulting in further taxation on the Spleen Qi as it struggles to transform, transport and manufacture Blood. This is a circuitous or spiraling situation addressed by breaking the pattern with moxa and diet.

- is pale, with tight, slow pulses and no deep rapid pulses, there may be internal Cold.
- has an area that is pale, there may be a Qi deficiency and circulation is inadequate, or there may be excess Damp controlling Heat.
- has red sides with the rest of the tongue covered in a greasy coat, Heat is trapped in the organs. The body is trying to push the Heat to the exterior, but the Dampness that is responding to that Heat is trapping the Heat on the interior and preventing its expression to the exterior.
- is red around the perimeter, Heat is moving up and out.
- is tending to dark red with a greasy coat, the Heat is in the Qi level; it has gone to Yang Ming and is in the channels. There are fevers, rapid breathing, great thirst. If the pulse is wiry, the condition could be in Shao Yang.
- is deep red with little or no coat, there may be advanced Yin deficiency due to dryness.
- is deep red and dry, with complaints of no saliva, Heat has damaged the Jing-Essence. Cool Blood to protect the Jing-Essence. I use the Luo Channels for this purpose.
- is deep red, verging on purple, the Heat is in the Ying level, causing high fevers, insomnia, tremors. The pulse is rapid and thin by this time.
- is deep red and shriveled, Jing-Essence has been consumed to a dangerous level.
- is deep red with a white coat, Heat is trapped, smothered by Dampness.
- is dark and moist, there is Blood stagnation.
- is dull, there is a Blood and Fluid deficiency.
- is purple to some degree, there may be stagnation in the Spleen Primary Channel, the Kidney Primary Channel, or the Heart Luo Channel, preventing free flow of mediumship to the tongue.
- is pale purple, there may be insufficient circulation of blood or a deficiency of Blood.
- is pale purple, with slow tight pulses, there may be internal Cold.
- is purple, the Blood may be occluded due to Qi stagnation. This can be a Heart Luo issue—not being able to vocalize what one wishes to express.
- is purple and appears bruised and shiny, there is consumption of Qi and reckless Blood. Blood is being lost or consumed. The patient may have had high fevers and has grave illness.
- is purplish-red, the Blood has become hot and stagnated due to long-term Heat.

• is red-crimson, there may be too much Blood, or Heat is moving Blood too quickly. Heat can crack a tongue this color, and protrusions can erupt on the tongue. The tongue may ulcerate as Heat becomes explosive.

• is pale purple or blue, and flaccid, there is tremendous Cold as Heat has consumed Qi. Blood is not moving well due to constraint by Cold and due to Qi deficiency.

• is blue, the body is trying to move Cold stasis or the Cold stasis is simply chronic.

• is black, long-term Heat has burnt the tongue. If fear is the root of the stagnation in the Blood, the entire tongue will become dark as Triple Heater acts to express fear held in the Kidneys.

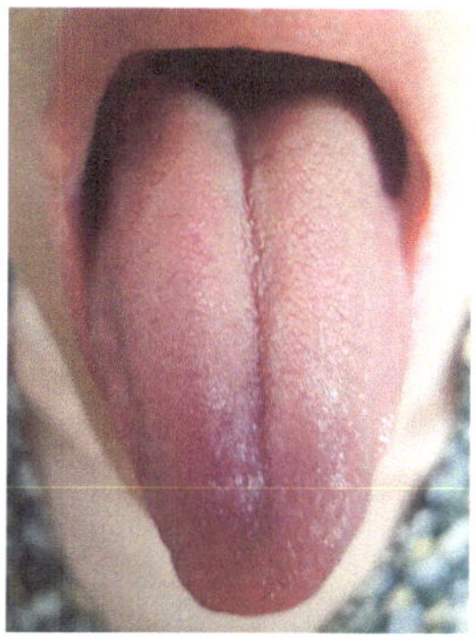

Pink

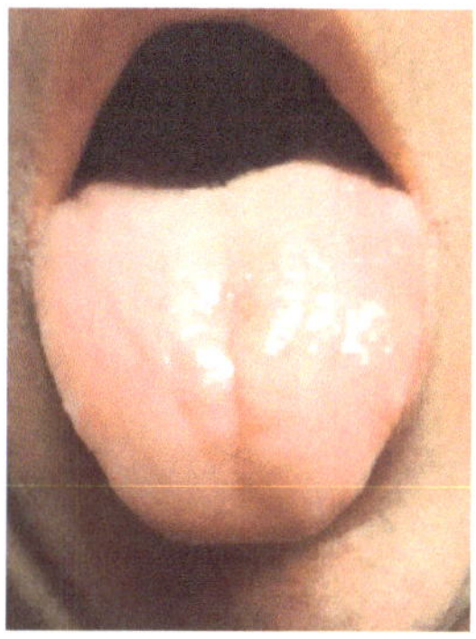

Pale

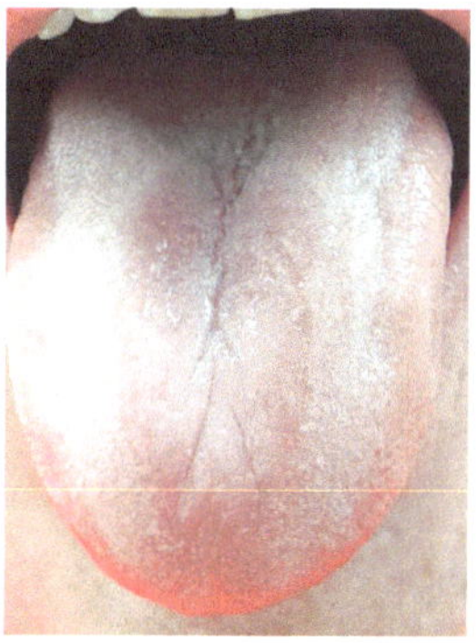

An area that is pale

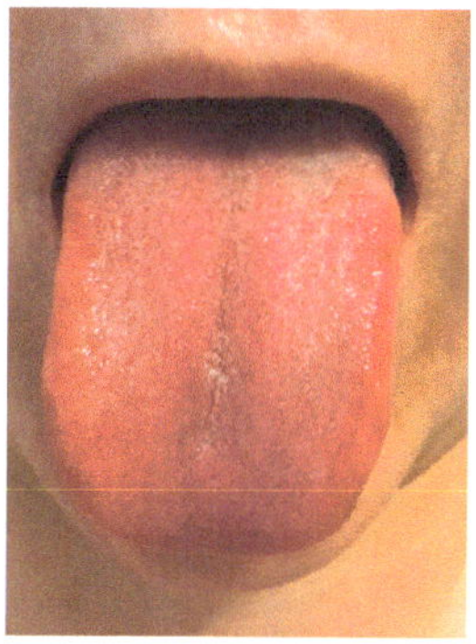

Red sides with the rest of the tongue covered in a greasy coat

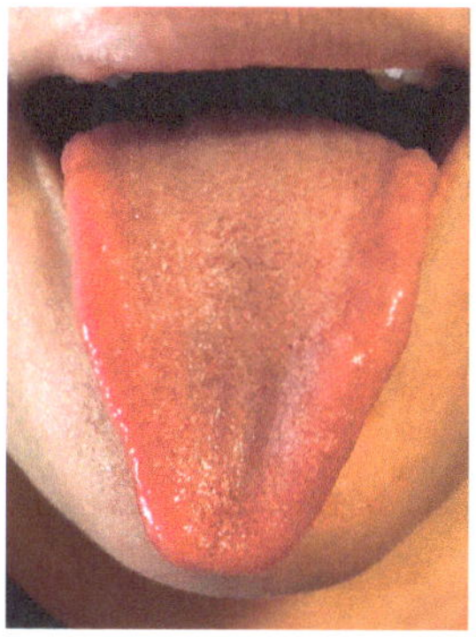

Red around the perimeter

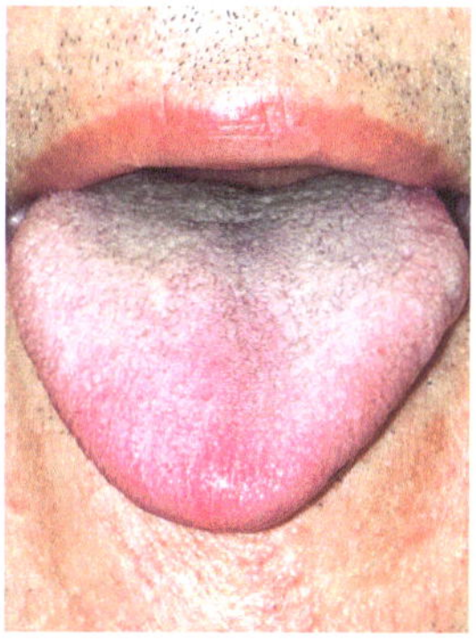

Tending to dark red with a greasy coat

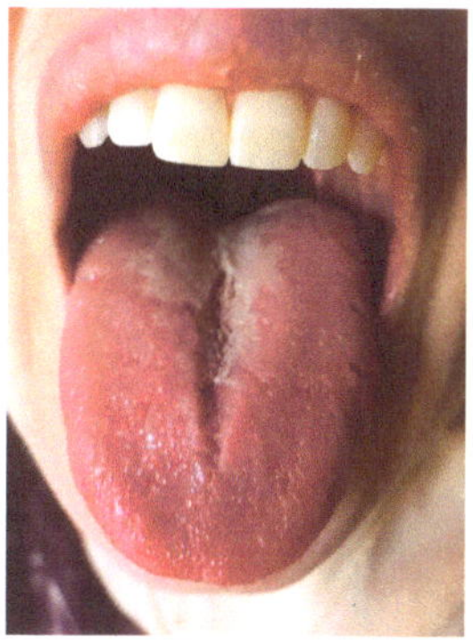

Deep red with little or no coat

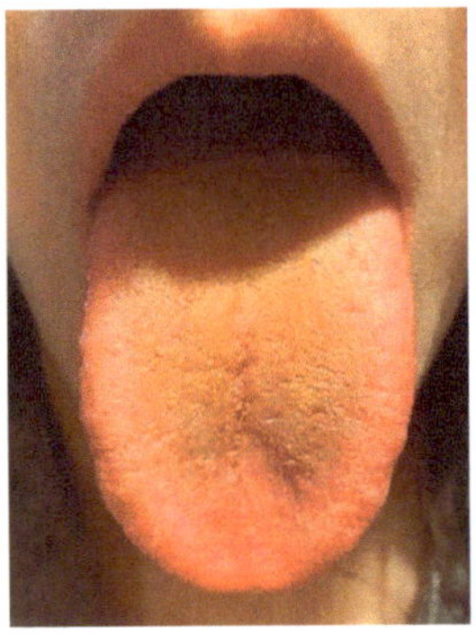

Deep red and dry, with complaints of no saliva

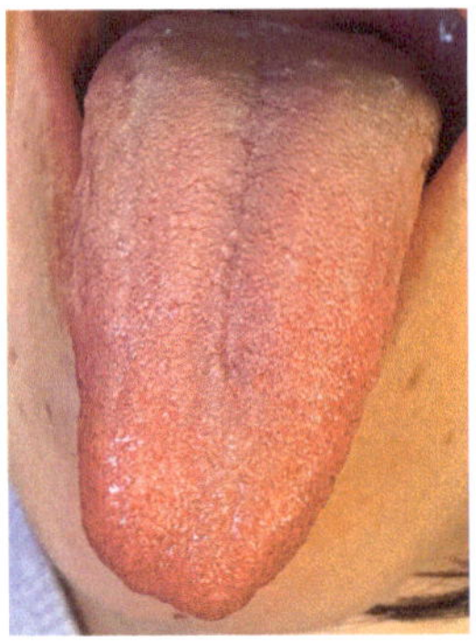

Deep red, verging on purple

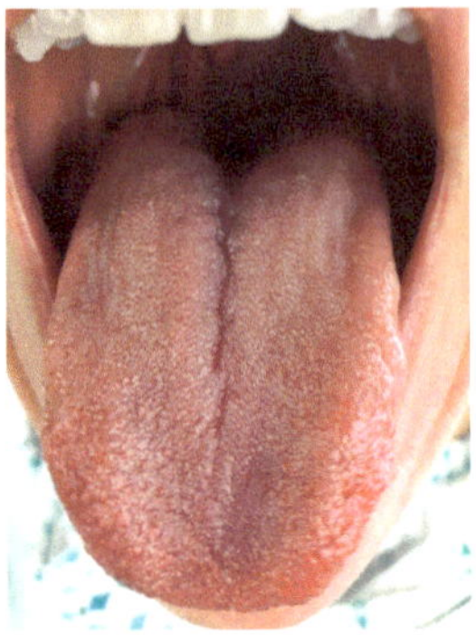

Deep red and shriveled

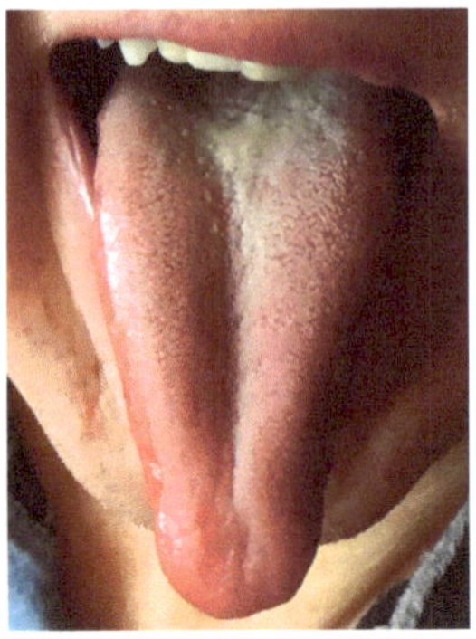

Deep red with a white coat

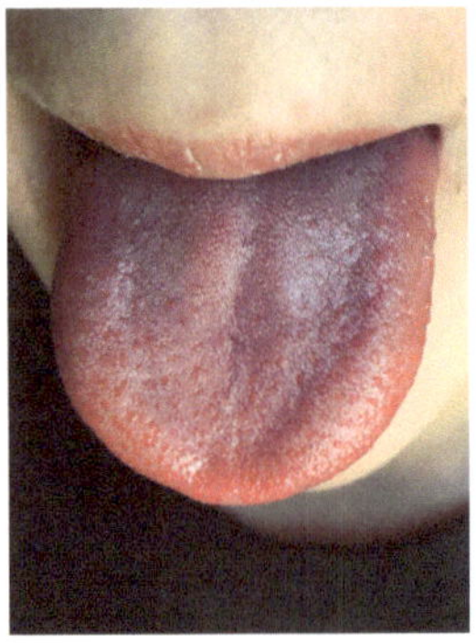

Dark and moist

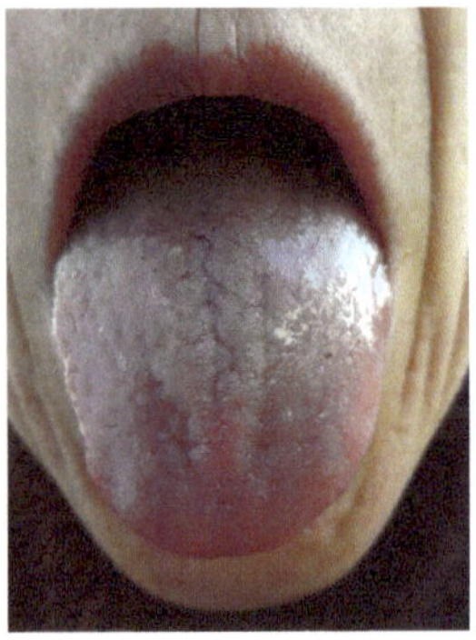

Dull

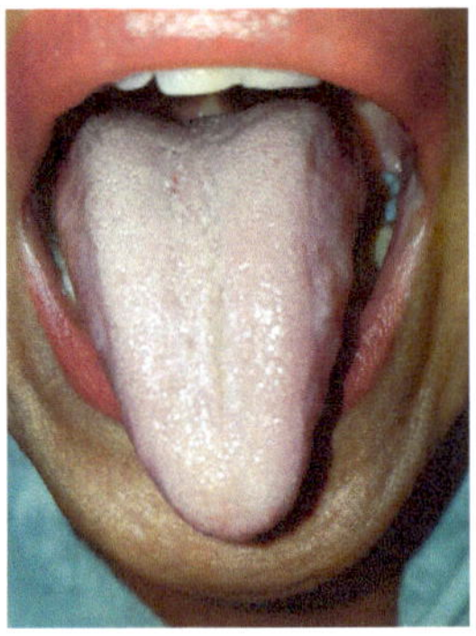

Pale purple

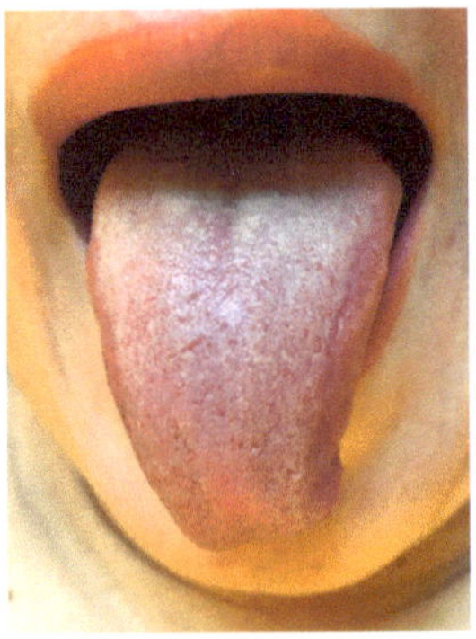

Purple

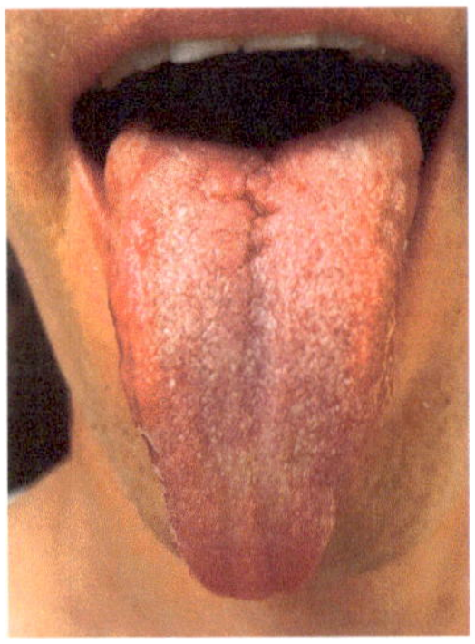

Purple and appears bruised and shiny

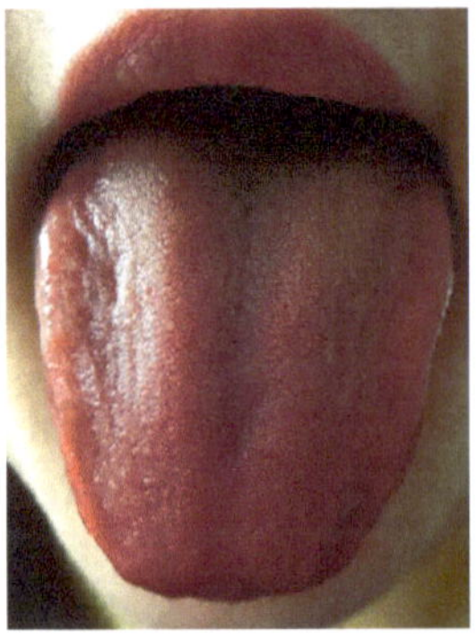

Purplish-red

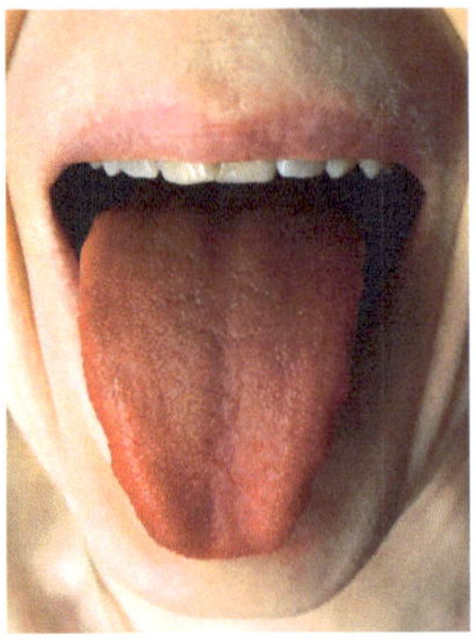

Red-crimson

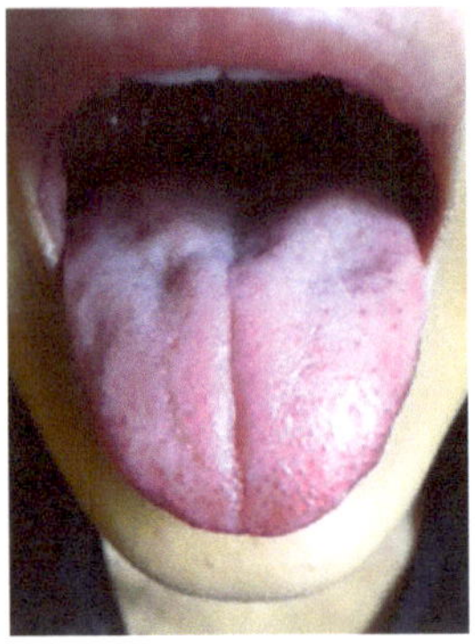

Pale purple or blue, and flaccid

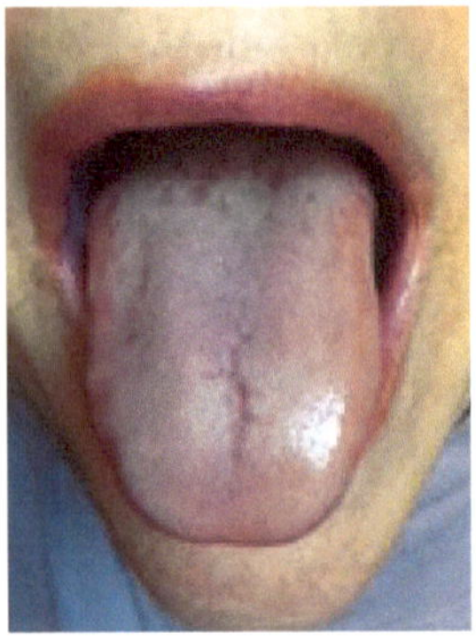

Blue

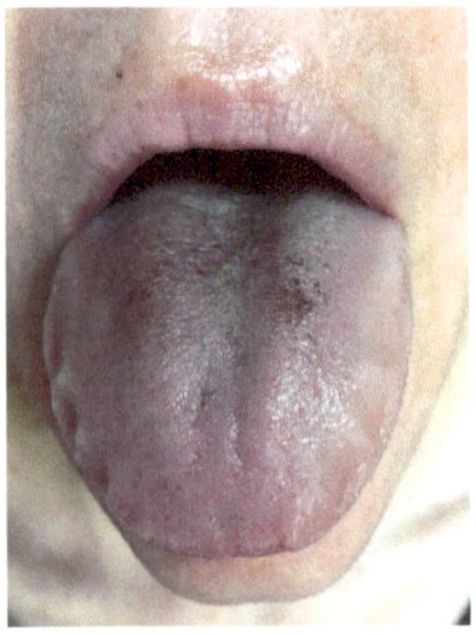

Blackening

Small Spots on the Tongue

This short section is about small spots, even specks, on the tongue, (not protrusions, lumps or swellings). Spots on the tongue indicate stagnation. Something is not moving adequately or is trapped. These days, I am seeing a lot of stagnation. Even people who claim not to eat much sugar are eating so many hidden sugars that their blood can be seriously sticky. Add to that the toxic fats converted from toxic sugars and we see widespread slowing of Blood in the channels and in the Heart.

But spots can also occur when the body intentionally stagnates Qi as it senses too much Heat. This is why spots often accompany tight pulses. At any stage of Heat progression, the body may feel it has enough strength to mount an attempt to stagnate or restrain Qi to prevent further invasion of that Heat. This prevents the subsequent consumption of a medium (Blood or Fluids). The stagnation will show in the tongue as spots, the color of which enables you to hone your diagnosis.

If the tongue has:

- pale spots, there is insufficient Blood to move pathology out.
- red spots, heat is trapped in the interior, due to stagnation.
- purple spots, there is blood stagnation and often emotional trauma.
- dark spots, toxins are beginning to form. There is damage to tissue.
- black spots, Heat is trapped and affecting or consuming Yuan Qi.
- white spots, fire toxins (free-radicals) are being expressed. There is often advanced damage or widespread damage to tissue.

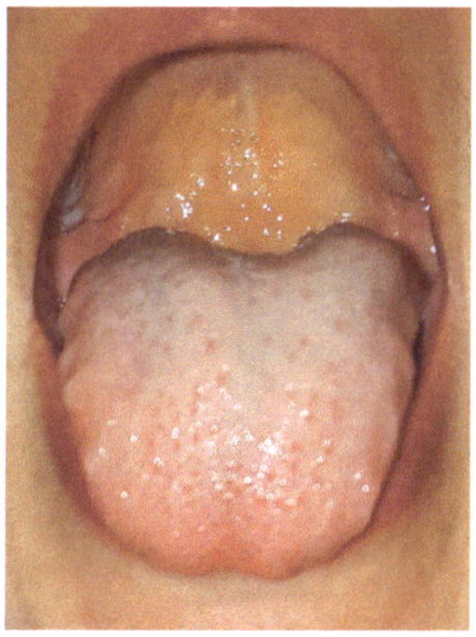

Pale Spots

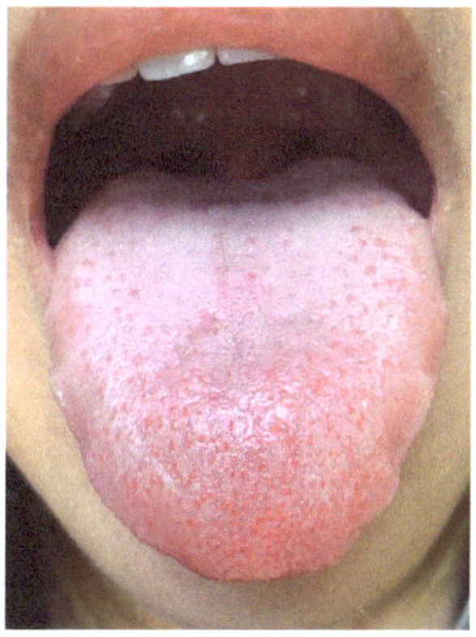

Red spots

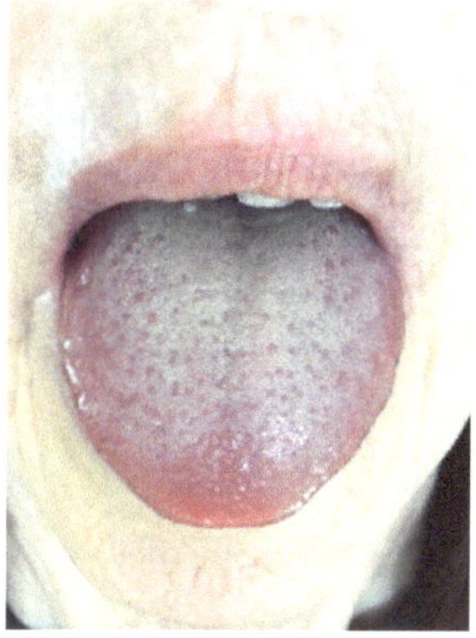

Purple spots

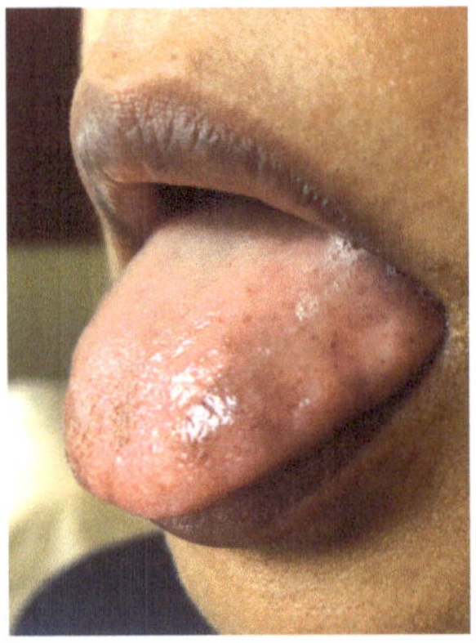
Dark spots

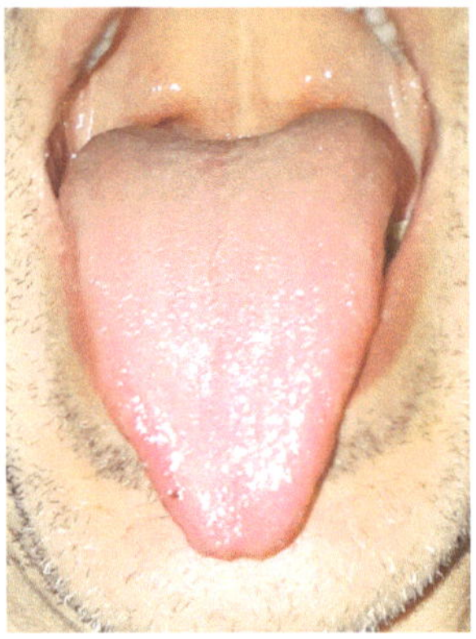
Black spots

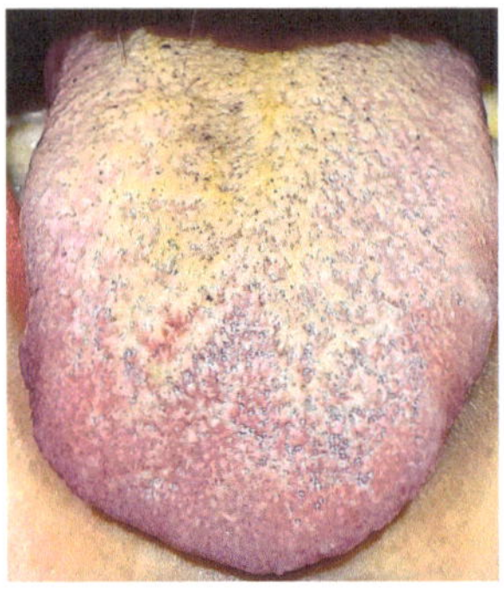
White spots

If you superimpose the location of the spots on the map in chapter 9, it's possible to diagnose the location of the stagnation and the resulting responses to that stagnation. In other words, the trail of spots can tell a story about the body's response to pathology. More about this in chapter 9.

Other Observations About the Tongue Body

If the tongue body is:

- shiny, Heat is consuming Qi and the Qi is escaping, projecting outward with a luminescence given by the Heat. You might think that a peculiar shine from the tongue is an aspect of the coat, or a sign of growing inner illumination. However, it's likely to be an indication of Yang Qi escaping. Assess for long-term Yin depletion and nourish Yin. Sometimes new qigong, yoga or meditation students accelerate their practice prematurely, over-heating and drawing their Yang upward in an uncontrolled way. This also can show in a shiny tongue body. The clinician can help by nourishing Yin to anchor Yang to prevent further Yang escaping.

- peeled, geographic, and shiny, there is a Yang deficiency due to the prolonged escaping of Yang and the consumption of Yin. Heat is now uncontrolled and the pathogen cannot be contained. Consolidate Qi in the Kidneys by anchoring the Qi down and nourishing Yin to provide ballast. KI-3 and KI-21 do this beautifully.

- dry and small, there is exhaustion of Qi and Fluids

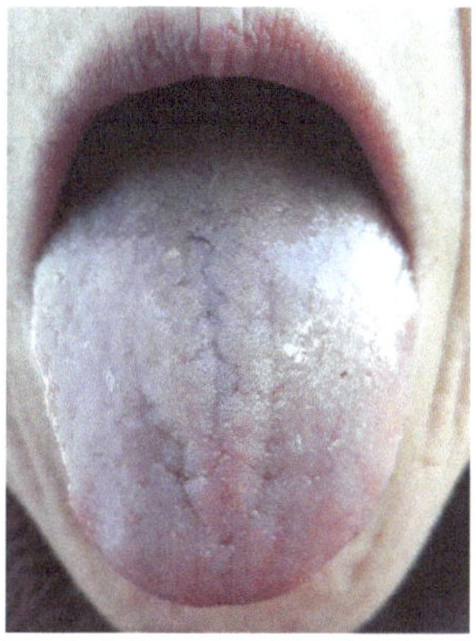

Shiny

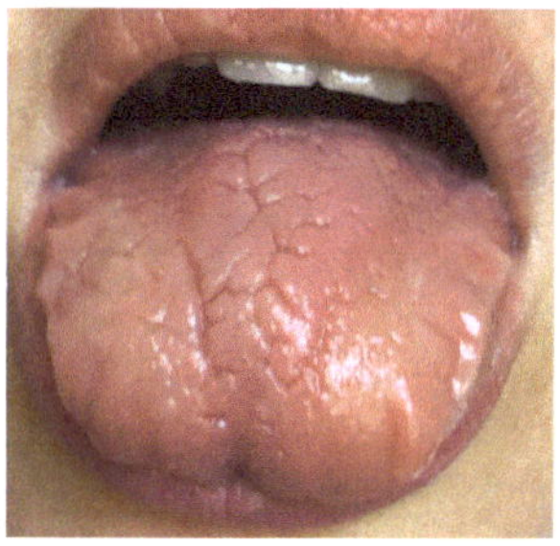

Peeled, geographic and shiny

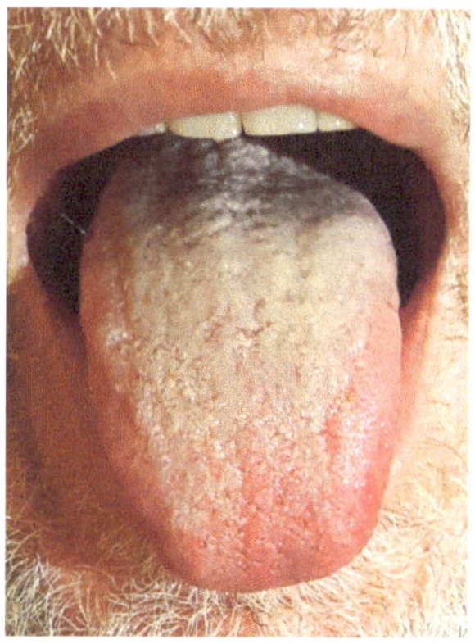

Dry and small

Erosion

Erosion of the tongue (actual missing flesh, gouges) occur when Yin is damaged, exhausted, or consumed.

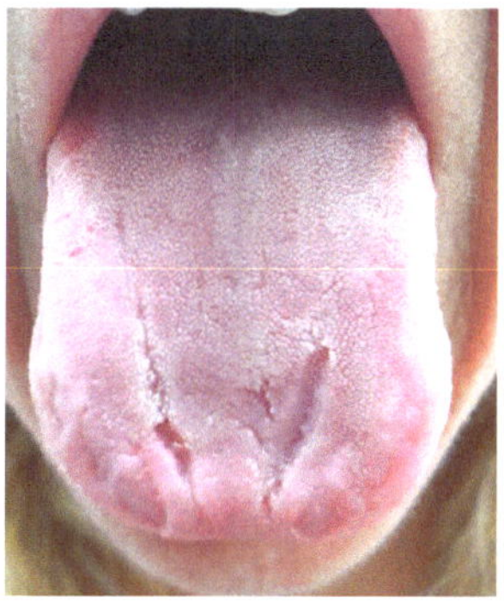

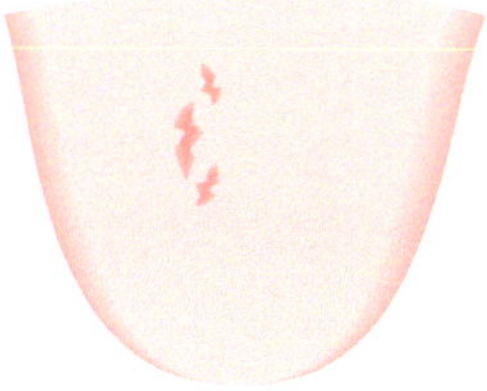

Missing flesh can indicate the location of the erosion of Yin and tissues. Erosion in the photo above (left) would likely indicate a Lung Yin deficiency. Erosion in the diagram (right) would likely indicate a severe or long-standing Stomach Yin deficiency, perhaps erosion of the Stomach lining, or an esophageal fissure. In either case clear the Heat that is causing the erosion.

7
The Sublingual Area and Sublingual Veins Reflect Yuan Qi

The sublingual area should be clear and have an openness to it. The veins should be clearly visible, but not swollen. When they are otherwise, the sublingual area provides information about:

1. long-term pathology affecting the Yuan-Constitutional level
2. pathology of the Heart Luo Channel and/or Shen disturbance
3. how much the Pericardium is controlling Blood
4. how well blood is returning to the Heart
5. how well the Spleen is managing Blood
6. toxicity of the blood
7. the Kidney Primary Channel
8. the Divergent Channels
9. the Eight Extraordinary Channels
10. the Transverse Luo Channels

1. Long-term pathology affects the Yuan-Constitutional level

Untreated long-term pathological accumulations in the Middle Jiao eventually affect the Yuan level. This happens because Spleen ascension is then often compromised and the management of Blood weakened. As this post-natal Qi becomes exhausted trying to cope with pathology, the body reaches more deeply, calling upon Yuan-Source Qi to finance more management of the pathology. At some point, the Yuan level itself assumes the pathology, attempting to keep it latent. As pathology shifts from the Ying level (the gut) to the Yuan level, the signs that had been appearing in the central area of the tongue usually drain through the tongue, into the sublingual area. In other words, what was seen in the middle of the tongue will sink to the sublingual area as the pathology deepens. Often after that happens, strangely, the top surface of the tongue can improve in appearance, or even assume an almost normal appearance. It's important to clear toxins from the constitutional level at the same time the gut is treated. (Bleeding TH-5 and GB-37 is extremely effective for this purpose and can change the appearance of the sublingual veins speedily.)

The sublingual is divided into regions representing the three Jiaos. Many signs of chronic pathology sit at the most posterior part of the sublingual area because pathology has settled into the Lower Jiao, the seat of Yuan Qi.

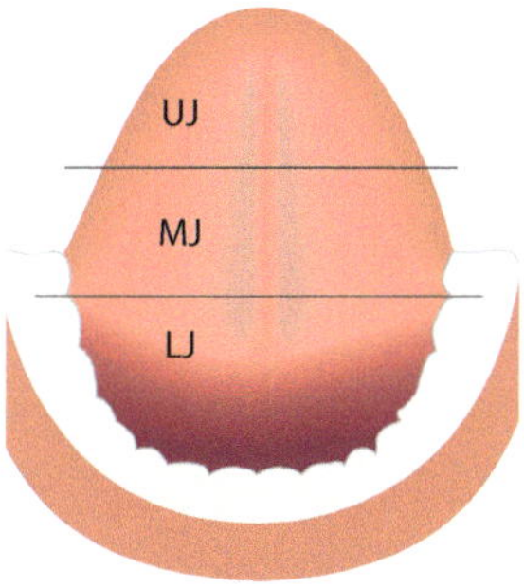

- Sometimes the tongue can appear relatively normal or very slightly purple or purplish-red while the sublingual veins look distended and deep purple. Purpling reflects occlusion of Blood. Anytime something is slowed down, the body will respond with Heat to try to move it. Long-term Heat, however, curdles the Blood and consumes the Qi. As the body is unable to vent that Heat, it becomes more internalized. On the tongue, the Heat that was visible sinks into the sublingual veins, reflecting its advancing internalization. This leaves the body of the tongue looking less overheated. As Qi is consumed, ascension of Qi is also compromised, leaving the Lungs deprived of Qi. This, combined with the compromised management and consumption of Blood, can create emotional volatility. Ultimately, the body is unable to restrain the Heat from the Yuan level, compromising the constitution. The underside (the sublingual area and/or the posterior underside of the tongue) then shows pathology.

- Redness at the base of the sublingual area of the tongue indicates Heat affecting the constitution.

- A general dark and dull hue at the base of the sublingual area indicates deep trauma at the level of the Kidneys.
- If the veins are dark and swollen, Dampness is smothering internal Heat and affecting the Yuan level.

- Very dark veins are a sign of profound stagnation and Heat in the Kidneys (the constitution).

- Veins that appear varicose-like can arise when the Lungs fail to move Blood, because Lung Qi has been consumed by Heat. This Heat may be coming from the Stomach. As the body is unable to vent the Heat, it tries to deposit the Heat in the Luo Channels to protect the organs. When the Luo Channels are overwhelmed with pathology, their pathology moves to the Source level, to the constitution. Bleed Luo points, especially ST-40, to treat this.

- If the sublingual area has a yellow hue, the Spleen is unable to control Blood, and its transportation function is weakened.
- If the sublingual area is pale, there is not enough Blood supporting the Kidneys.
- If the sublingual area is pale and flaccid, with noticeable pallor in the frenulum, there may be insufficient Qi and Blood at the level of the constitution.
- If the sublingual veins are not showing, Blood has been depleted by emotional stress to such an extent that Jing-Essence is having to break down to finance Blood in the hope of containing the emotion.

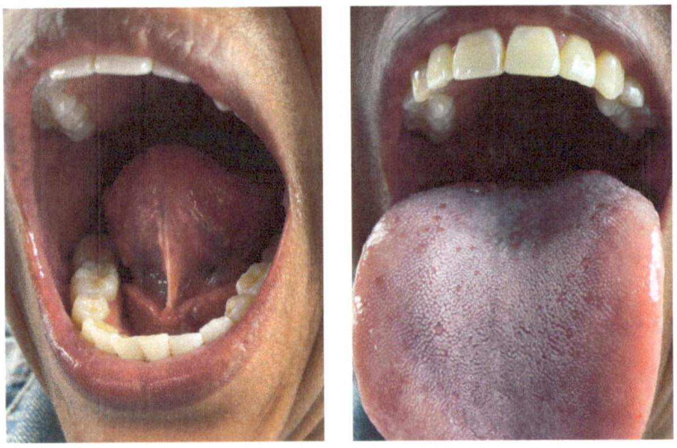

Distended and deep purple

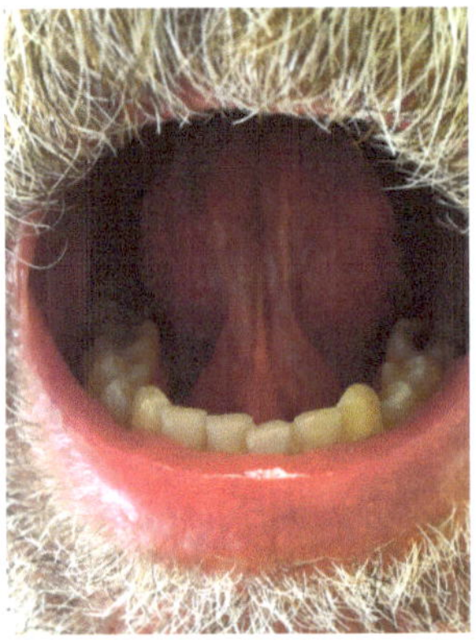

Redness. A patient with early Kidney failure.

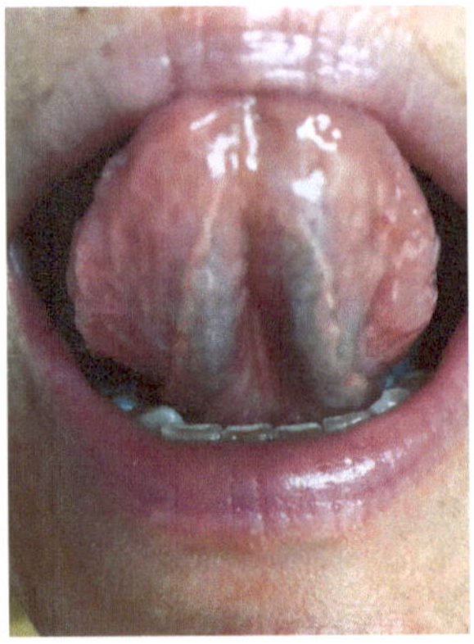

Dark and dull hue. Heroin and amphetamines ravage the Kidneys.

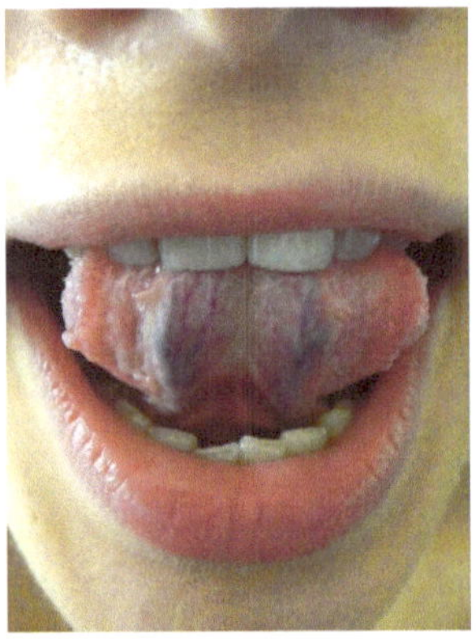

Dark and swollen

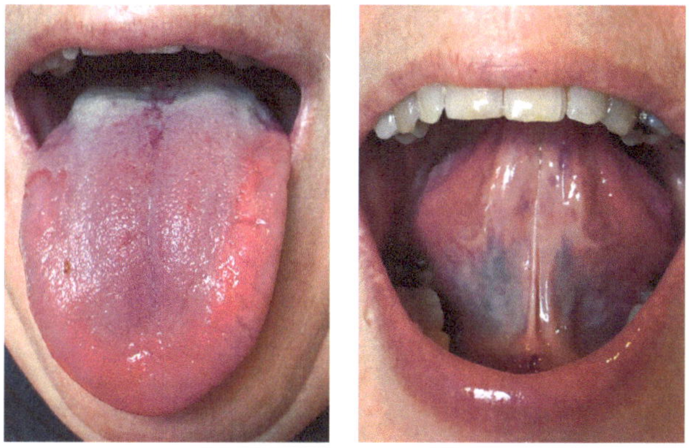

Very dark. Heat accumulated in the Kidneys due to stagnation. Note the thick coat at the rear that has formed to protect the Kidneys and the constitution. It is essential that this Dampness not be drained until the Heat clears, otherwise fire toxins may form.

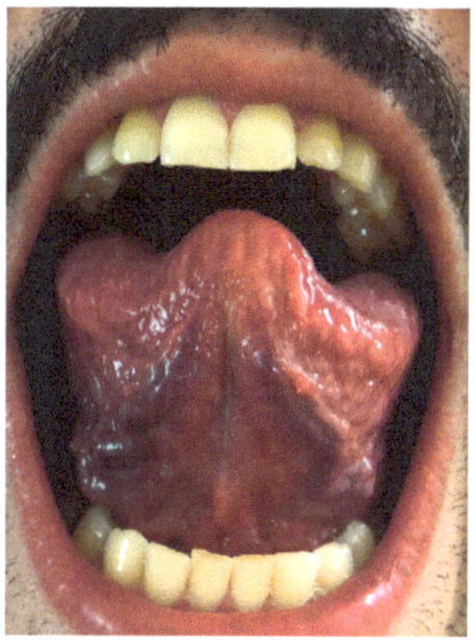

Varicose-like

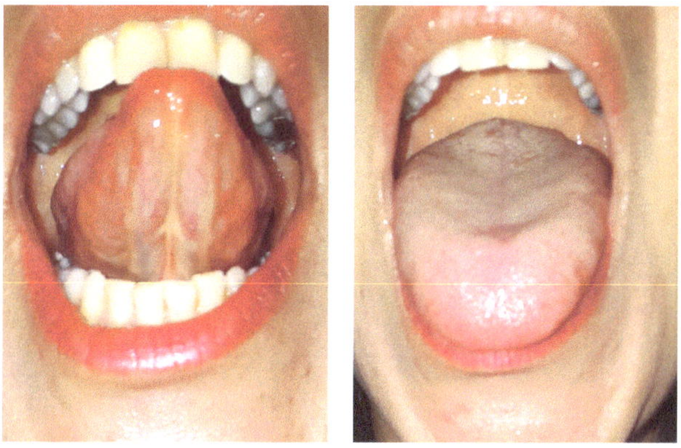

Yellow. The Spleen is weak, failing to control transportation and Blood.

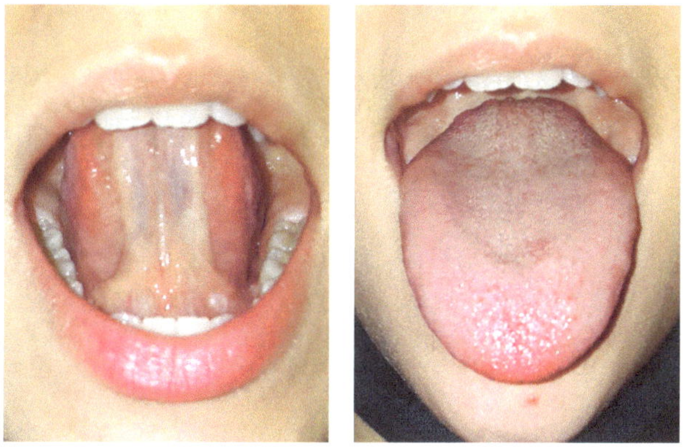

Pale. Blood fails to support the Kidneys.

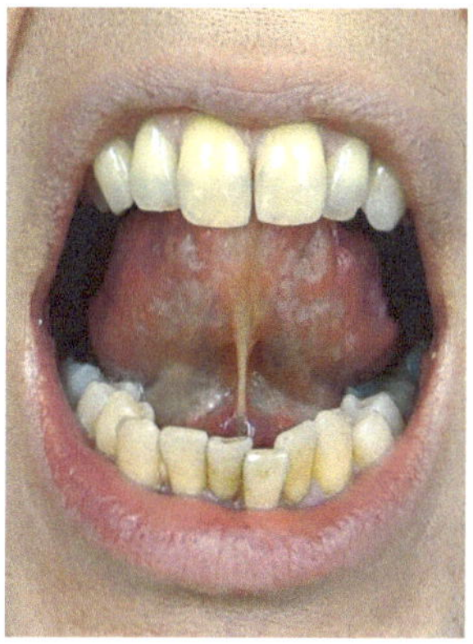

Qi and Blood deficiency originating from a lack of dissemination of Yin and Yang from the constitution (stagnant Jing-Essence)

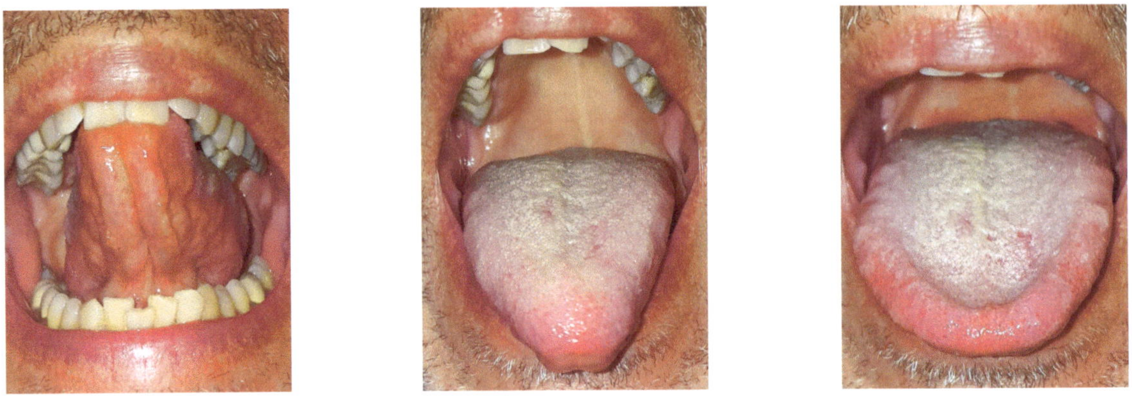

Sublingual veins not showing. This patient arrived with suicidal tendencies at my colleague's office. Unable to maintain the posture in the middle photo, the tongue relaxed, revealing a distinct pallor on the sides at the Middle Jiao and thick yellow phlegm, accumulating in an attempt to build pathological Yin as Jing-Essence is being depleted. The combination of deep Blood deficiency, its resulting Wind, and thick Phlegm can further affect the Shen. (He is now doing well after a series of Luo treatments, especially treatment of the Great Luo of the Spleen.)

2. Pathology of the Heart Luo Channel and/or Shen disturbance

The Heart Luo Channel connects to the tongue, enabling articulation of one's emotions. Repressed emotions resulting in Shen disturbance will show as stagnant purple veins. When Blood stagnation in the sublingual area concurs with symptoms of the Heart Luo Channel, the Heart Luo should be treated by letting a tiny amount of blood from HT-5 with a lancet. Symptoms include having a sense of being betrayed, yearning for someone or striving for something that is no longer available, and feeling that one's dreams have been broken. Advanced signs include loss of speech following trauma or disappointment, denial of the reality of a disappointing situation, inability to talk about trauma, and a reactive attachment to intellectual thought. Treatment of advanced signs requires bleeding and immediate moxa at HT-5. (See *Advanced Acupuncture, a Clinic Manual* for more detailed instruction.)

Heart Luo Channel is implicated in the swelling of the sublingual veins if there is speech difficulty with nervousness, impeded tongue movement and reduced moisture.

3. Pericardium fails to adequately control Blood

If the tip of the tongue is constrained and raised, the sublingual area looks tight and restricted, and the patient is timid, shy, or depressed, the Pericardium is tightening to protect the Heart, limiting the flow of Blood to the Heart. Emotions then become internalized (to the Heart Luo).

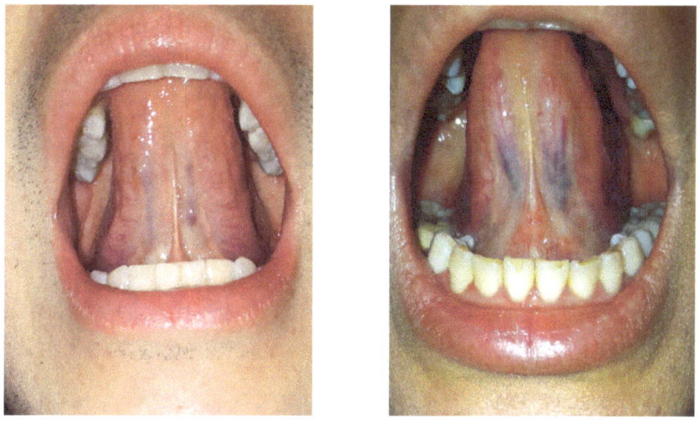

Tight and Restricted

4. Blood fails to return smoothly to the Heart

If constraint in the Kidneys or the Liver is occluding Blood, preventing its return to the Heart and causing chest pain, the sublingual veins become very swollen. Wind-Stroke can result.

5. Spleen fails to manage Blood

The tonus of the tongue is governed by the Spleen's ascension of Blood to the end of its channel—the tongue. A floppy tongue demonstrates that Spleen Qi is inadequate to create good ascension. If there is stagnation of Blood because Blood is not being moved sufficiently, the Spleen will react by constantly trying to control Blood, resulting in dark sublingual veins. Note also that the Spleen can react similarly when there is a Blood deficiency. The pulses will clarify this for you; if the pulse is thin or narrow at the moderate level of the Spleen or Liver positions, there is a Blood deficiency. If the same pulses are wiry, there is stagnation of Blood.

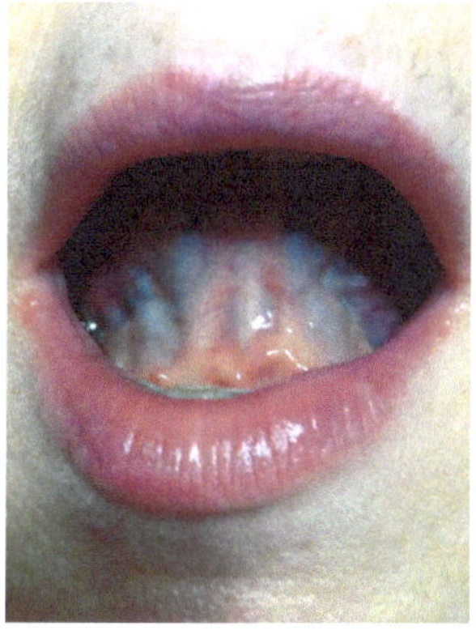

Swollen

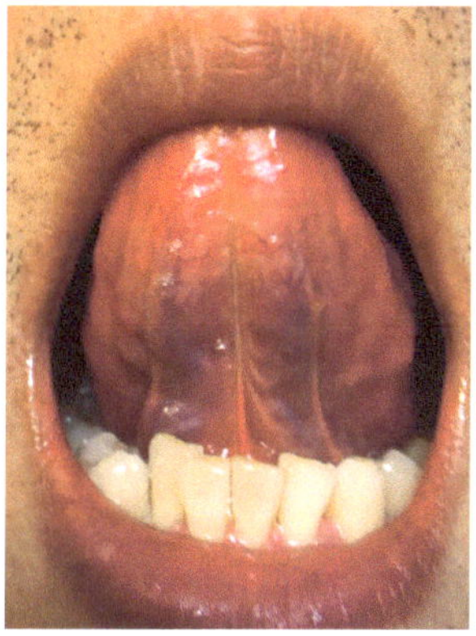

Spleen fails to manage Blood

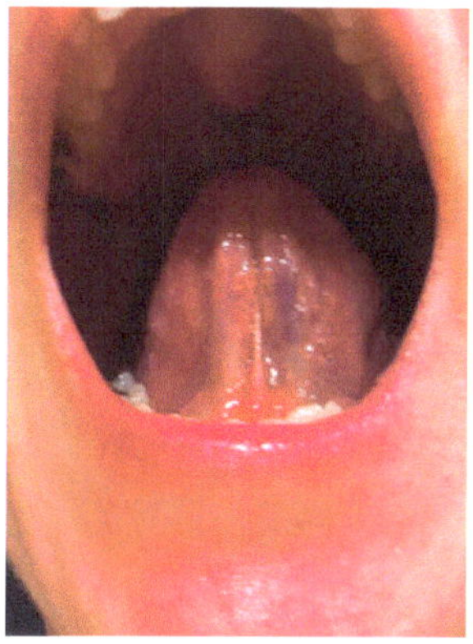

Toxicity

6. Toxicity Affecting the Blood

If the sublingual area is deep red and the body of the tongue is purple, there is substantial toxicity in the Blood. Bleed the Luo points.

7. The status of the Kidney Primary Channel

The Kidney Primary Channel connects to the root of the tongue, where it spreads its Qi.[16] If the sublingual veins are distended (swollen) and the underside of the tongue is pale, there is a Yang deficiency allowing the vessels to collapse. If the sublingual area is very shiny and glistening in an unusual way, Kidney Yang is escaping. Nourish Yin to anchor it, or consolidate it at KI-21 or KI-3.

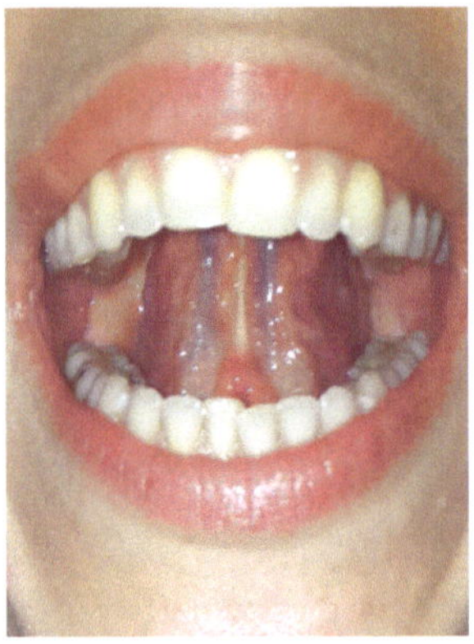

This patient presented with a chief complaint of alopecia and irritable bowels. Yang was rising to the point of burning the hair follicles.

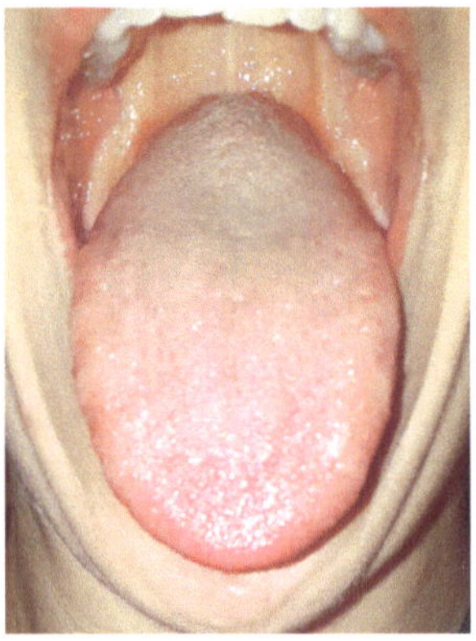

Note that the back of the tongue is narrow and tight, trying to astringe Kidney Yin to prevent more Kidney Yang escaping.

8. Divergent Channel Activity

The Divergent Channels connect Wei Qi and the Yuan level to bring to latency a pathogenic factor that the body is not equipped to handle. They hide away pathology that would otherwise harm the organs. If the Divergent Channels fail to contain pathology, toxins begin to leak and affect Jing-Essence. If the sublingual veins are distended and have small protrusions on them, fire toxins (including free radicals) are present and active, escaping from the Jing. These protrusions can be various colors, including white. If there are petechiae (small red spots) on the posterior underside of the tongue, fire toxins may be active or brewing. Treat using Triple Heater Divergent Channel or another method of equal potency.

[16] In Qigong, you would say this area stimulates the golden nectar, Jin Ye (Thick and Thin Fluids) and Yu Ye (Jade Nectar), as stimulation and movement of the tongue affects salivation.

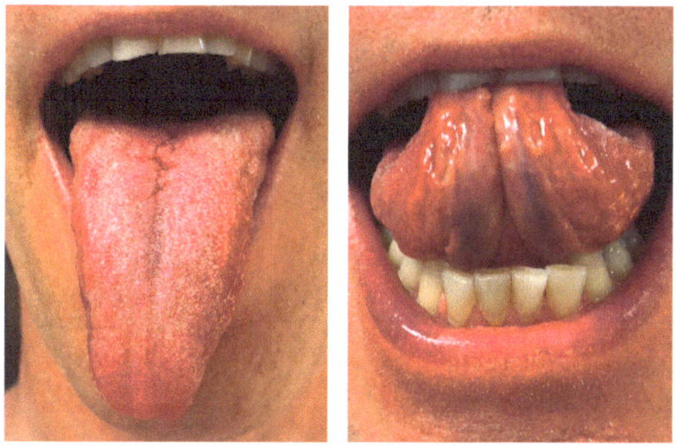

Deep cracks moving into the rear of the top of the tongue indicate Heat moving into the Lower Jiao threatening to breach the constitution. The cinching of Dai Mai, as it tries valiantly to protect the constitution, is evident at the level of the deepest part of the crack. The cracks are horizontal, indicating this man has been engaged in dehydrating practices. The sublingual area shows the presence of fire toxins (free radicals) manifesting as thorns.

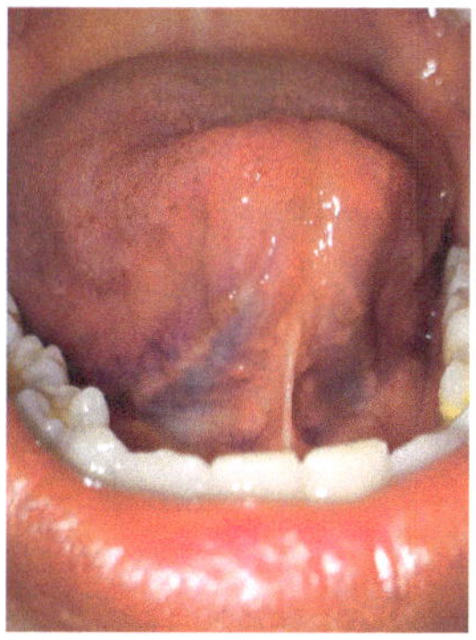

Toxins leach from the blood as petechiae and thorns form on the sublingual surface. Accumulations are also seen here in Dai Mai, at the posterior aspect of the sublingual area.

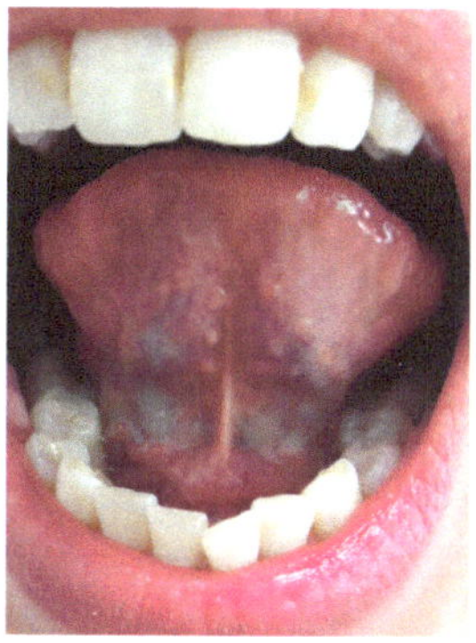

Heat affects the constitution, as seen in the emergence of thorns and the deep reddening of the posterior sublingual area.

9. Eight Extraordinary Channel Pathology

The Eight Extraordinary Channels can contain pathology.

- Chong Mai, in particular, is responsible for the replication of RNA and DNA and the management of factors that can impede that function. These include all carcinogens, xenobiotics, all plastics, heavy metals, vaccines, saccharine, aspartame, and petroleum derivatives. The Eight Extras either hold the pathogenic factor in the Jing-Essence, or they produce changes in the DNA in an attempt to enable the body to tolerate the pathogen. If the Chong or other Eight Extra Channels fail to hold such challenges, some kind of eruption occurs on the sublingual surface, since this is a window into the constitution. These eruptions can include white dots, white patches, unusual localized swellings, and blackened lesions.

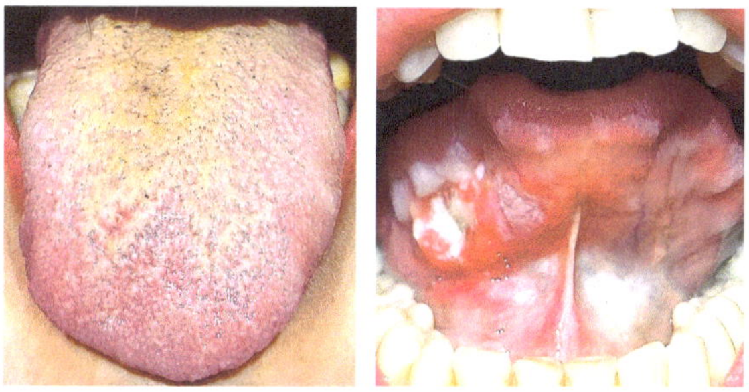

This patient received a Western diagnosis of fourth stage cancer. The Jing-Essence, which is under the command of Chong, is corrupted.

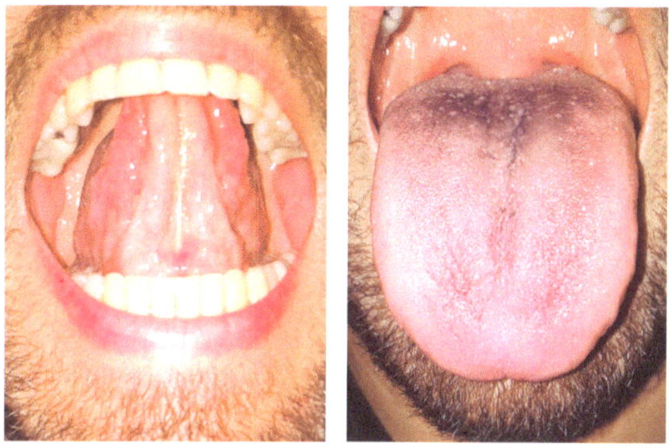

This person is a runner. Overexertion of Kidney Yang has overheated the Kidneys and affected Chong Mai, as seen in the overall bumpy underside of the tongue and the Heat at the posterior aspect of the sublingual area.

• Qiao Mai pathology is characterized by purple sublingual veins. This is because the Yang Luo Channels terminate or empty into Yang Qiao Mai and the Yin Luos terminate or empty into Yin Qiao Mai. Since Luo pathology is contained in the Blood, the deposits of Blood level pathology in the Yuan level—in this case, the Qiao's—will appear purple as the body tries to stagnate the toxicity. Confirm your diagnosis by finding *moving* pulses (pulses that move alternating laterally and medially from beat to beat).

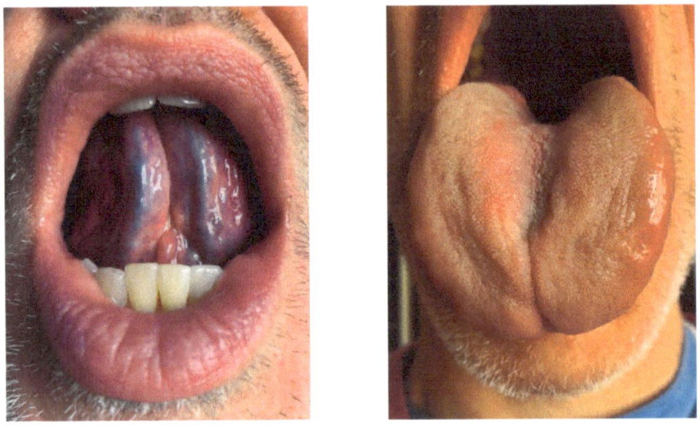

Stagnation in the Middle Jiao, and Blood stagnation from emotional pathogenic factors, over time result in deposits in the Qiaos and affect the sublingual area.

• When the frenulum is the feature of the sublingual area, you might consider Ren Mai (the channel of bonding) or Du Mai (the channel of separation).

• Dai Mai "belt channel" pathology is characterized by swelling in the rear (the posterior area) of the sublingual area.

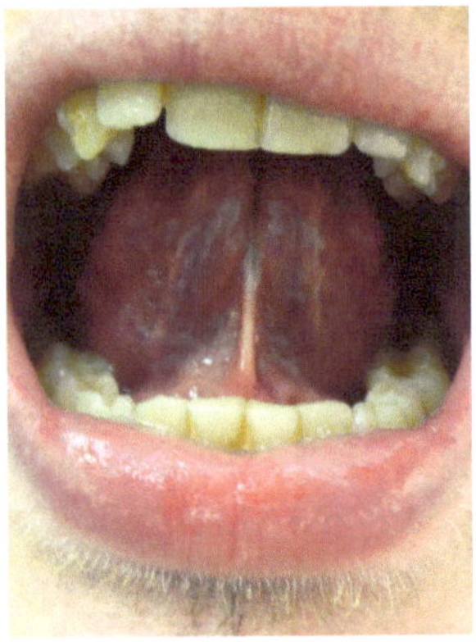

Ren/Du Mai

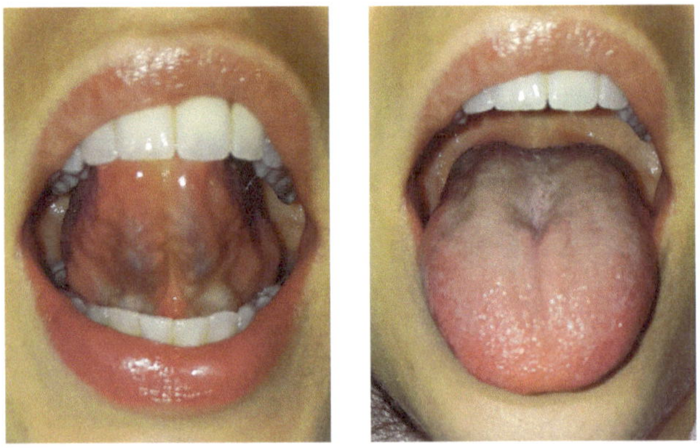

A deficiency of Kidney Yang precipitated the collapse of Spleen Yang, leaving the Spleen unable to transform and transport. A diet high in salads, cold foods, and cold water complicated the weakness and caused Dai Mai to react to contain the Cold, leaving the posterior sublingual area pale and swollen.

10. The Transverse Luo Channels

If the sublingual area becomes dark red and inflamed, Heat is moving via the Blood (using the Luo Channels) to the interior (the Yuan-Source level), via the Transverse Luos—the internal branches of the Primary Channels. Tremendous Heat is threatening to enter the organs and the constitution. The condition is potentially terminal and must be treated.

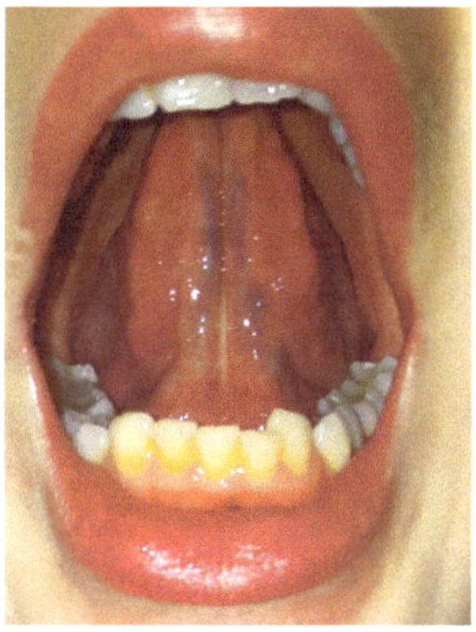

Anxiety has taxed the Blood and affected the Transverse Luos

8

The Tongue and the Transformation of Jing-Essence into into Shen-Spirit

Much of my practice is centered on personal transformation. Many people come asking to work on the full and peaceful unfolding of their Destiny, their purpose in life. This is such an honor, to be a steward in the patient's awakening and the emerging awareness of their role in this lifetime.

As I work, I enjoy putting different perspectives on things. For example, one can read pulses through any of many lenses: the channels, the fluids, the levels of Qi, the anatomical regions. And within each of these categories there are sublenses—infinitely deep layers. The tongue is far less complicated but it, too, has an interesting alternative take—reading about the unfolding of Jing, the unfolding of personal Destiny.

The tapering of the tongue can be seen as a representation of the density of the various humors. The rear of the tongue is wide and thick, since the Kidneys store Jing-Essence, the thickest, densest medium in the body. The middle section of the tongue represents the first stage of transformation of Jing-Essence since it unfolds into Blood and Qi. The distal third of the tongue is the narrowest, since the Shen is pure light and has no density.

So looking at the tongue through this lens alone, one can get a sense of the Eight Extraordinary Channels. A questions to ask while examining the tongue is, "What can I see in the tongue that describes resistance to the unfolding of Destiny? What can I see in the tongue that describes resistance to the world? What can I see in the tongue that describes resistance to this life?"

The shape of the tongue is key. Is it widest at the rear? Or is the rear of the tongue narrower than the middle? Let's start there. If the tongue is narrow at the rear, Jing-Essence is depleted or restricted. The container of Jing-Essence—the storage of the mediumship that contains Destiny—is broken.

The realization of Destiny occurs via the constant conversation the Heart has with the Kidneys. The Heart inquires of the Kidneys about the nature of the Qi it is to carry through to its branches: the tongue and the eyes. The Kidneys respond with instruction that manifests as inspiration. If the rear of the tongue is narrow, there is not sufficient ballast in the Lower Jiao to receive Heart Qi as part of the communication of Heart and Kidneys. While I think that it is not the business of the practitioner to announce this, I do think that the practitioner can notice it and then, through careful choice of channel, or simple awareness, allow the space for increased interaction between those two organs. It's important for the practitioner to be mindful that even the resistance to the unfolding of one's nature is inherently part of one's destined path.

When using this kind of lens, the Eight Extraordinary Channels are indispensable. You will need the permission of the patient, however, so as not to be intrusive. The patient must be in the driver's seat. Having said that, if you feel called to view a tongue this way, it's likely that this is precisely what the patient has arrived to explore.

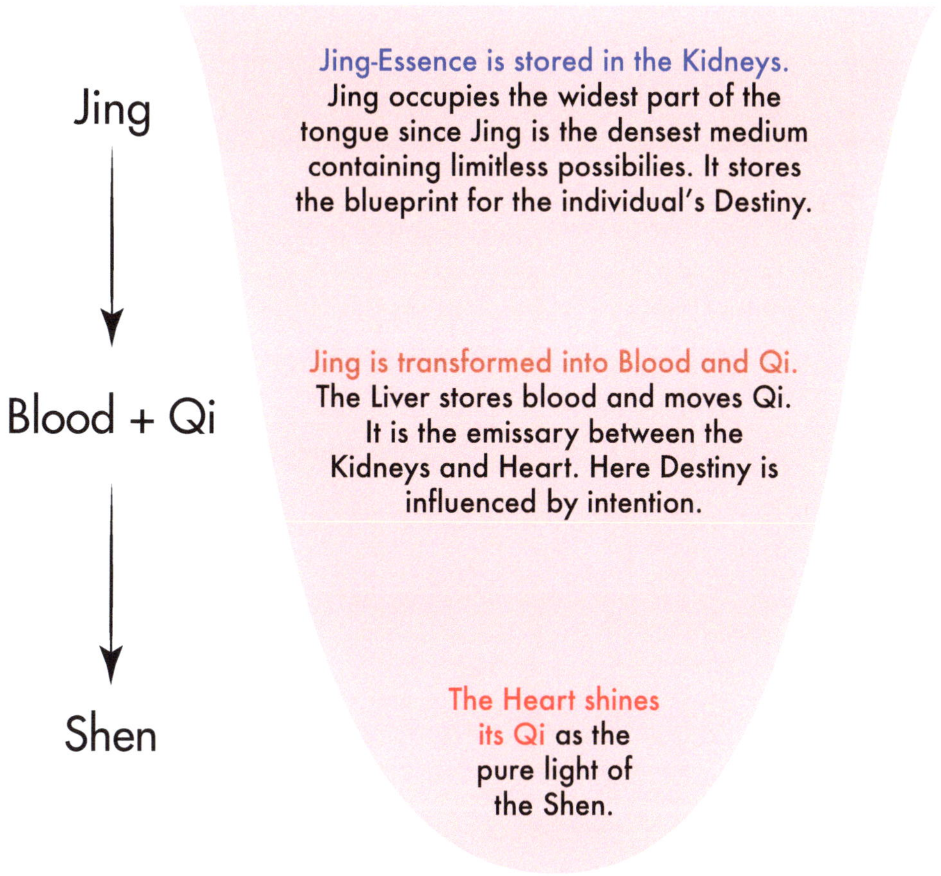

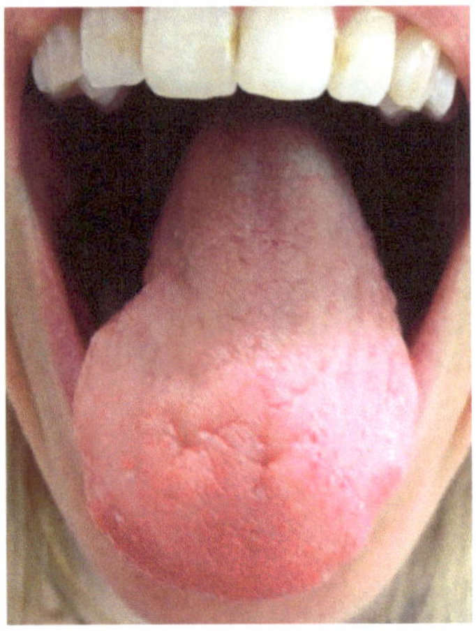

This tongue belongs to a person insistent on fighting and suing her way through life, holding grudges, walling herself off from most people, and ultimately making herself ill by refusing all invitations from the Divine to follow her gut instincts and stay her own course. Her astute practitioner attached a note to the photo, directing me to a parallel between the patient's life and her tongue: "As I reflected on the patient in this photo, I was suddenly struck by how she had painted herself into a corner in the years I knew her. It was as though she kept drawing lines in the sand until she had no room left, nowhere to go. Her determination was enormous, but like a tourniquet. She had an unhappy childhood and was so weathered by life that she was battened down in the chest, could only be warm to select people, and had a need to be perceived as strong, put-together and perfect." This tongue shows not just a Dai Mai constriction, but constriction of the entire Lower Jiao, pushing it upward toward the palate. The pressure is causing restless leg problems, a general inability to slow down, deep tiredness, and, years ago, contributed to excess bleeding after childbirth. Communication between the Jiaos is utterly lost, allowing Qi to accumulate in the Upper Jiao, resulting in fire toxins in the breast (cancer), rage, insomnia, sinus infections, and an inability to cry. Instead of cultivating the journey—allowing Jing to become Shen—she has stifled the natural expression of her Jing, causing it to wither, while the Shen, eager to sparkle, is trapped by the Mind. I would use Yin Wei Mai to release the obstacles to the realization of Jing in this case.

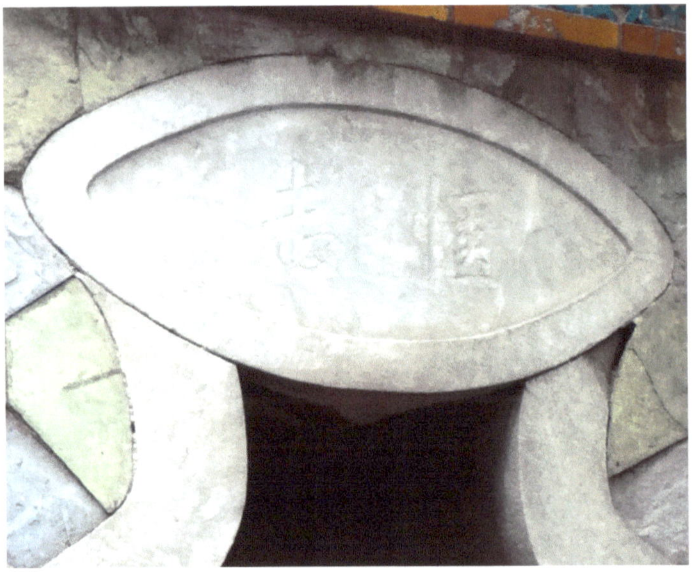

A doorway in Beijing. "Thy Heart be Satisfied."

9

Tongue Reflexology

The Tongue Map

It is only after determining the status of Fluids and Heat that we can responsibly be interested in the tongue map. The **first consideration** in tongue diagnosis is moisture, since hydration is crucial to all aspects of physiology. Even slight dehydration impairs every physiological function; damage to or deficiency of fluids must be addressed if health is to be restored. The status of Fluids is evident on the tongue coat and in the flesh of the tongue body. This can manifest as excess fluids on the tongue, accumulations of pathological fluids (coagulated coating) on the tongue, the absence of any coat at all, swelling of the tongue body, and the actual shriveling of the tongue body. The **second consideration** is color, as its technicolor display adds to our understanding of the severity of illness.

Although many clinicians look at the tongue map first, it's most useful as the third consideration. The tongue map is not a complete diagnostic key; it is a specific guide to the pathologies of Heat and of Fluids. The tongue map reflects where Heat has transferred. Heat is generated in the Stomach in response to a pathogen, but Heat can transfer anywhere, creating damage to fluids, tissues, and organs. It could rise to the Lungs, descend to the Large Intestine, transfer over to the Liver, affect the Spleen, inflame the Liver, try to vent through the skin or sensory orifices, etc. If you are using the Primary Channels to clear Heat, the tongue map is key to keeping treatments specific to the patient.[17]

Organ Pathology

Heart

The most forward region of the tongue reflects the Heart.

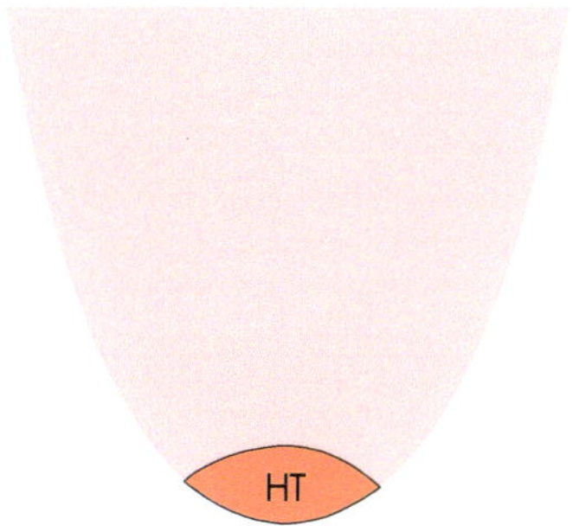

[17] In my practice, if I find pathological Heat I will often bleed the Stomach Luo (ST-40). This is an efficient way to clear Heat using the Complement Channels.

The Heart moves Blood, expresses the Shen by opening to the tongue and the eyes. It shares love and joy, and controls relationships. The Heart must be relaxed to honor its resident, the Shen, whose expression is the purpose of life. Connecting through the eyes and tongue, the Heart must be allowed to shine its light outward through the eyes, speak its truth, and circulate its enthusiasm. Heat showing in the Heart area may affect any of these functions.

Common observations about the Heart area and possible implications include the following:

If you see a:

- red tip,
  - Stress—stagnation due to the mind's resistance to what is—is creating tension in the Heart region.
  - There is a lack of control in relationships or difficulty in interactions, since the Heart identifies people and situations destined for its engagement.
  - Impaired circulation is causing Kidney Yang to be summoned to move Heart Qi, potentially causing (renal) hypertension.
  - There is difficulty with speech, an inability to communicate adequately, clearly, confidently, or with certainty. Emotional trauma is often the root. There may be difficulty articulating feelings.
  - There may be constraint in communication to the point of stuttering.
  - Excess Heat is ascending to the eyes, head, or Upper Jiao.
  - The Shen is suppressed and Qi is accumulated at the Heart.
  - The Pericardium is restricting the patient's expression of the Heart and emotions, causing Heat to build up in the Heart region. When it's felt that something cannot be expressed or spoken, the Pericardium restricts the flow of Blood and Qi flowing from the Heart to the tongue, but also, the Pericardium region on the tongue itself reflects this restriction. As unexpressed emotions percolate in the body, creating pressure and then steam upward, hypertension and Heat diseases can result. Over time, the tip remains red as the body brings Heat to try to move this stagnation. The sublingual veins then swell and darken with the lack of movement and with complications involving the Heart Luo Channel.
- raised tip,
  - A raised tight area, often appearing like a small pyramid lying on its side, indicates that the Heart is constrained while the Pericardium fiercely defends it.

- missing tip,
  - A tip that is curved inward indicates the Heart is so restrained, stagnated, or deficient, its region appears missing. A key point here is that all Heart Qi and Heart Blood is utterly reliant on the Liver being able to provide Qi and Blood to the Heart. When the Liver is unable to provide sustenance to the Heart, the Liver's Jue Yin partner—the Pericardium—tightens in sympathy. This results in retraction of the Heart region.
- retracted tip,
  - A tip that is retracted is either reflecting that there is insufficient Qi either to move Blood from the Liver up to the Heart, or to move Spleen Qi up to the Lungs.
- turned under,
  - Very often, when the tip is turned under, there is disappointment involved. The Heart is not flourishing and retreats.
- blanched,
  - Constraint in the Heart has taxed Yang Qi.

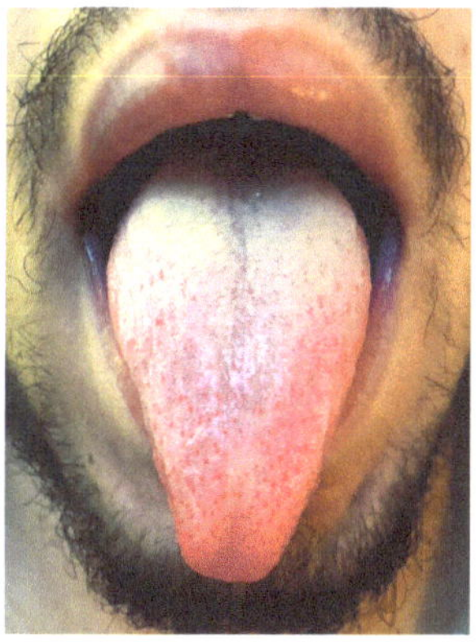

Red

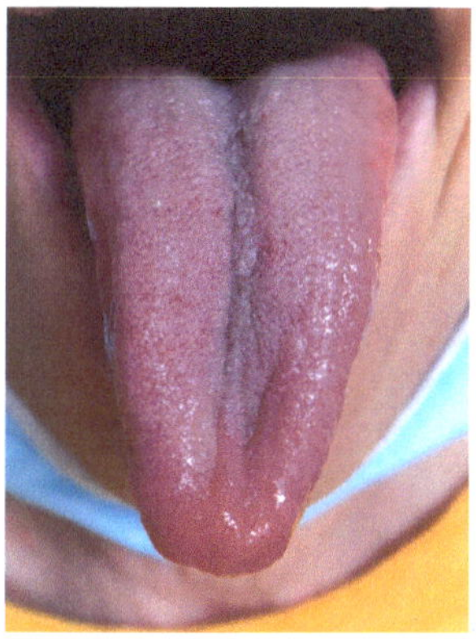

Raised

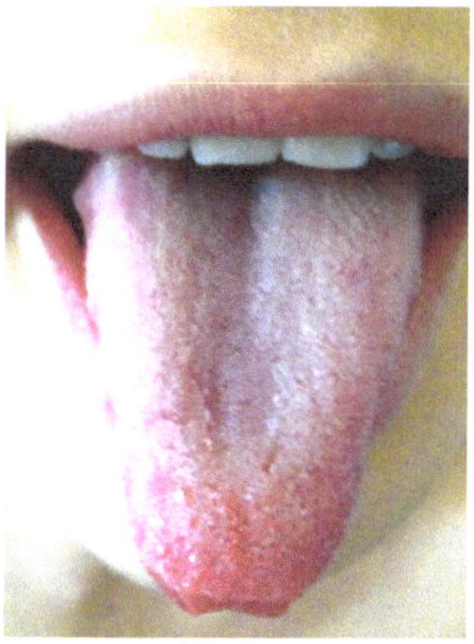

Missing

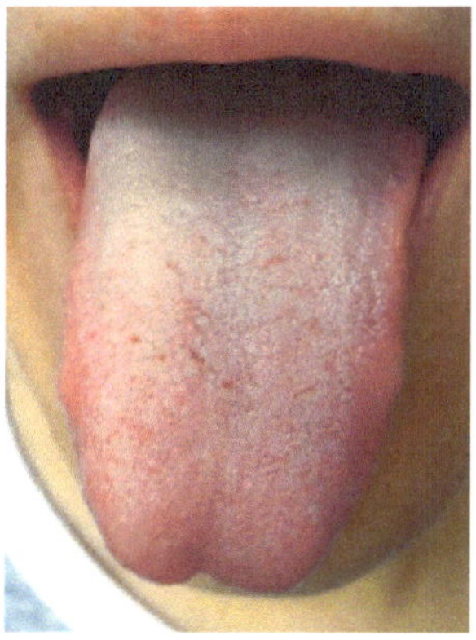

Retracted

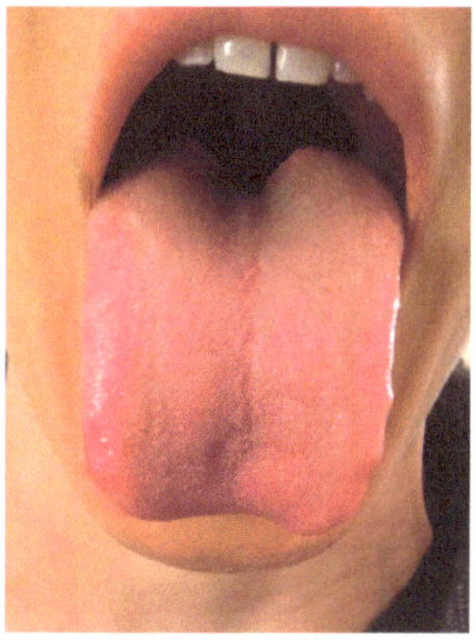

Turned under

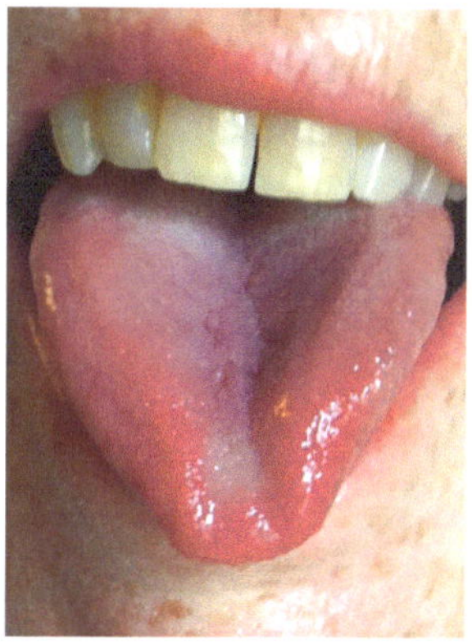

Blanched

Pericardium

Just posterior to the tip of the tongue is the Pericardium area.

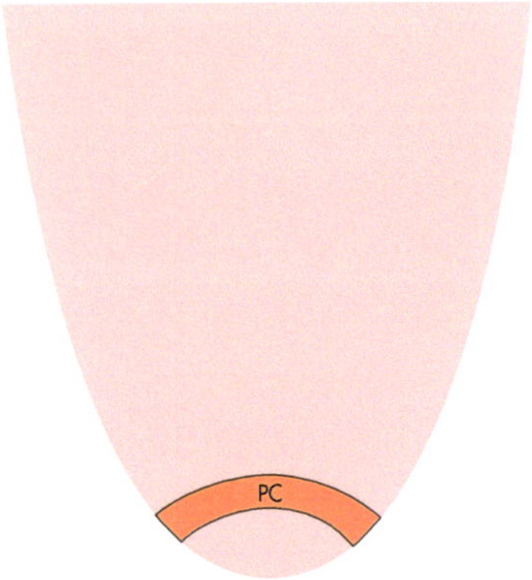

The Pericardium commands the very internal circulation of Blood, but its key function is to protect the Heart and honor its vulnerability. The Heart's mission is to remain completely open, knowing that the Pericardium can catch it at any time. The Pericardium tenses if it feels there are potential or actual influences threatening the Heart's freedom. This tension shows in a band that isolates the Heart.

Common observations about the Pericardium area and the body's responses to pathology involving the Pericardium include the following:

If, in the Pericardium region there is a:

- red band,
  - The Pericardium is reacting to protect the Heart, causing stagnation of Qi. When Qi stagnates, Heat builds. The Pericardium then works harder to hold that Heat away from the Heart.
  - The Liver may be constrained and the resulting pent-up Heat is transferring to its Jue Yin partner, the Pericardium.
- gripping around the tip,
  - The Pericardium may be defending the Heart against protracted emotional insult.
- swelling in the Pericardium region,
  - The body is trying to defend the Heart from Heat in the Stomach or Liver.
- tightness creating a waist around Heart region while the sides are very tight,
  - The Pericardium is defending the Heart against Heat rising from the Liver.
- pallor,
  - The Heart is not receiving sufficient Blood from the Liver due to insufficiency of Blood.

• tight or elevated band,

• The Pericardium is protecting the Heart, and therefore restricting the expression of emotions.

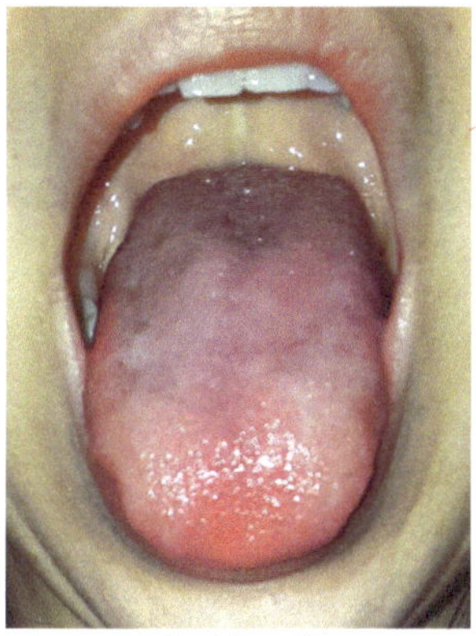
Red band

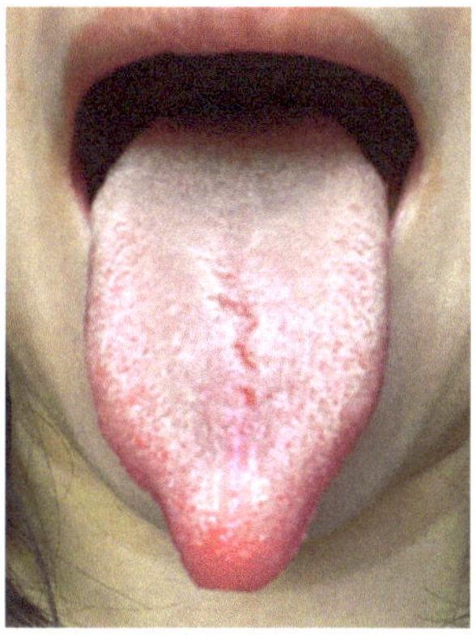
Gripping

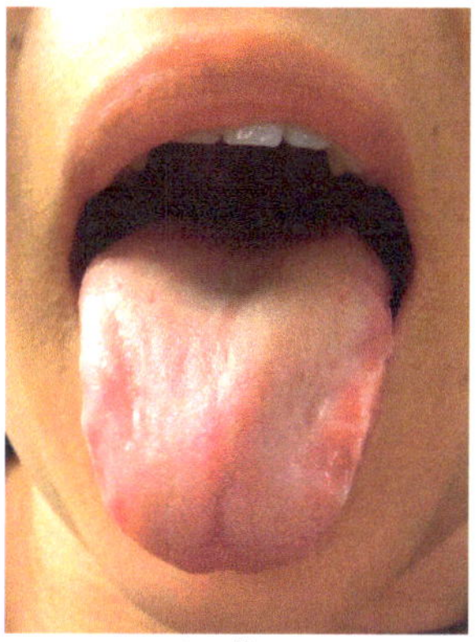
Swelling

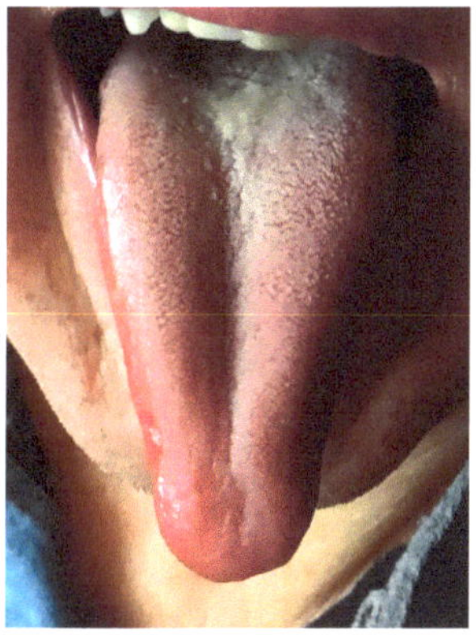
Liver-Pericardium

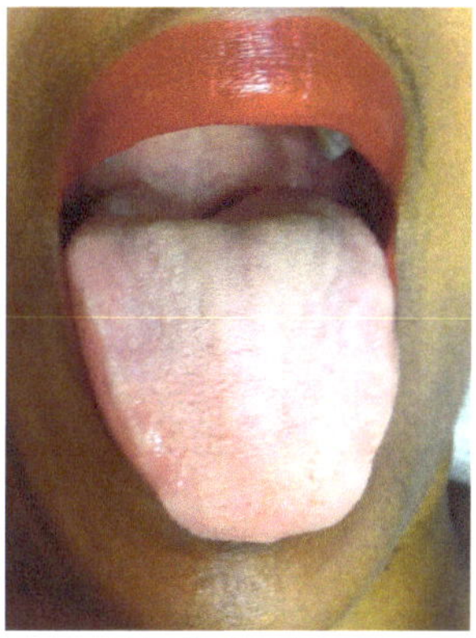
Pale Pericardium

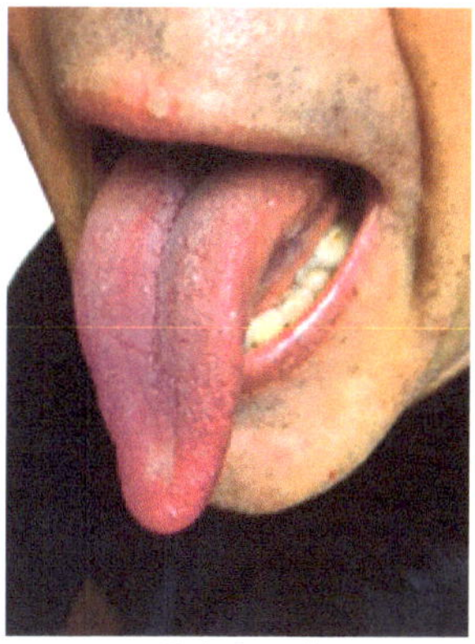
Tight band

Lungs

The Lung or chest area appears just behind the Pericardium band.

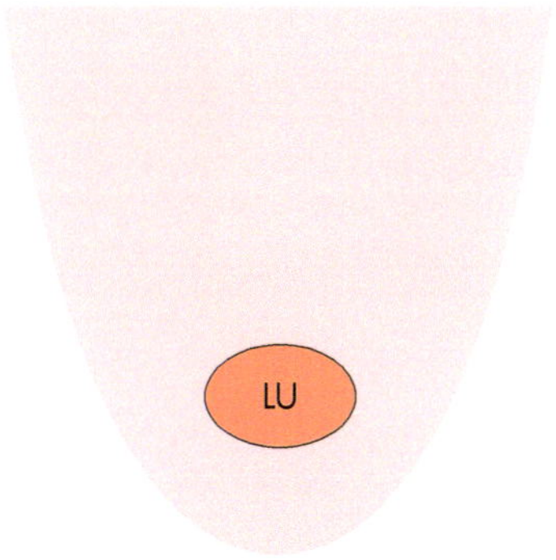

The Lungs command the Qi to move Blood and descend Qi and Blood. Hence Lung Qi controls cardiac sufficiency, menstruation, fertility, and bowel movements. The Lungs diffuse Wei Qi to defend against pathogens and to ensure adequacy of Wei Qi for movement of the musculoskeletal system. The Lungs moisten by moving Blood and Fluids. Heat showing in the Lung area may affect any of these functions.

Common observations about this area and the responses include the following:

If, in the Lung region, there is:

- swelling or elevation,
  - The Lungs are weak and unable to expel a pathogenic factor, causing stagnation of Qi.
  - The Lungs are weak and unable to expel Phlegm.
  - The Upper Jiao is stagnated; the lymphatic system is sluggish, not moving enough to drain efficiently through the Bladder.
  - The tongue might be swollen at the middle, as food and fluids are not properly transformed. The Spleen sends these pathological Fluids upward to the Lungs, creating stagnation in both Upper and Middle Jiaos.
  - The diaphragm is blocked or stagnated.
- a depression or dip in the area,
  - The patient may be depressed. Lung Qi is not dispersing.
  - There may be an inherent deficiency of Lung Qi or an issue in the chain of manufacture of Lung Qi including a deficiency of Spleen Qi, failure of Spleen Qi to ascend, or a weakness in Kidney Yang—the ultimate foundation of Lung Qi.
  - The patient may be confused about their Destiny, what it is they are here to do. This impedes the free communication from Kidneys to Lungs and from Lungs to Kidneys. There may be a reluctance to breathe in freely and allow Lung Qi to connect to the Kidneys to reveal that Destiny.
- a depression or dip in a tongue with engorged sides,
  - Liver Qi constraint may be insulting the Lungs, preventing the free flow of Qi from the end of the Primary Channel sequence at LR-14, to the beginning of that sequence, at LU-1.
- redness, dryness, irritation,
  - Heat is present. This area will become inflamed and irritated if Dryness is present.

- red dots with a crack in the mid-tongue,
    - Heat is rising from the Middle Jiao to the Upper Jiao, affecting the junction of the two, irritating the diaphragmatic area, and reflecting in the tongue as red dots. This may be a sign of reflux, diaphragmatic constriction, hiatal hernia, or other pathology of that region. There may be an accompanying centerline crack extending from the Middle to the Upper Jiao in the tongue.
- a purple appearance,
    - The Lungs are unable to move Blood well. Blood may be stagnating due to unresolved emotions, especially grief or sadness.
- a pale appearance,
    - Dampness is present in the Lungs. Dampness impedes or slows the free flow of Qi and Blood, resulting in pallor. Look for slippery pulses in the right cun and guan pulses.
- blanching (appears whitened),
    - There is long-term Dampness in the Lungs. This is a curious phenomenon. Sometimes you'll suspect the area is slightly paler than the rest of the tongue and sometimes there appears to be a very distinct patch of white in the Lung region. When this happens, often you'll see that the rest of the tongue is quite stiff, and the sides look as though they are stretched out. This can mean there is so much stagnation from repressed emotions that the patient can no longer take a very deep breath. The blanching is showing you the absence of the free flow of Qi and Blood through the Lungs and the Lungs' inability to move Blood adequately.

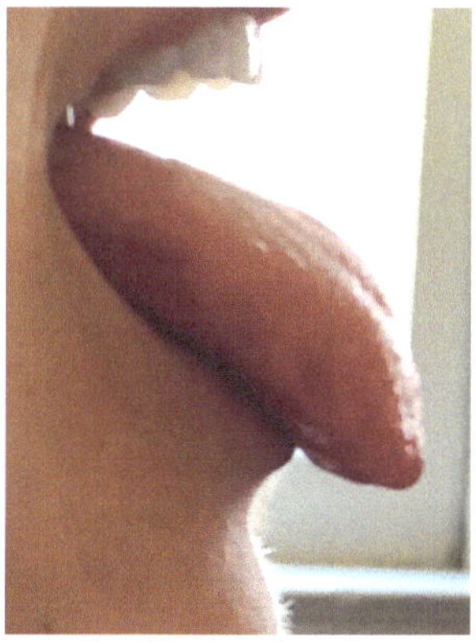
Swelling or elevation

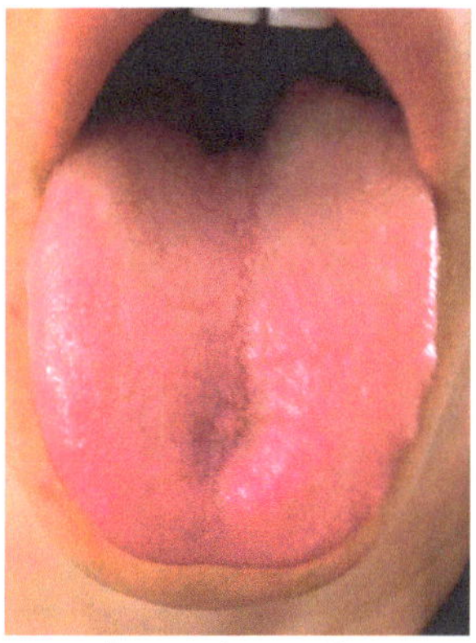
Depression or dip

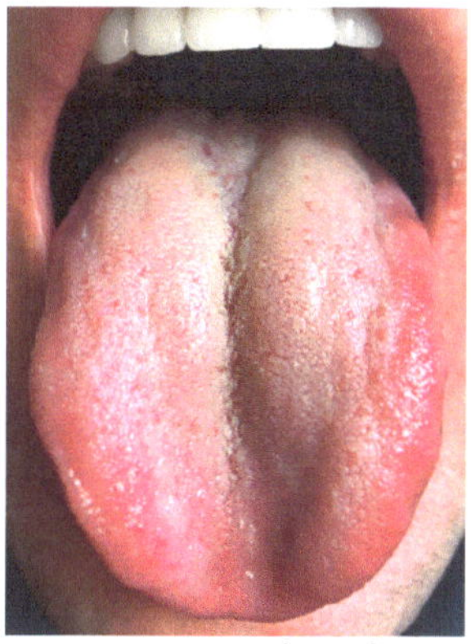
Depression or dip with engorged sides

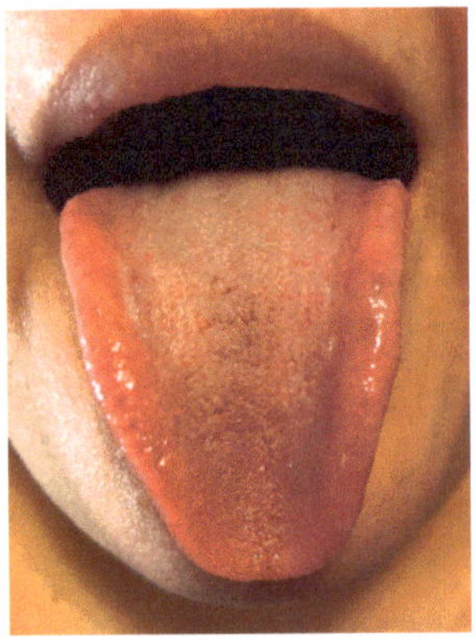

Redness dryness irritation

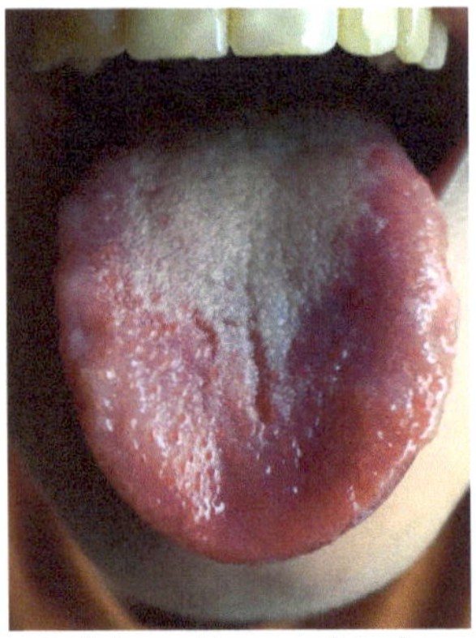

Red dots with a crack in the mid tongue

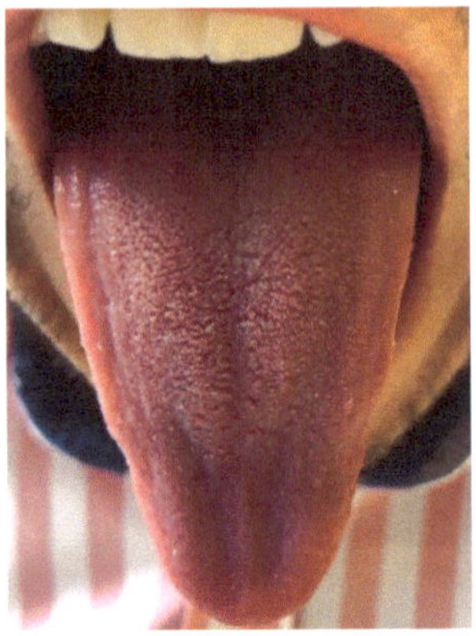

Purple

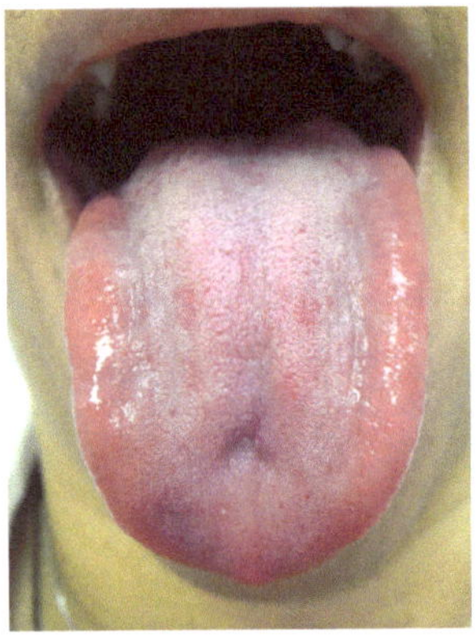

Pale

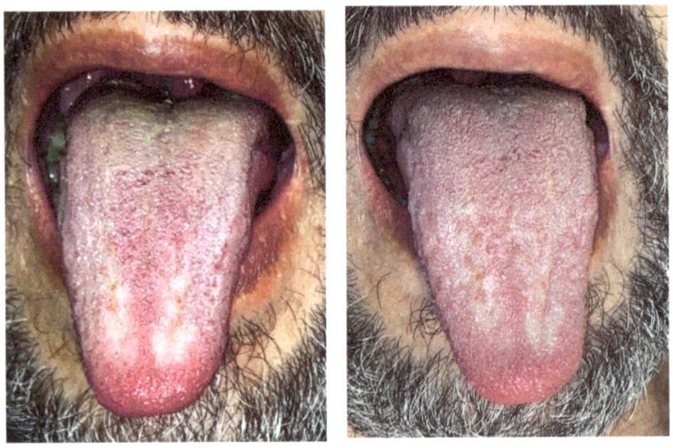

Blanching.
This person has a long history of pessimism about himself, narcissism, emotional volatility, frustration, and feeling a victim. Since emotions are held in the Blood and depletes it, and since the Liver's function is to store Blood, tremendous tension arises in the Liver, since it finds there is not enough Blood to store. Tension in the Liver constrained the diaphragm which in turn constrained the Lungs. If Lung Qi cannot cross the diaphragm, their Qi cannot reach the Lower Jiao to clear it via the stool. The Lungs themselves—wearied from the effort—then become further impeded. The results are dire, since the Lungs are unable to move Wei-Defensive Qi effectively to the exterior to create sweat. The patient is also a smoker. The failure of these mechanisms, combined with the smoking, resulted in facial paralysis, eczema in the Lower Jiao, lumps in the skin, constipation, and ultimately, fire toxins in the Lower Jiao. Upon his recent diagnosis of prostate cancer, he sought acupuncture. The second photograph was taken a month later after treatment by a colleague.

Asymmetry and the Map

Often you'll see a discernible asymmetry in the tongue where the left and right sides are not mirror images of each other. To determine left-right differentiations in the tongue, note that the right side of the tongue reflects Yin and, therefore, the Yin organs. The left side of the tongue reflects the Yang and the Yang organs. Use this information if the tongue is asymmetrical to reveal the meaning of the differences showing in the two halves. For example, if the two halves of the center area of the tongue appear different from each other, the right side of center will give you more information about the Spleen. The left side of center will give you more information about the Stomach. If the sides of the tongue are different from each other, the right side of the tongue will give you more information about the Liver, the left about the Gallbladder.

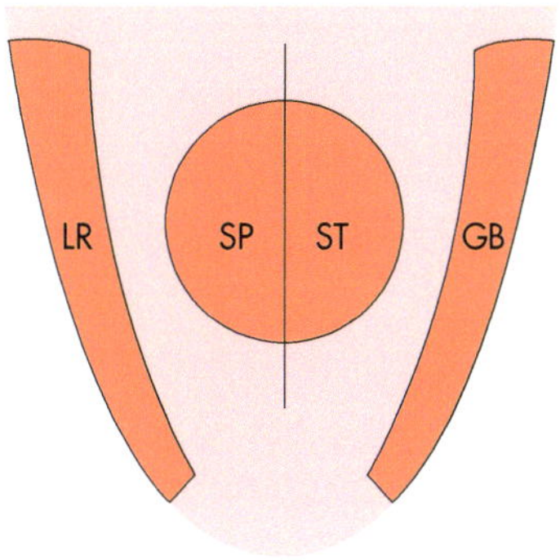

Spleen and Stomach

The Spleen and Stomach area is in the center of the tongue, just posterior to the Lungs.

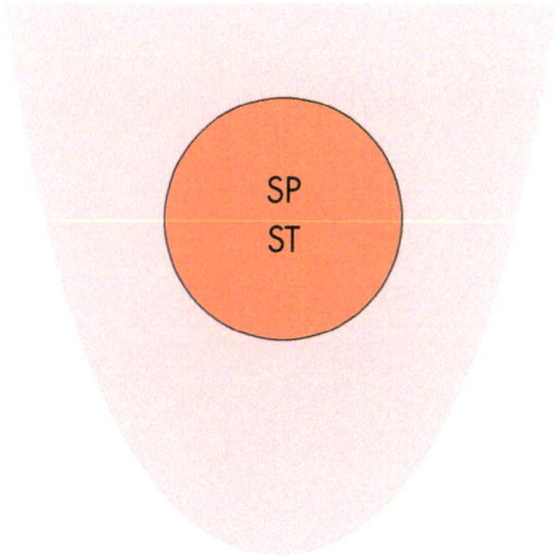

The Spleen's functions include transformation and transportation of nourishment, ascension of Kidney Yang, ascension of Blood, management of Blood, control of the Mind, resolution of Dampness, control of the four limbs, and harmonization with the Stomach. The Stomach is the origin of Fluids and Blood and rots food. Heat showing at the center of the tongue may be affecting any function of the Spleen and Stomach.

If you see:

- swelling or elevation at the center,
    - This is very often a cultural issue, since so many people eat a diet that is Damp, Cold, and processed without even knowing it. As a result of these habits, the Spleen is weak, its transformative function unable to keep up with the daily onslaught. A swelling at the center can over time expand to swell the entire tongue, resulting in a dramatic roundness in all directions.

- scalloping due to swelling that is clearly emanating from a swollen center,
  - The Spleen and Pancreas are weakened and unable to digest efficiently. The Dampness that is accumulating has become so systemic that it has engulfed the sides of the tongue.
- a moist, pale, purple center,
  - Cold and Damp have accumulated. Heat may have been extinguished as Yang is consumed or depleted.
- redness at the center of the tongue,
  - There is Heat (inflammation) in the digestive tract. This is most often due to inflaming elements in the diet, but since the Stomach is the origin of all Heat, central tongue redness may indicate a response to pathology anywhere in the interior.
- purple at the center of the tongue,
  - There is blood stagnation in the Stomach.
- a collapsed center,
  - The Yang Qi of the Spleen may be collapsed. In these cases, often Kidney Yang (the source of this Yang), is also collapsed.

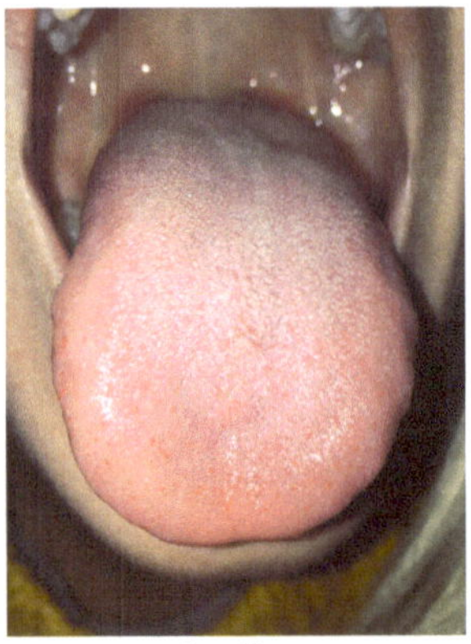
Swollen

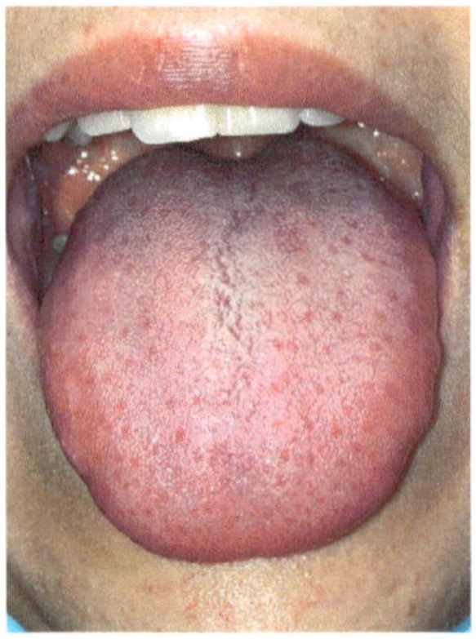
Scalloped

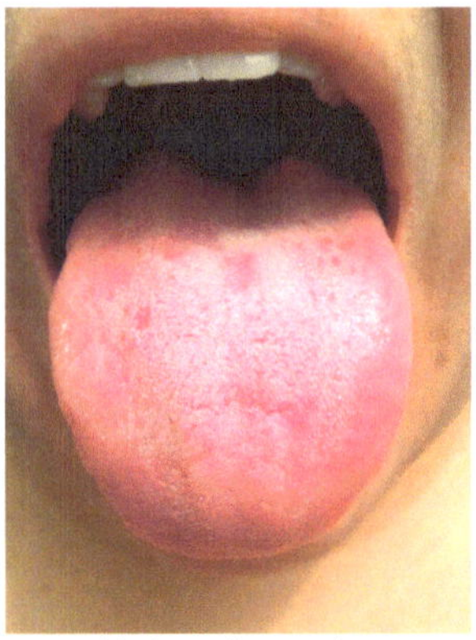
Moist pale purple

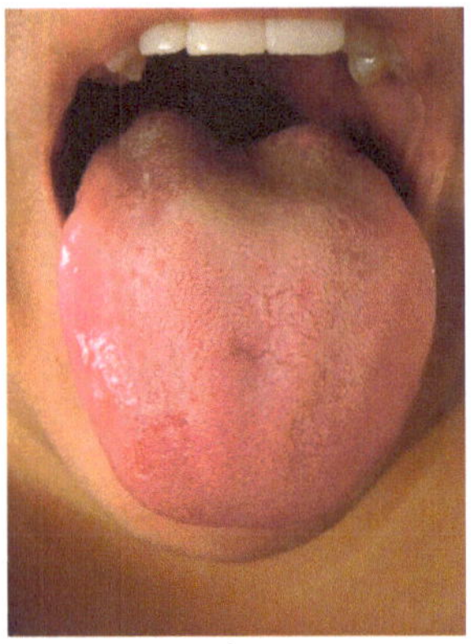
Redness

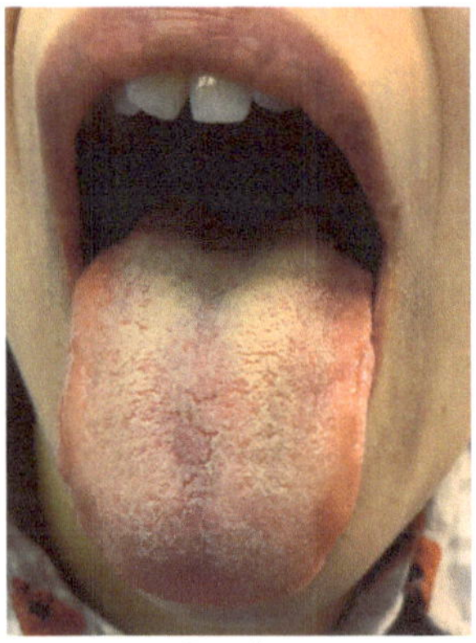
Purple

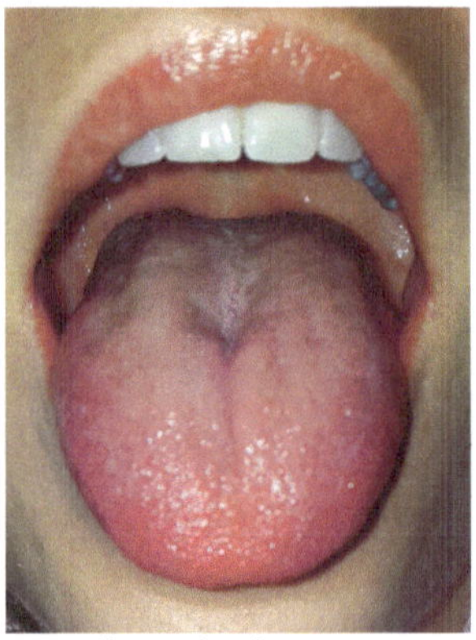
Collapsed Spleen Yang

Liver and Gallbladder

The Gallbladder is reflected on the left lateral band of the tongue; the Liver on the right lateral band. (The right side of the body reflects Yin and the left side of the body reflects Yang.)

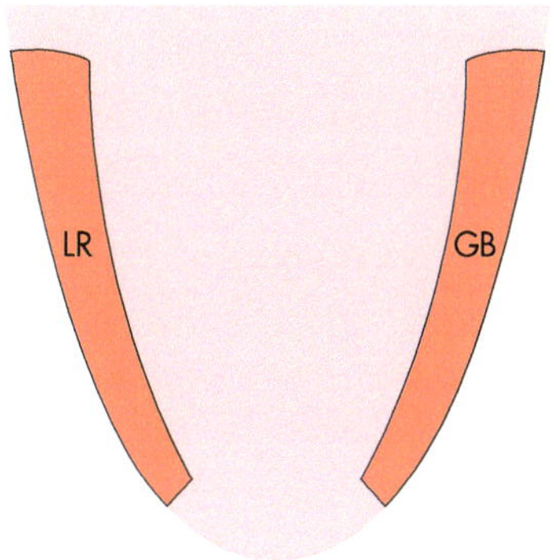

The Liver regulates and ensures the smooth flow of Qi, stores Blood, engenders Heart Qi and Blood, brings Blood to the sinews and brain, opens to the eyes, houses the Hun, enables planning, nourishes the Kidneys, hair and nails, nourishes the Lower Jiao, and harmonizes the emotions. The Gallbladder controls the bone and is the link between the post-natal arena and the Curious Organs.

When the sides of the tongue call your attention, the Liver and Gallbladder will be included in the thought process leading to diagnosis. Either there is Liver or Gallbladder pathology, or—if there is Heat showing along the sides of the tongue—the Liver and Gallbladder are engaged in responding to pathology. The right side will show more strain if the Liver is more taxed than the Gallbladder; the left side will show more strain if the Gallbladder is overtaxed as it strains to support the Liver.

Stages of Liver Qi Constraint

Many factors have been in play for a while by the time Qi constraint affects the Liver, including some or all of the following:

- The diet has been deficient in Blood-building foods: saturated fat, soups, stews, nuts, and seeds.
- The diet is high in coffee, chocolate, sugar, alcohol, hot spices, garlic, and onion.
- Late bedtime has become a habit.
- Emotional stress is unmanaged.
- The patient overworks.

After these factors set in, the results begin to show in the tongue, in the following order:

1

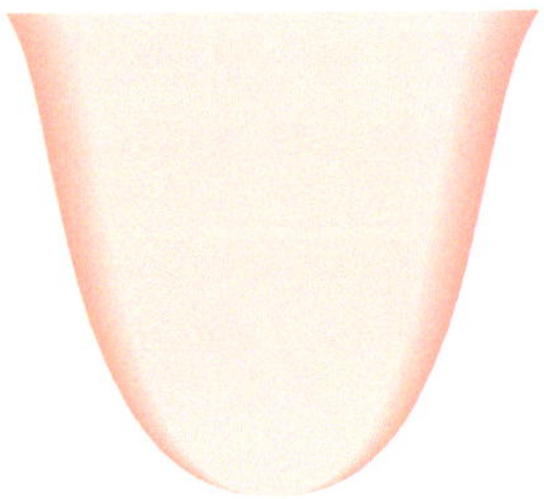

Normal

2

A deficiency of Blood pales the sides.

3

The sides swell and scallop as the Liver tries to store Blood.

4

The sides flatten, reflecting the developing constraint.

5

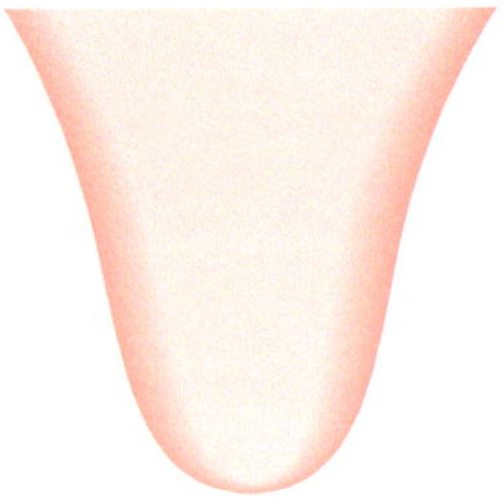

The sides continue to tighten as diet and lifestyle remain unchanged.

6

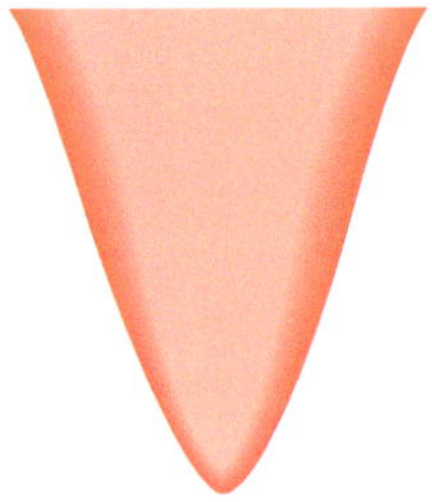

The tongue lengthens as the tension stretches the sides out.

7

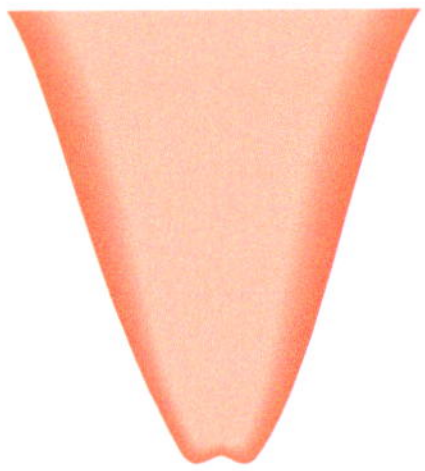

The Liver's Jue Yin pair, the Pericardium, tightens to shield the Heart. The Heart is distanced from the Liver, preventing Liver Blood from engendering Heart Qi and Blood.

8

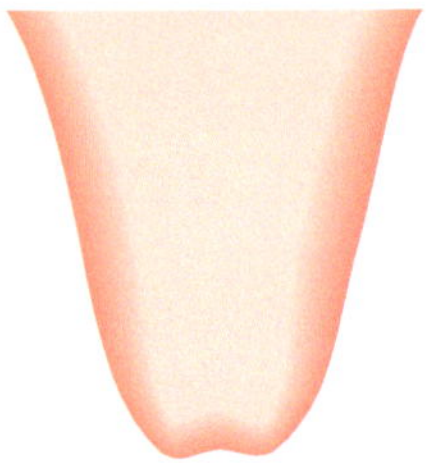

The Spleen accumulates Dampness to quell the Heat.

9

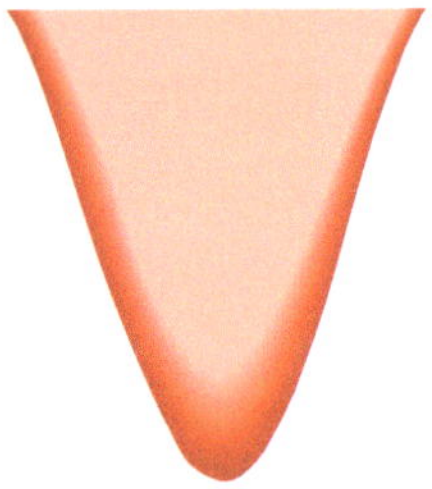

Heat in the Upper Jiao becomes severe.

If you see that the sides of the tongue are:

- different in color from the tongue tip,
    - If the Liver pulse is more than slightly tight, the Liver is trying to store more Blood. Often the tip will be red or pink while the sides are noticeably paler or slightly purple. This is helping you differentiate where the body is prioritizing. If the sides are pale, there may be a Blood deficiency. If they are slightly purple, the body is stagnating Blood to reserve it. It's important to remember that the Liver holds on to Blood, not only to store it but also to contain emotions that are unprocessed in the hope of harmonizing them, or to keep them

from unwelcome expression. The longer this process goes on, the deeper the purple hue in the sides. It's not uncommon to see a purple-hued translucency in the sides, which indicates a complex mix of all the above elements.

- dry,
  - There is insufficient mediumship in the Liver. The Liver is not adequately storing Blood.
- pale,
  - Long-term constraint and resulting Heat has exhausted Yang Qi. The Liver may be damaged.
- translucent, pale, and glass-like,
  - There is a deficiency of Blood and possibly systemic Cold.
- pale and dry,
  - There is insufficient Blood to store.
- peeled,
  - There is a Liver Yin deficiency (Blood deficiency.)
- dry and red,
  - There is Qi constraint, but not long-term. The body is producing Heat to try to move Qi. The rest of the tongue could be wet concurrently, since it harbors Dampness in compensation.
- purple,
  - There is pain. Qi stagnation is causing Blood to stagnate. The pulses will be wiry.
- very red or quite purple,
  - There is long-term Qi constraint. The body responded by creating Heat to shift that constraint, but the constraint was intransigent and trapped the Heat, creating damage.
- smoky brown or orange,
  - There is very long-term Heat due to overstimulation of the Gallbladder. There may be hepatitis or gallstones. Dampness (in this case, cholesterol levels) might be high, since the body creates vital protective Dampness in response to that Heat.

- dry and orange,
  - Heat has damaged the Liver. There may be cirrhosis or fibrosis of the Liver.
- wet and orange,
  - Dampness smothered long-term Heat, resulting in Damp-Heat. This can become a Hot-Phlegm condition, such as lymphoma.
- dark,
  - Blood deficiency is chronic. Qi is trying to conserve what Blood there is by stagnating it.
- noticeably darker than the rest of the tongue,
  - The emotions are not harmonized. The Liver is trying to store Blood which contains emotions, in order to harmonize those emotions.
- long and stretched out,
  - Heat in the Liver is causing the tongue to lengthen and shoot forward.
- elevated and tense,
  - There is long-term stagnation of Liver Qi.
- swollen,
  - The Liver is struggling to store Blood, while Blood is deficient. The tongue sides swell as the Liver draws Qi to itself for the function of consolidation. If this goes on long enough, pathological accumulations of Blood will form in locations nourished directly by Liver Blood; fibroids may form in the uterus, for example.
- scalloped but the scalloping is independent of the center (the swelling at the sides is clearly separated from the center or the center is not swollen),
  - The Liver is unable to store sufficient Blood or there is insufficient Blood to store, or Liver Qi is stagnating to prevent deep penetration of a pathogenic factor.
- scalloped on the left and swollen, with no scalloping on the right,
  - The Liver is working to store blood and the Gallbladder is straining to deliver enough. The patient is likely going to bed too late.
- cracked,
  - Dryness is advanced due to Heat.

- very swollen with many cracks,
    - There may be food stagnation with chronic constipation.
- severely cracked,

  There is emotional disturbance possibly to the level of panic as the Liver is unable to contain and harmonize the emotions.
- rough,

  Smooth movement of Qi is absent. Long-term stagnation of Qi is preventing pathology being pushed to the Upper Jiao (the tip of the tongue). There is diaphragmatic constriction and frustration with life as the Heart is constricted. The patient feels powerless.
- swollen with red petechiae,

  Qi stagnation in the Liver caused Heat to accumulate.
- chopped up, rough,

  The Liver is unable to store Blood or to harmonize the emotions and Blood deficiency is becoming advanced.
- tight,

  While the rear of the tongue appears narrow, the Liver is tightening to bring resources back to the Kidneys. As it does so, it overwhelms the Spleen, causing Spleen signs and symptoms, resulting in anger, sugar cravings and bloating. Nourish Blood.
- tight sides with elevation in the Lung area of the tongue,

  Frustration has affected the Lungs resulting in envy or resentment.
- tight sides with elevation of the Pericardium region (the band around the Heart region) of the tongue,

  Frustration has tightened the Liver. Its Jue Yin pair—the Pericardium—is assuming some of the tension to prevent the Heart being affected.
- tight sides with elevation of the tip of the tongue,

  frustration has affected the Heart, resulting in jealousy or rage.
- tight sides that are red and flat,

  there is a blood deficiency but enough Qi to tighten the Liver to conserve Blood. This causes Heat to accumulate in the Liver and Gallbladder.

- pinched along the edge like a pie crust,

  there is a long history of deficiency of Blood, and the Liver is very constrained, trying to hold on to what blood it can. The edges were once swollen as the Liver tried to astringe Blood, but over time the edges became scalloped.

- curled around the perimeter,

  Liver Qi constraint is advanced and curling the front of the tongue.

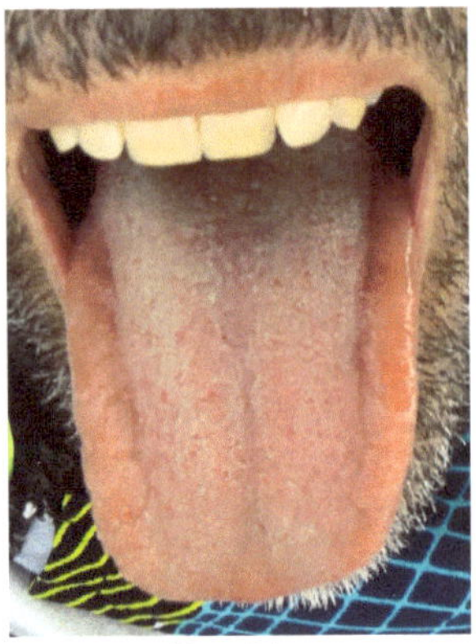
Dry sides

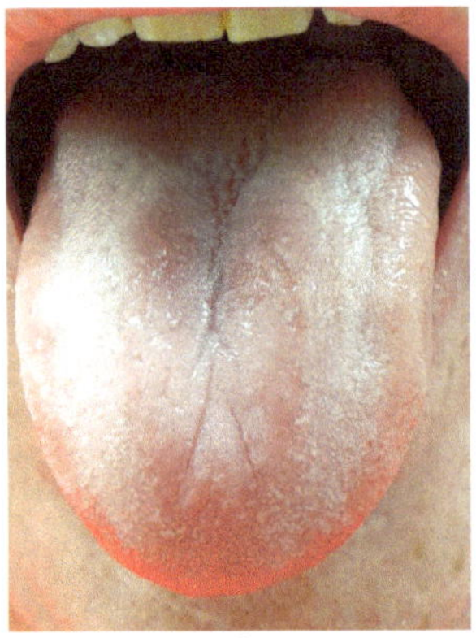
Pale

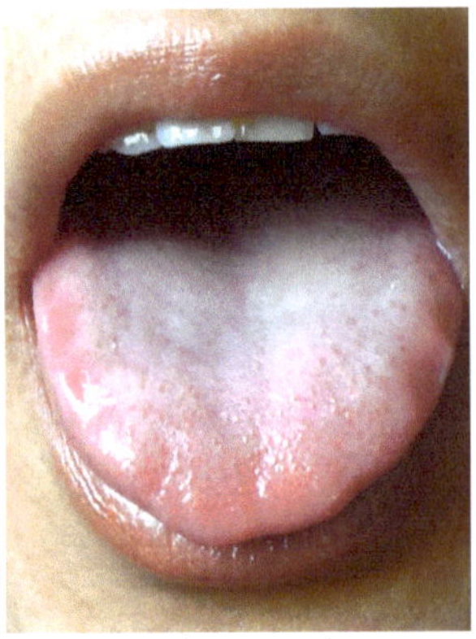
Translucent, pale and glass-like

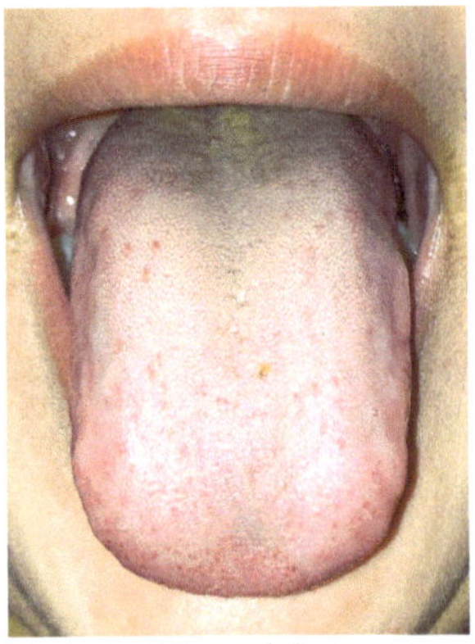
Pale and dry

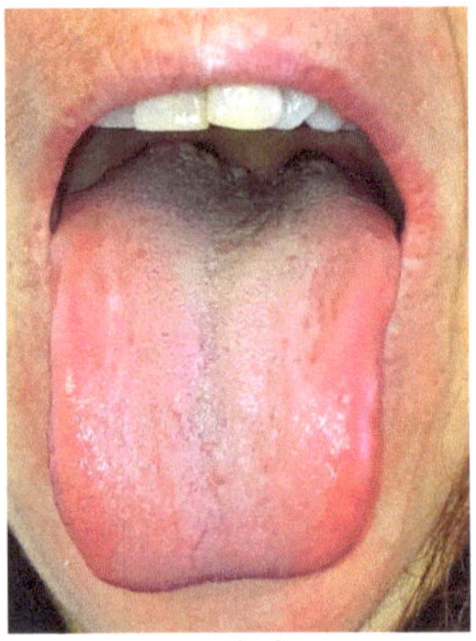
Peeled

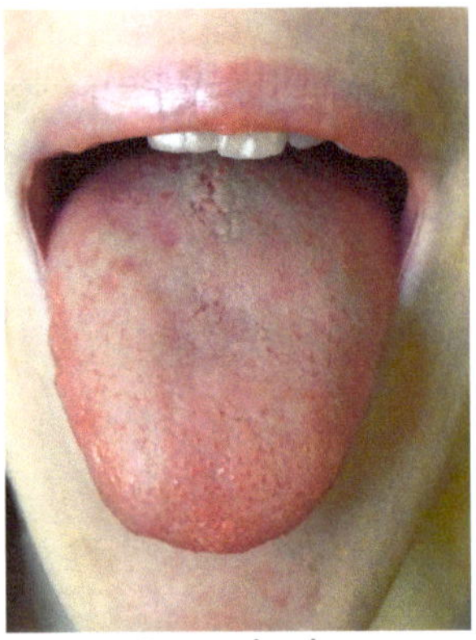
Dry and red

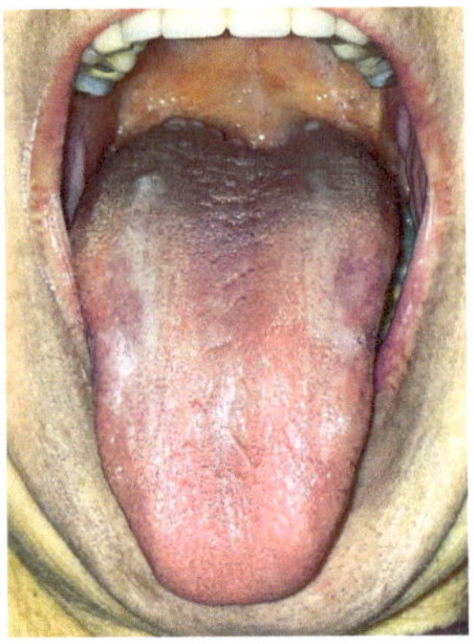
Purple

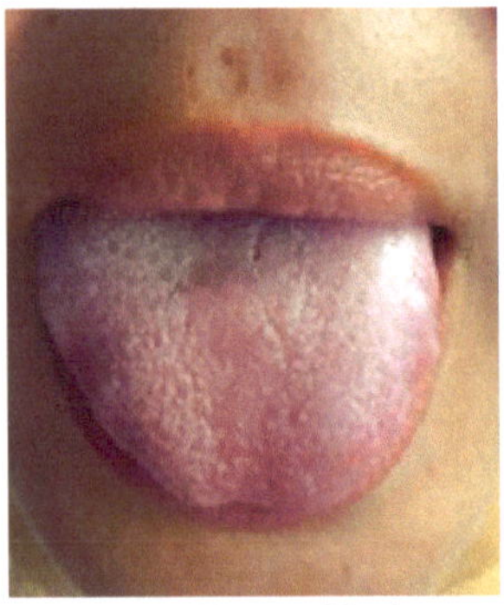
Purple and bruised looking

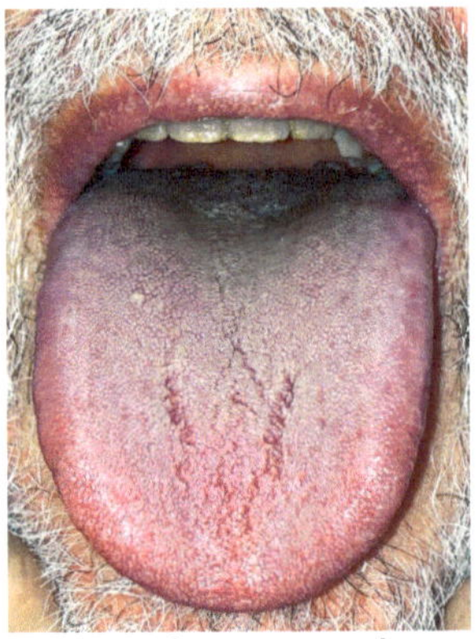
Very red or quite purple

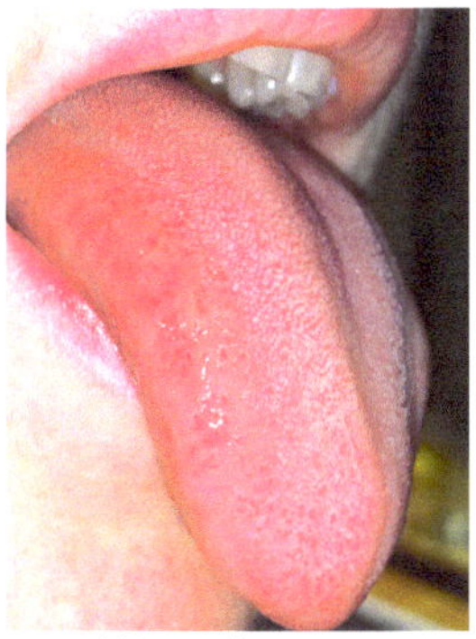

Wet and orange

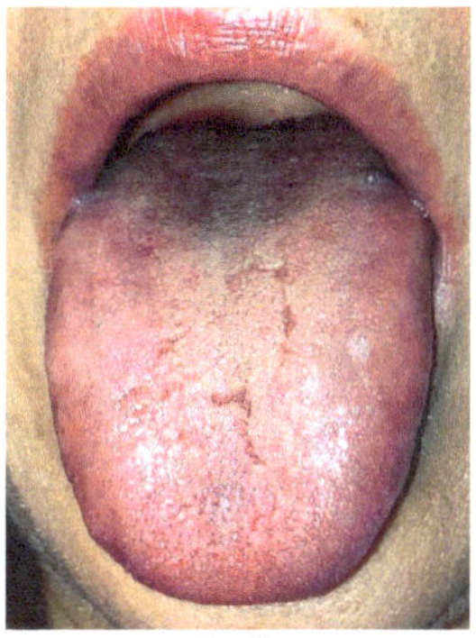

Dark

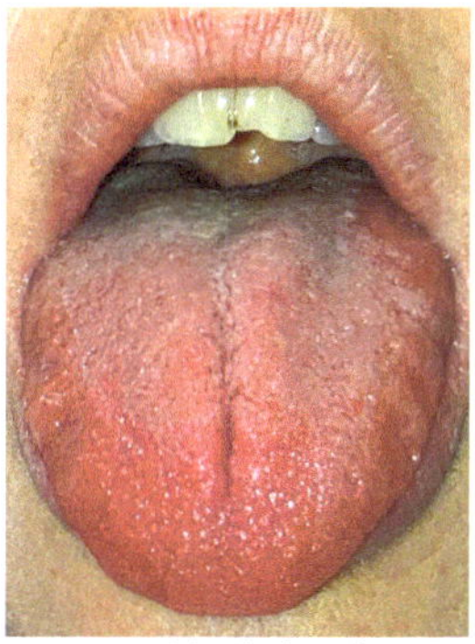

Noticeably darker than the rest of the tongue

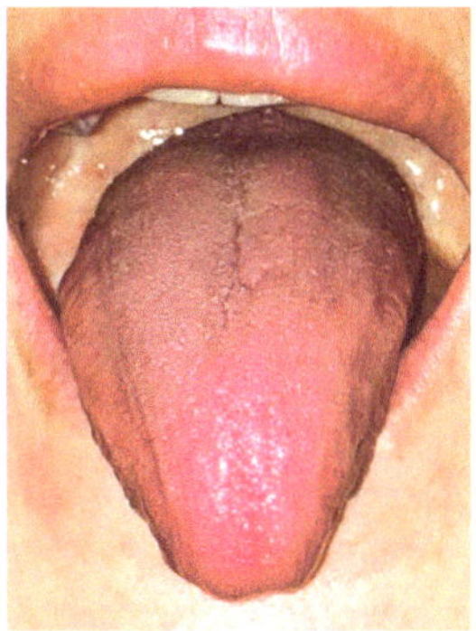

Long and stretched out

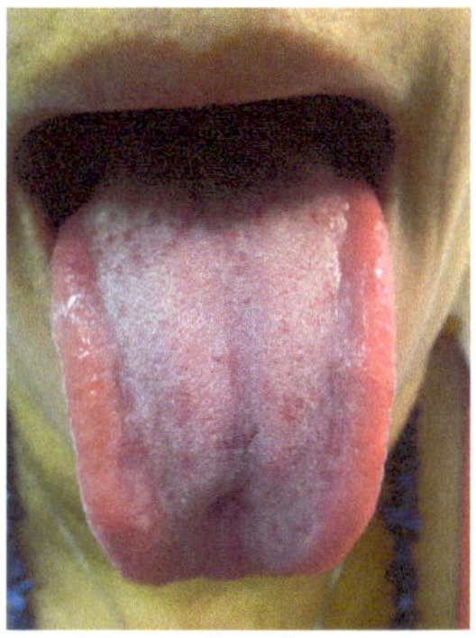

Elevated and tense

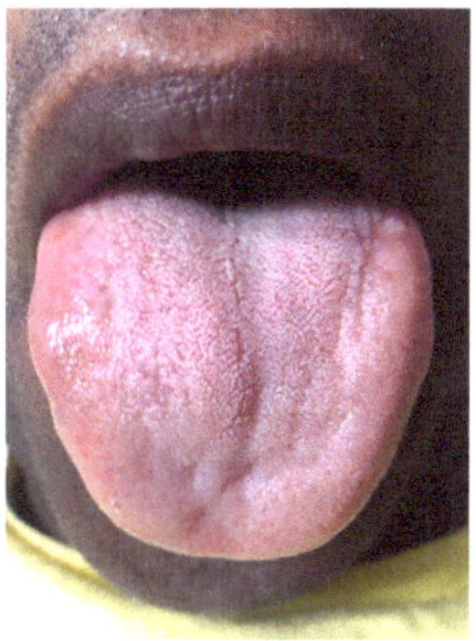

Swollen

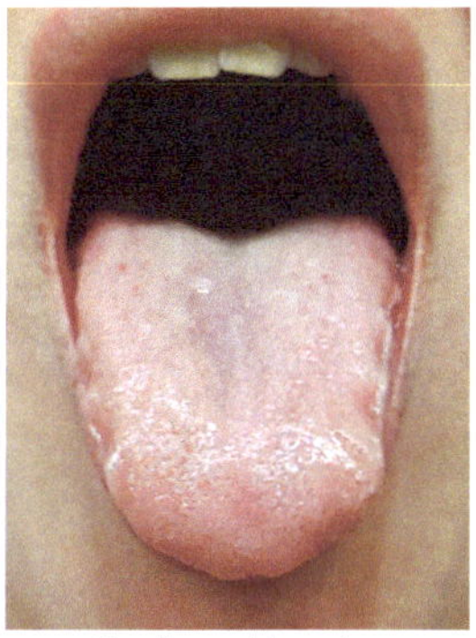

Scalloped but the scalloping is independent of the center

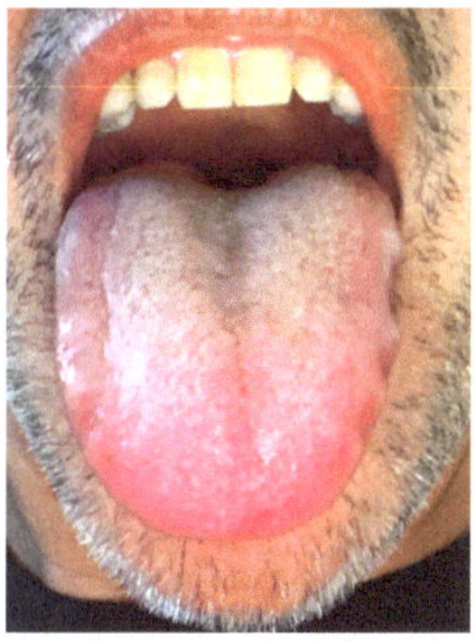

Scalloped on the left and swollen with no scalloping on the right

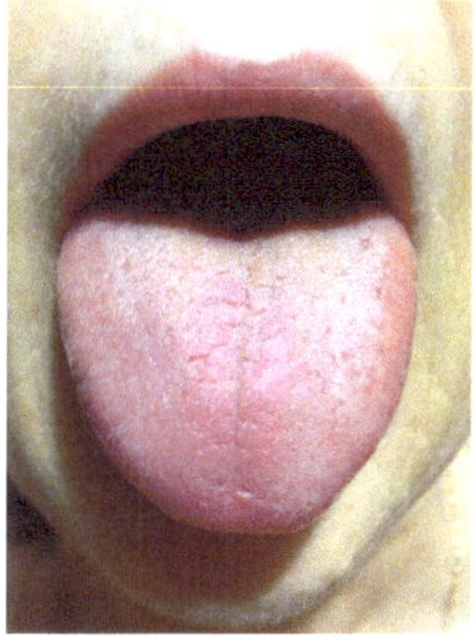

Cracked

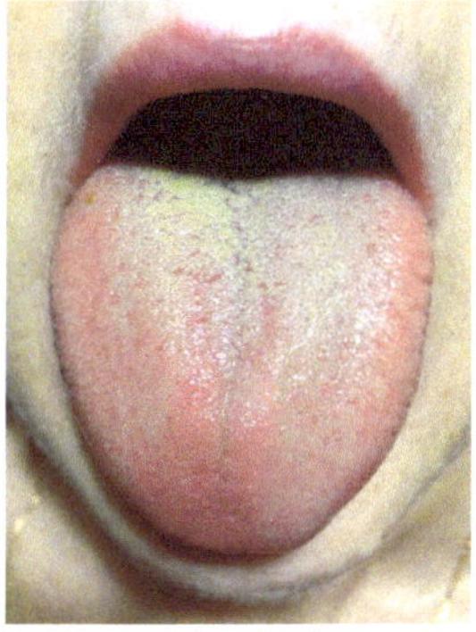

Very swollen with many cracks

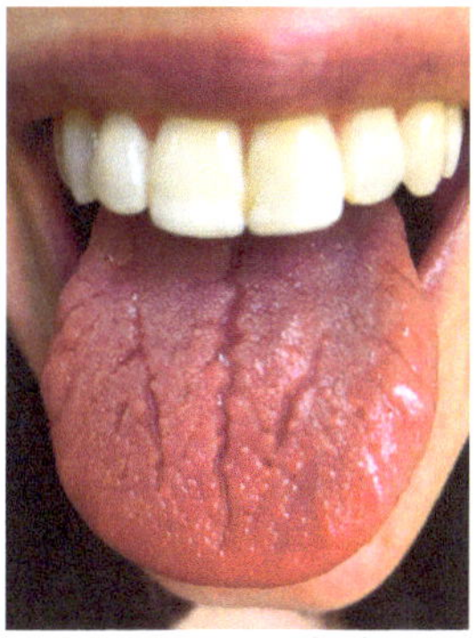

Severely cracked

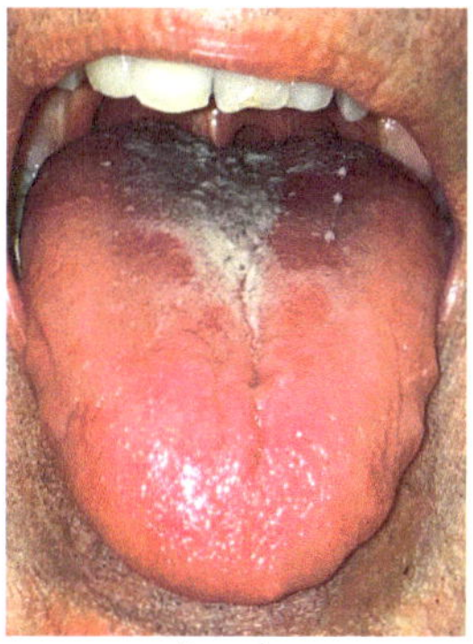

Rough

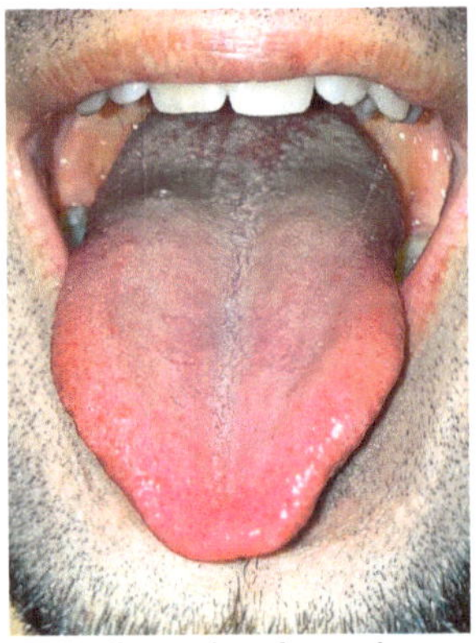
Swollen with red petechiae

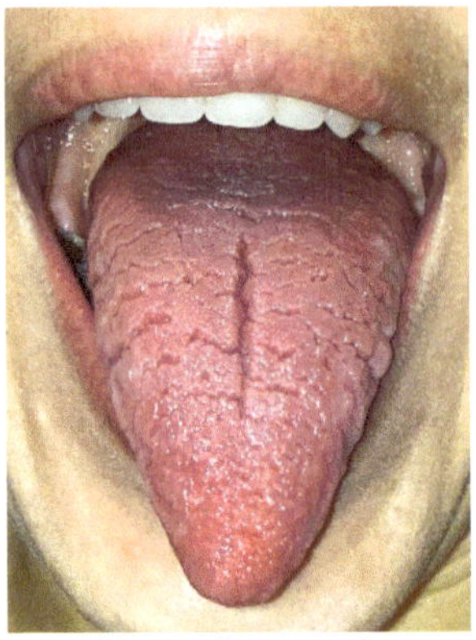
Chopped up, rough

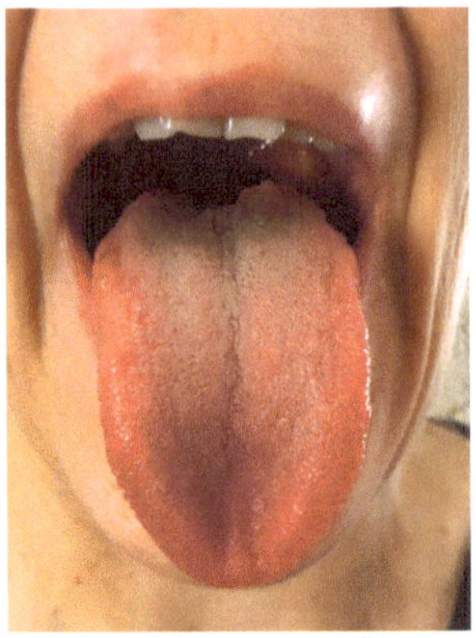
Tight, while the rear of the tongue appears narrow

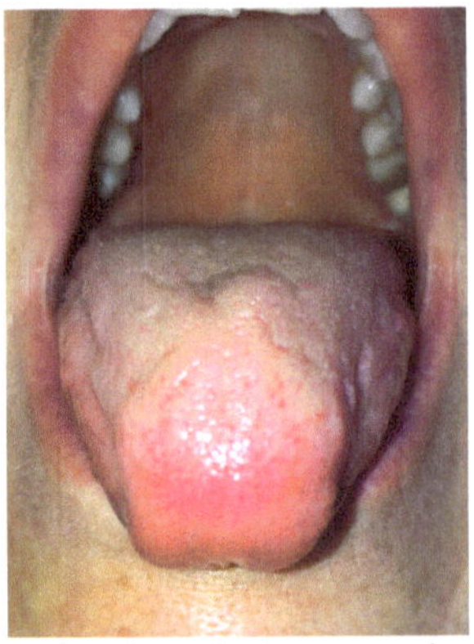
Tight sides with elevation in the Lung area of the tongue

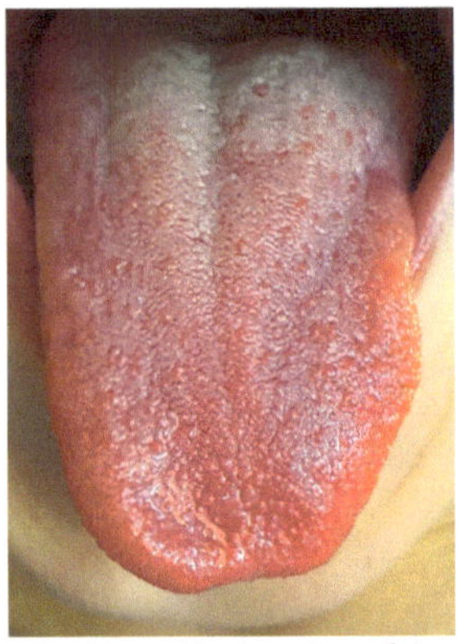
Tight sides with elevation of the Pericardium region

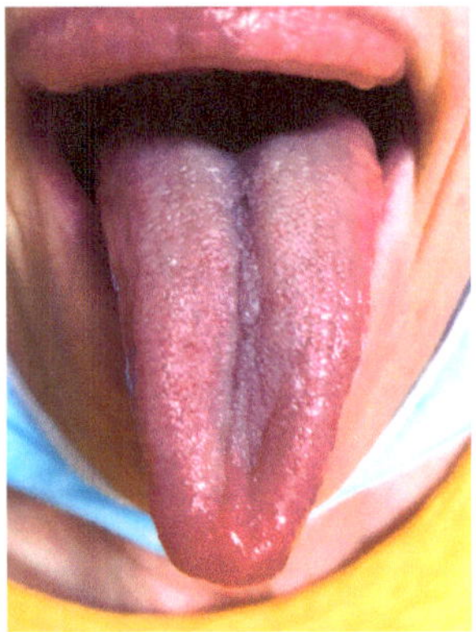
Tight sides with elevation of the tip of the tongue

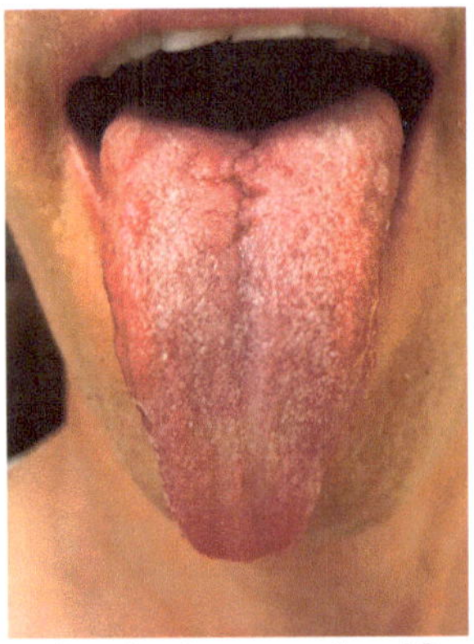
Tight sides that are red and flat

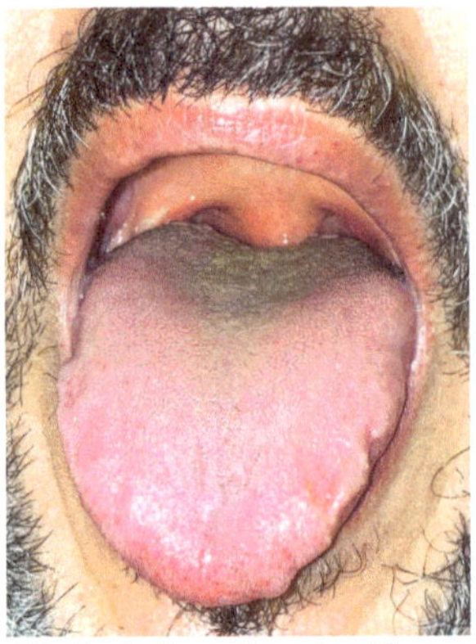
Pinched along the edge like a pie crust

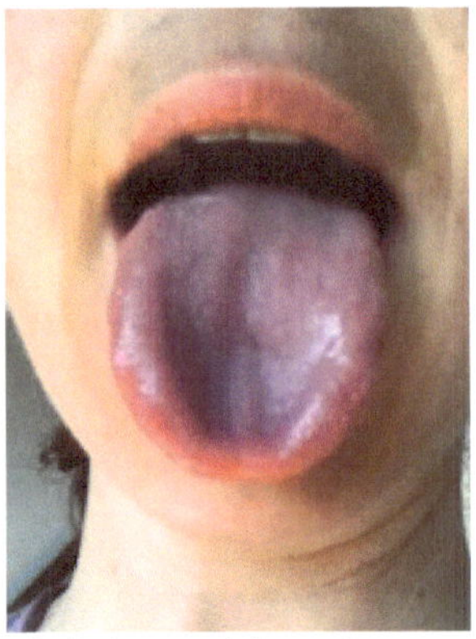
Curled around the perimeter

Kidneys, Bladder, and Small and Large Intestines

The Central Area of the Back of the Tongue

The central area of the back of the tongue reflects the Kidneys. The Bladder is also at the rear but, being the Yang partner, sits anterior to the Kidneys.

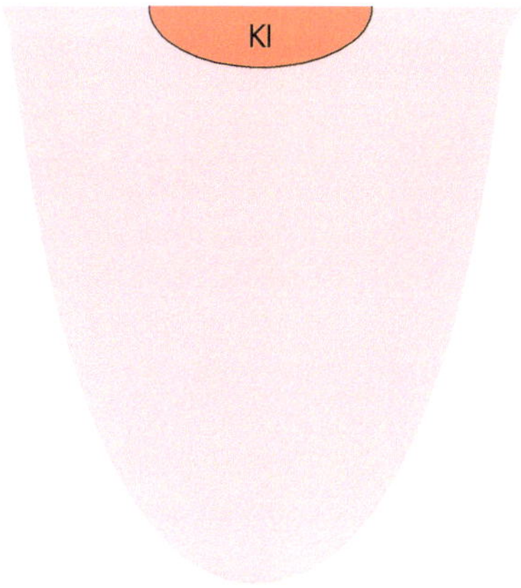

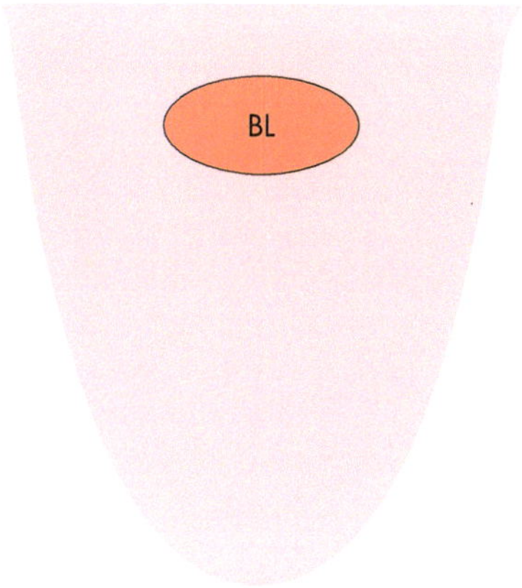

The Kidneys store Yin and Yang and are the root of the constitution.

The Bladder flushes out the lower burner, controls the sinews, and conveys thought to movement and posture.

When the center of the rear of the tongue features in your diagnosis, the Kidneys are dealing with pathology.

Observations at the rear of the tongue are focused on moisture.

- If the rear of the tongue is dry or dry and cracked, the Bladder's ability to move Fluids in the Lower Jiao—both pathological and not— is compromised.
- If the coat at the rear of the tongue is not rooted to the tongue (if you feel you would be able to wipe it off with a cloth if you tried—don't try!), the body's ability to hold on to Fluids is compromised. This could be due to constitutional weakness, severe disease or drug use that has weakened the constitution. Yang is then unable to hold the Yin in its place.
- If the rear of the tongue is very "cheesy-looking", or very damp, the body is likely trying to build back Yin.
    - The body could be trying to hold onto Fluids.
    - The Liver could be trying to hold onto Yin to share with the Kidneys, as post-natal Qi nourishes prenatal Qi.

- The Lungs could be trying to move Yin down to the Kidneys, as post-natal Qi nourishes prenatal Qi.
- If the coat at the rear is thickening, fluids in the Lower Jiao are becoming more turbid or phlegmatic.
- If the rear of the tongue is dark, the body is trying to reserve Blood, creating stagnation in the Lower Jiao.

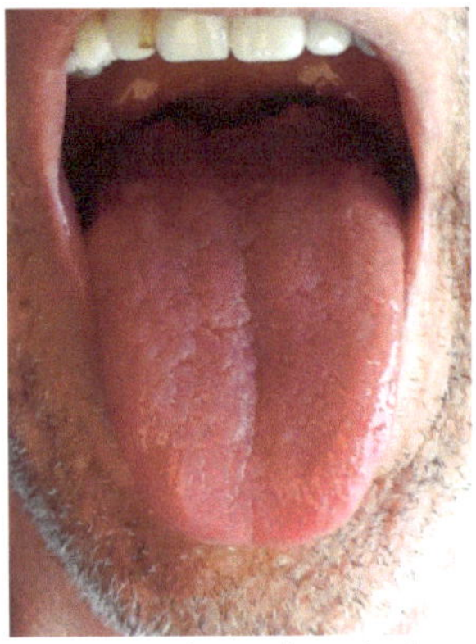
Dry or dry and cracked

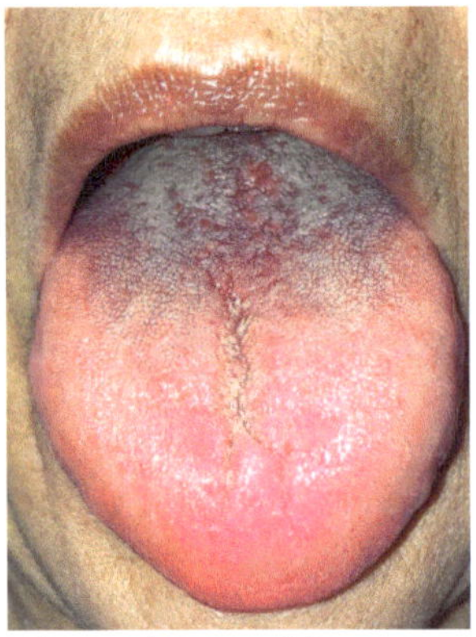
Coat at the rear of the tongue is not rooted

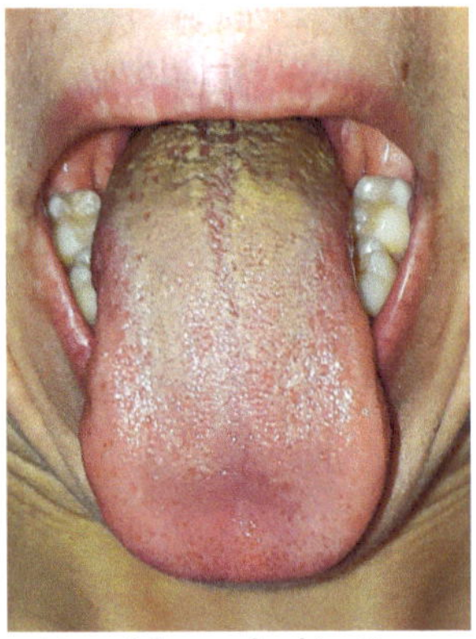
Very "cheesy-looking" or very damp

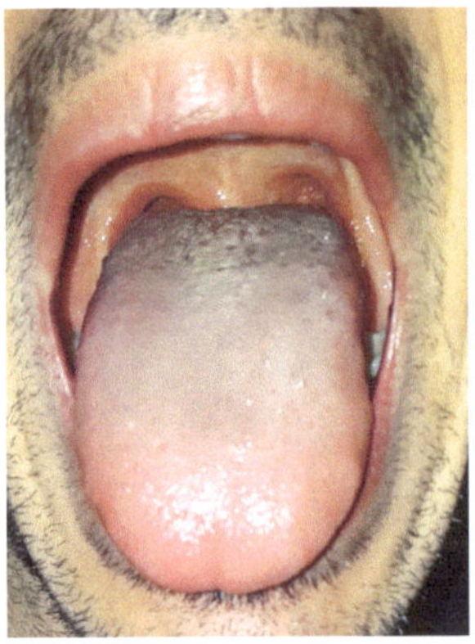
Coat at the rear is thickening

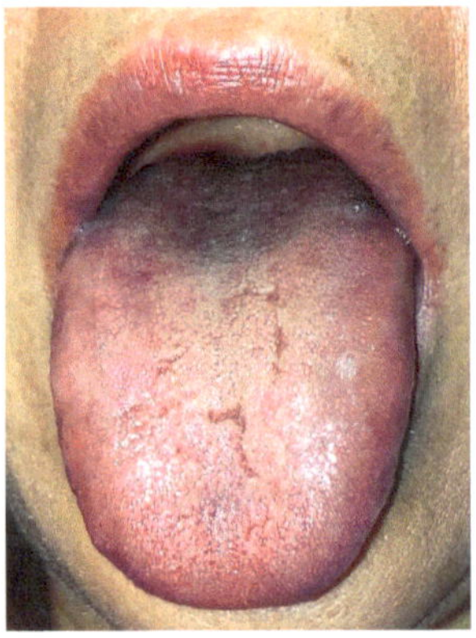
Rear of the tongue is dark

The Sides of the Back of the Tongue

The sides of the back of the tongue reflect the Large Intestine and the Small Intestine.

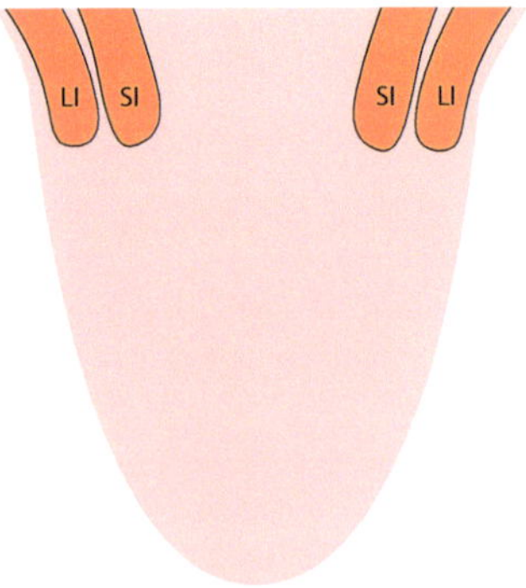

The Large Intestine controls Jin-Thin fluids. Since it has an outward vector, it is reflected in the outer edge of the sides of the rear of the tongue.

The Small Intestine separates pure and impure. It internalizes pathology using the Fluid it controls, the Ye-Thick Fluids. It has an inward vector; therefore it occupies the inner region of the sides of the rear of the tongue.

When the sides of the rear area of the tongue feature in your diagnosis, the Intestines are dealing with pathology.

Observations at the side of the rear of the tongue are also focused on moisture. The differentiation between Small and Large Intestine on the sides of the rear of the tongue is quite subtle. It can be difficult to see back there, but even a general impression of the sides of the rear is useful.

- If the sides of the rear of the tongue are dry, or dry and cracked, the Large Intestine's ability to control systemic Fluids is compromised.
- If sides of the rear of the tongue are very cheesy-looking, or very damp, the body is likely trying to build or hold on to Fluids.
- If the sides of the rear of the tongue are dark, the body is reserving Blood in lieu of Yin.
- If the sides of the rear of the tongue are withered or narrowing, Yin has been depleted and may be insufficient to finance the latency of pathology.
- If the coat at the sides of the rear is thickening, fluids in the Lower Jiao are becoming more turbid or phlegmatic. Fluids are depleted, leading to systemic dehydration.
- If the sides of the rear of the tongue are collapsed, Yang is not articulating within the Lower Jiao.
- If the sides of the rear of the tongue are swollen and red, there is Dampness responding to Heat in the Lower Jiao. Be careful not to drain Dampness until the Heat is cleared.
- If the medial aspect of the sides of the rear of the tongue are swollen, there is pathology of the Small Intestine (jejunum or ilium).
- If the sides of the rear of the tongue are absent, that is, if the tongue narrows at the rear, there is a serious deficiency of Yin. In general, this means that Fluids on a deep level, including hormones, are not being generated as they should be. Most often, at least in this part of the world, this is a result of Yin not being cultivated. The patient declines to rest or make any part of their day calm. In our culture this is often the case in menopause: the patient is often stressed, failing to sleep or sleep early enough, and not eating enough saturated fat.

When Yin is so deficient that the rear of the tongue is wasting away, the ability to hold a pathogen in latency is severely compromised. This is because the body uses mediumship—including Yin—to hold away from the organs, pathogens, and pathogenic factors that it cannot eradicate or expel. When Yin is this depleted, there is no buffer between the pathogen and the organs. The pathogen becomes free to enter the peritoneum, then the organs, where the pathogen causes organ disease—the deepest form of pathology.

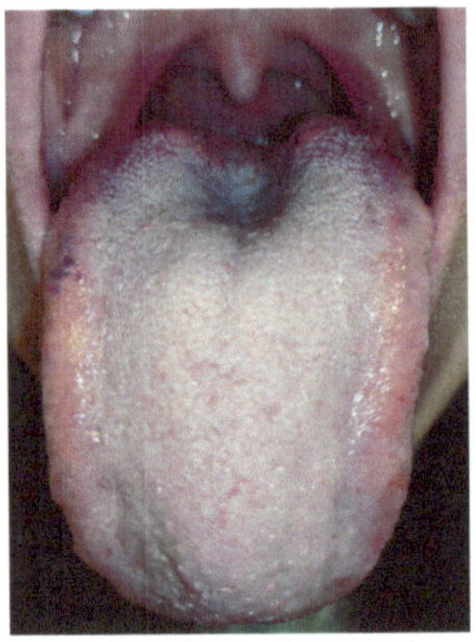

Dry, or dry and cracked

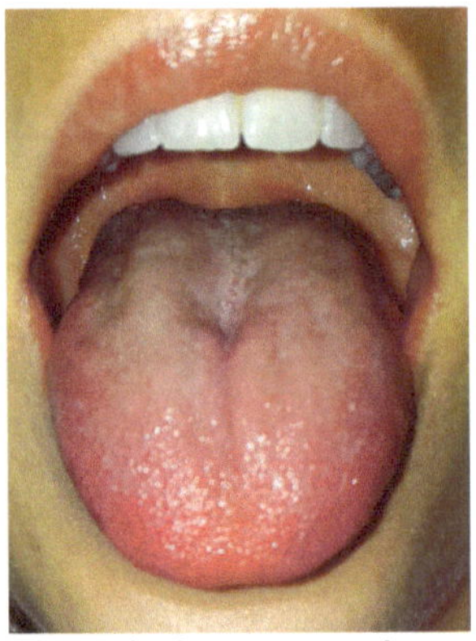

Cheesy-looking, or very damp

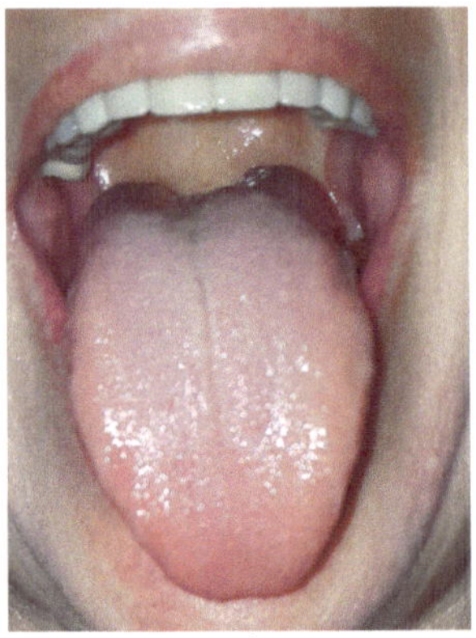

Dark

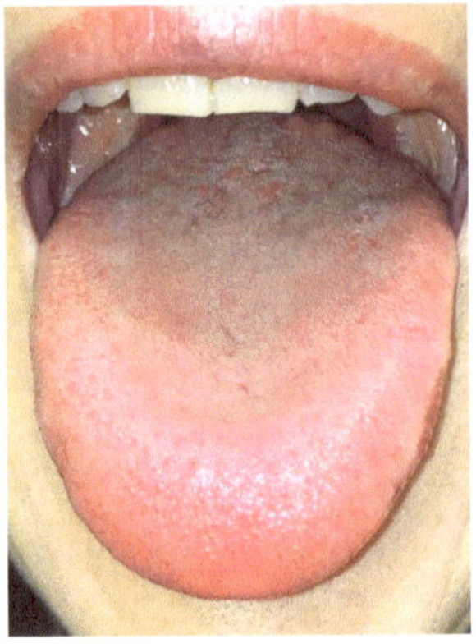

Withered or narrowing

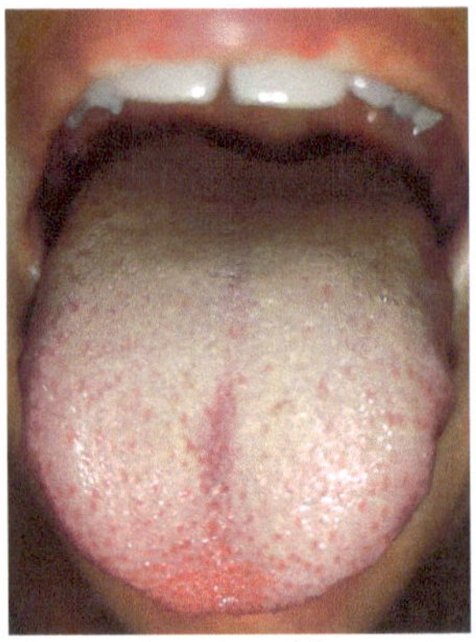

Coat at the sides of the rear is thickening

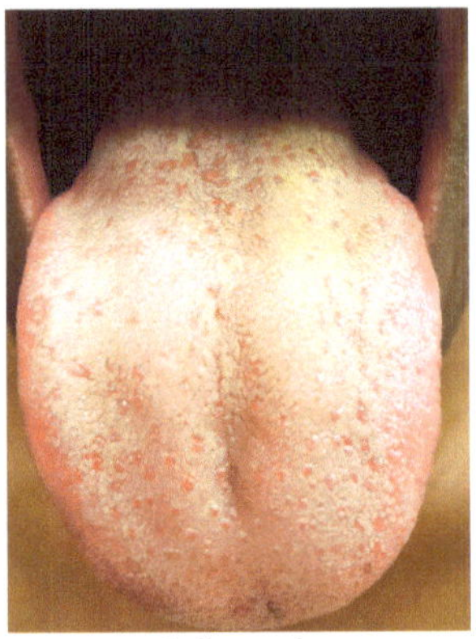

Collapsed

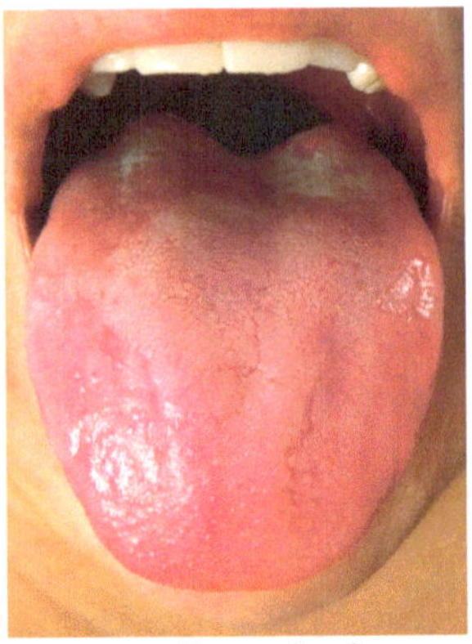

Swollen and red

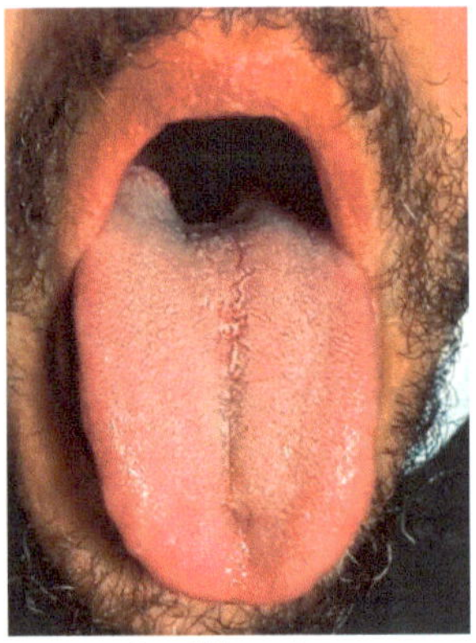

Small Intestine

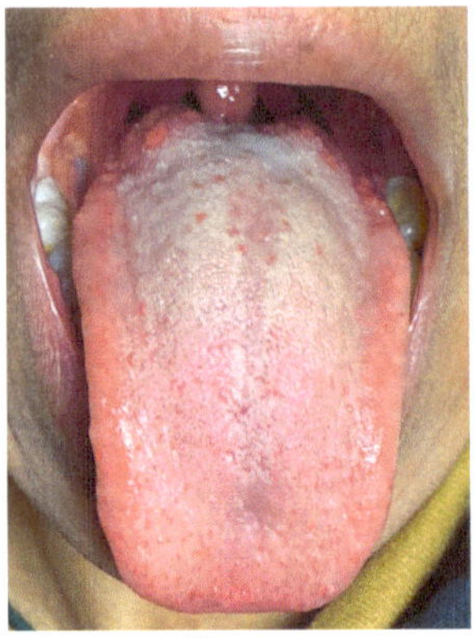

Absent

Areas Between Organ Regions

Triple Heater

Triple Heater is reflected in the area between the organs.

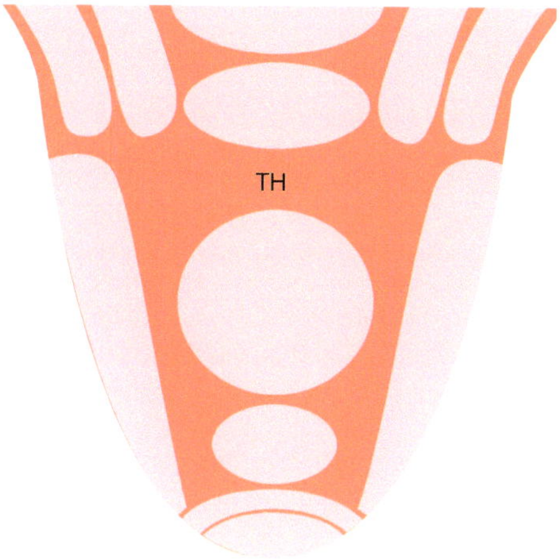

Triple Heater distributes Yuan Qi to the organs, clears Heat from the organs, controls latency and Qi, governs systemic irrigation, and manages surpluses of post-natal Qi to ensure longevity.

When the entire tongue is covered in protrusions or white spots, the Triple Heater is failing to control latency of a pathogenic factor. The Triple Heater is an immensely complex organ that governs the interaction of the three burners, the reception of Qi, and balances water and fire. Its region will redden as Heat becomes systemic.

Between the Spleen-Stomach Region and the Liver-Gallbladder Regions

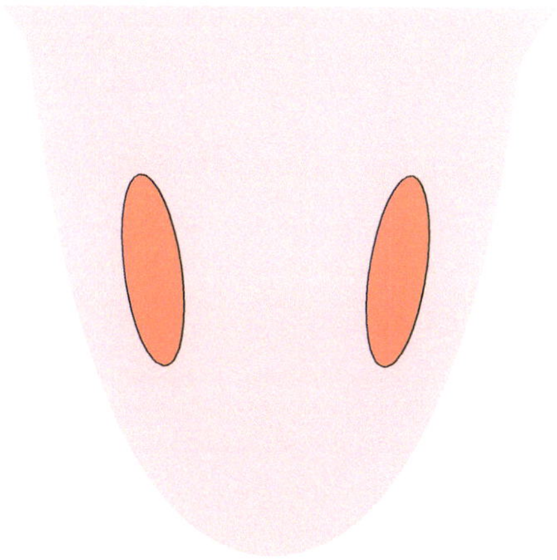

Between the Liver/Gallbladder region and the Spleen/ Stomach region, it's common to see dispersed or grouped little spots. They can be various colors: pink, purple, red. These indicate disharmony between Spleen and Liver. Some might call it Liver invading the Spleen, which means that the Spleen has become weakened and the Liver tries to come to its aid, potentially overwhelming it. Sometimes there can be vertical bands bisecting the halves of the tongue. There may be food stagnation, gas, bloating, distention. A patient presenting with these bands has compromised digestion or has poor food combining habits. They might be mixing cheese or fruit in with other foods, or eating too little or too much. Investigate by asking questions and gently suggest avoiding the factors that are weakening the Spleen.

The Coat and the Map

The tongue coat can vary from area to area. Find where there is a lack of moisture on the tongue. This is an important factor in diagnosis.

If there is dryness or absence of coat found:

- in the Lung area, Lung Yin is deficient. If the area is inflamed or irritated, there may be a dry cough, dry skin, or a dry throat.
- in the Spleen and Stomach area, Stomach Yin is deficient—the mucosal lining is thinning. There may be dry lips, gut sensitivities, allergies.
- on the rear of the tongue, there is a serious depletion of fluids in the Lower Jiao, including perhaps the fluids of the constitution—the Jing. Long-term Heat may have damaged the Lower Jiao. The Kidneys and the Intestines may be very dry and thinning as the illness has advanced far beyond simple constipation. There must be Yin available so that the Lower Jiao is able to flush and clear itself; otherwise, toxins accumulate, showing as bumps on the rear of the tongue. Eventually, these can reenter the bloodstream and cause disease. Clear toxins as you hydrate.

If the tongue has a clumping coat (often said to resemble cottage cheese), whether thick or just a hint:

- on the Lower Jiao area of the tongue, there may be Damp-Heat type inflammation in the intestines or genitalia.
- on the Middle Jiao area of the tongue, there may be Damp-Heat in the Liver or Gallbladder, or parasites in the gut (including candida), or a severe inadequacy in the digestive tract's capacity to separate pure from impure fluids.
- on the Upper Jiao area of the tongue, there may be Damp-Heat in the sinuses, the upper lymphatic system, or the brain (known in Western medicine as candida with brain fog).

Hollowing

Hollowing of the Jiaos shows that an organ related to that region is in a Qi or Yang deficient state.

- Hollowing of the Upper Jiao reflects a Qi deficiency of Lungs or Heart.
- Hollowing of the Middle Jiao reflects a Qi deficiency in the digestive tract, often a Spleen Qi deficiency.
- Hollowing of the Lower Jiao indicates a Kidney Yang deficiency.

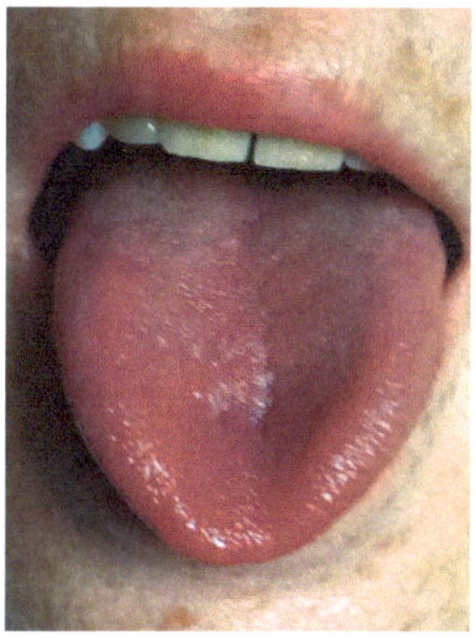

Upper Jiao Hollowing

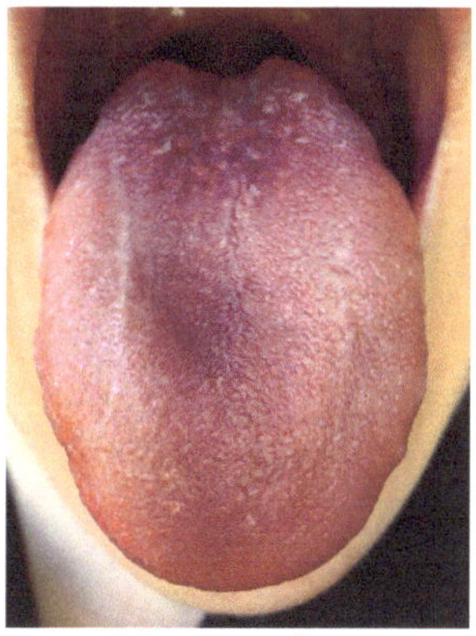

Middle Jiao Hollowing

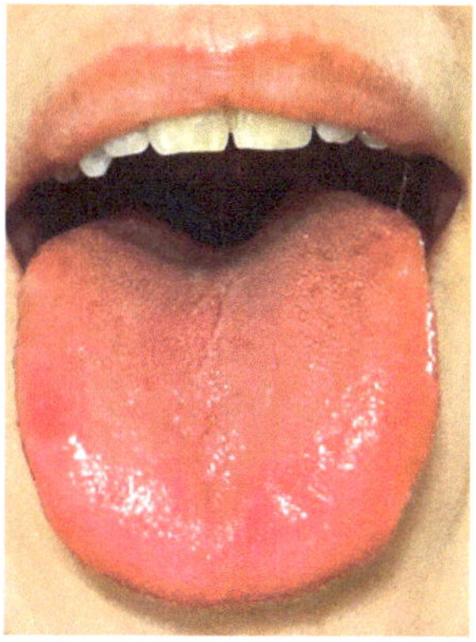

Lower Jiao Hollowing

Compensations

The tongue will swell when the body accumulates pathological Yin as it tries to compensate for missing mediumship or blocked communication between organs.

- The Lung region may swell as the Lungs gather Yin and send it to the Kidneys to nourish Kidney Yin. If communication between Jiaos is blocked, locate the blockage, release it, and then nourish Yin. The communication will start up again and the deficit will be restored.
- The Kidney region may be swollen as they restrain their own Yin, due to Yin deficiency. Nourish Yin so that they can resume their support of the Heart.
- The right side of the tongue may swell as the Liver struggles to store sufficient Blood. Nourish Blood.
- The left side of the tongue may swell as the Gallbladder tries to contain Dampness. To determine whether the Damp is pathological or responding to Heat, take the pulses. If the deep pulses are rapid, the Dampness is protective and must not be drained. The Gallbladder region may also swell if it is trying to buffer toxins from the Jing.

Trapped Heat

Blockages between organs and Jiaos can result in the buildup of Heat as movement of mediumship and Qi is stifled. Heat trapped in any area will consume Fluids, Yin, and eventually, the flesh. If not treated, it can lead to Wei Atrophy Syndrome. Petechiae (red dots) are early signs of trapped Heat. As the Heat stagnates further, the dots can become progressively darker, becoming crimson and even purple. If very long-term, petechiae can turn white, indicating the presence of fire toxins (in Western terms, free radicals, due to damage from inflammation). Needling Ying-Spring points, bleeding Luo points, and treating other points that release Heat are key to treatment, along with freeing the entrapment.

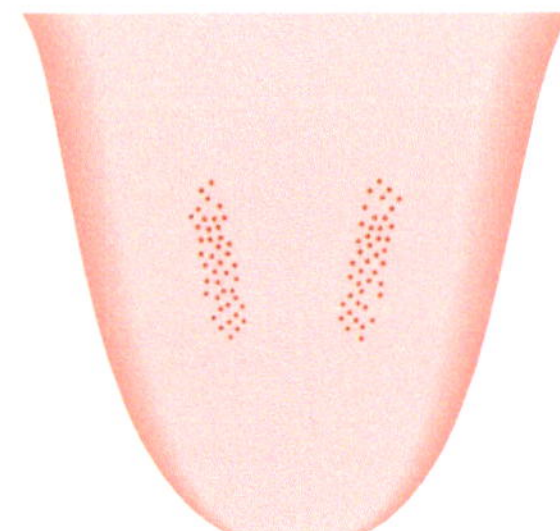

An imbalance between Liver and Spleen is shown here. As the Liver invades the Spleen, trying to support it, the area between the Liver and Spleen becomes constrained. The body responds by creating Heat to try to move the constrained Qi. If the cause is not resolved, the Heat itself then becomes trapped, and the product of constraint and Heat manifests as petechiae.

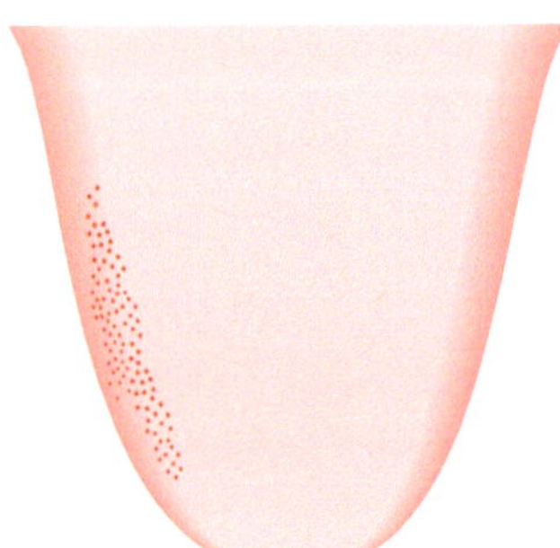

Heat trapped in the Liver

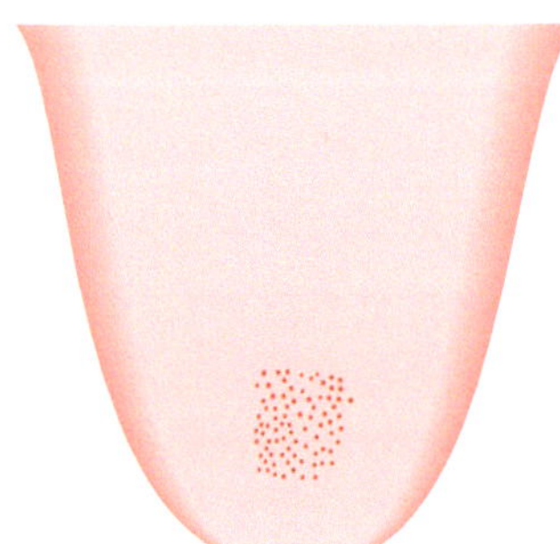

Heat trapped in the Lungs

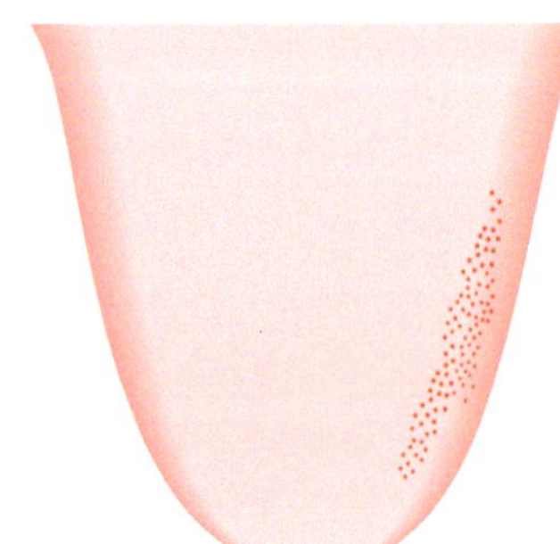

Heat trapped in the Gallbladder

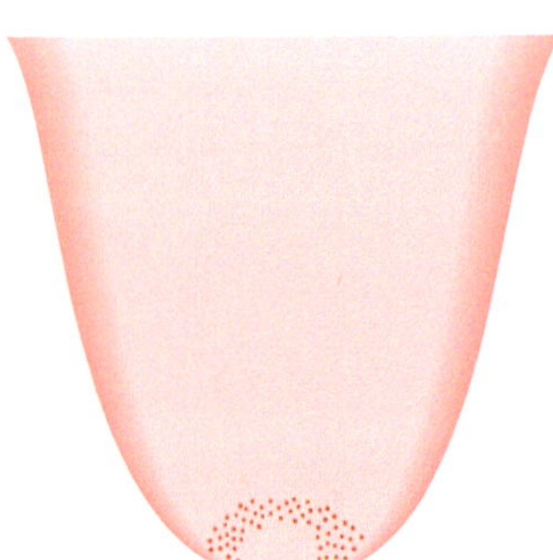

Heat trapped in the Pericardium

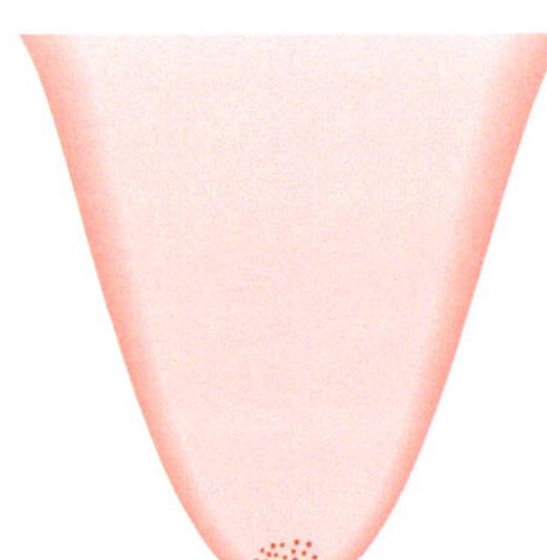

Heat trapped in the Heart

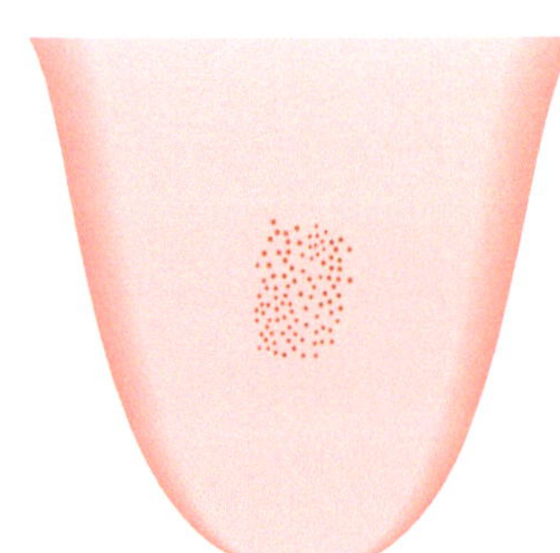

Heat trapped in the Spleen

Vectors

Vectors (the direction of communication from or between organs) are featured findings in the classical art of dynamic and directional pulse diagnosis. They show in the tongue as follows:

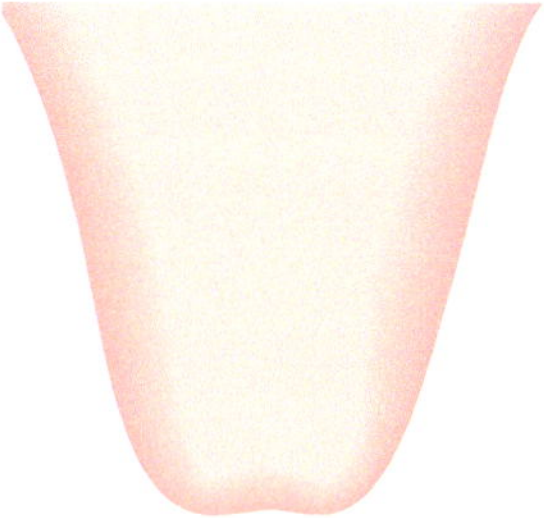

The Lungs are not dispersing Wei Qi.

The Spleen is not ascending.

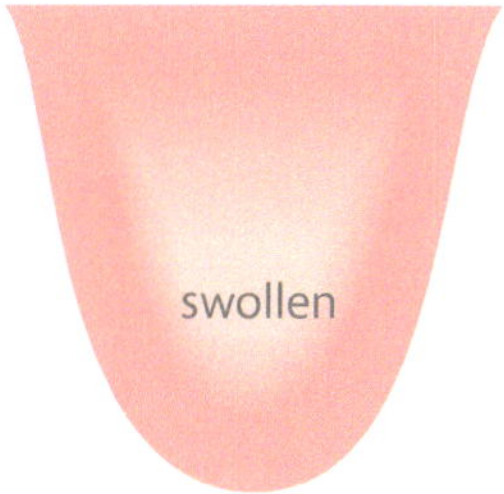

The Stomach is not descending.

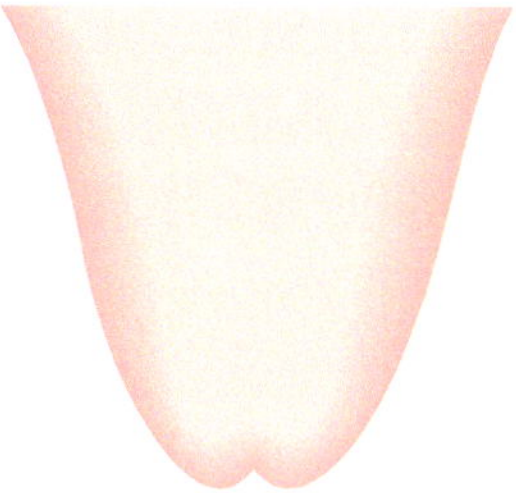

The Heart is not dispersing its Qi.

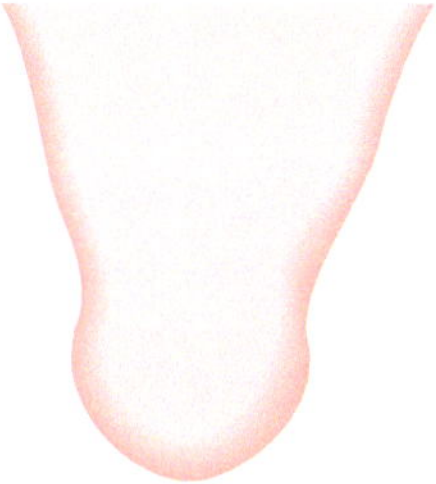

The Liver is neither ascending nor descending Blood and Qi.

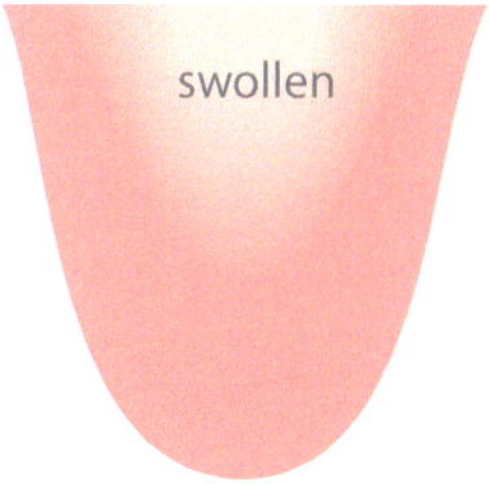

The Heart and Kidneys are not communicating.

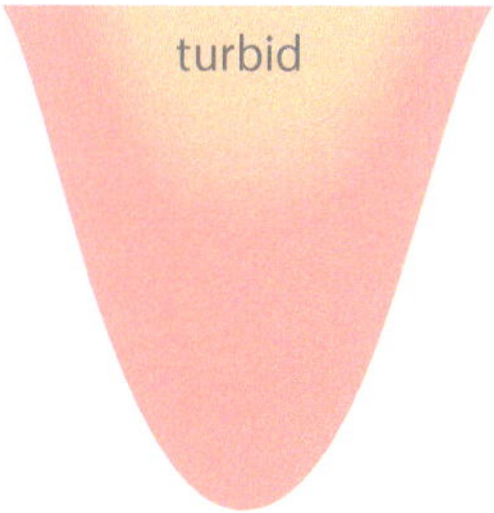

The Liver is not descending to the Kidneys.

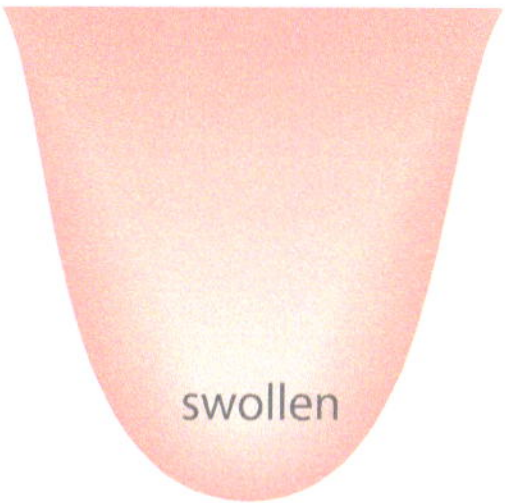

The Lungs are not descending to the Kidneys.

The Simplified Map

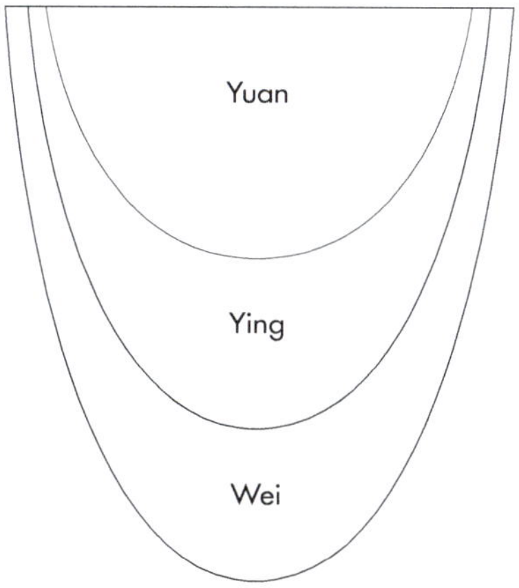

Sometimes the tongue sends a message best read using a simplified map. These messages should be read first, before noting complexities. The simplest (and oldest) tongue map consists of three areas corresponding to the three levels of Qi, drawn almost like ripples emerging forward from the rear of the tongue. The most posterior portion of the tongue shows the status of Yuan-Constitutional Qi, the first ripple (the middle region) shows the status of Ying-Nutritive Qi, and the second ripple—the edge of the tongue—shows the status of Wei-Defensive Qi. This maps is most useful when a tongue presents with a distinct redness all the way around the edge in the outermost ripple. I refer to such a tongue as a Wei-Qi tongue. It is common in people with skin issues including eczema and other rashes, allergies, autoimmune issues in an active phase, or any kind of inflammation affecting the exterior.

10
Lines and Cracks

Lines, cracks, and protrusions show that unresolved Heat is resulting in the consumption of Yin or that the diet and lifestyle are resulting in dryness.

Folding Lines in the Tongue

Heat originates in the Stomach, is reflected in the Center of the tongue, and expands outward. When dryness arises as a result of Heat, or when dryness is an underlying factor, the body tries to hold on to as much fluid as possible. Folding lines begin to arise in the tongue, demonstrating the effort of holding on to Fluids.

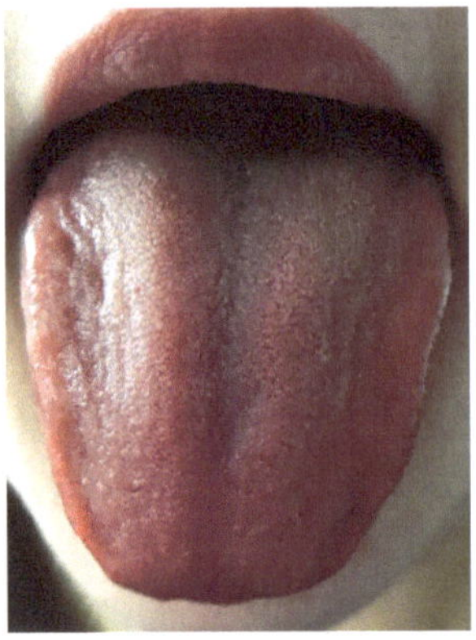

Folding lines

Roughness, Unevenness in the Tongue

Roughness or unevenness in the tongue can be thought of as a pre-crack. There is deficiency and a consequent stagnation as the body tries to hold on to what it can, but the tongue has not yet cracked.

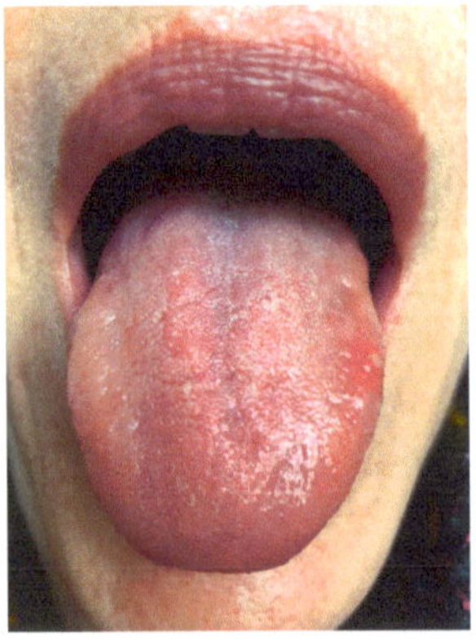

Roughness

Cracks in the Tongue

Cracks in the tongue are caused by Heat drying the tongue enough to crack the tongue flesh, just as the sun cracks desert earth. Sometimes it is said that cracks reflect consumption of Blood more than other media. Heat can be introduced in various ways, but it can also be generated by the body in response to pathology. Cracks can also appear in situations where there is a deficiency of Fluids, Blood, or Jing, and the body is not able to gather pathological Yin (Dampness) in response. This scenario occurs when there is a Qi or Yang deficiency.

Introduced Heat can come from:

- consuming substances that produce Heat (stimulants or irritants). These include: coffee, sugar, chocolate, garlic, onion, fried foods, cigarettes, alcohol, drugs, hot spices (such as black pepper and spicy hot red capsicum peppers), pesticides, herbicides, preservatives, and too much protein (especially overindulging in very Yang proteins such as beef, lamb, bison, venison, lobster, shrimp, and crab).
- engaging in a very Yang, rushed, stressing view of life
- engaging in heat-generating emotions: anger, anxiety and worry
- long-term infections, usually bacterial

Cracks caused by Heat are diagnosed by area. The tongue map generally reveals that cracks caused by:

- dietary factors, which will first show in the tongue center
- grief and smoking, which will show in the Lung region
- anger and toxins from drugs and alcohol, which will show on the tongue sides
- worry, which will show as a midline crack
- anxiety, which will show with tightening or withdrawal at the tip of the tongue
- long-term inflammation, which will show in the Lung or Liver areas since they control Wei-Defensive Qi
- constitutional factors, and sometimes fear, that has taxed the Kidneys, which will show in the Lower Jiao

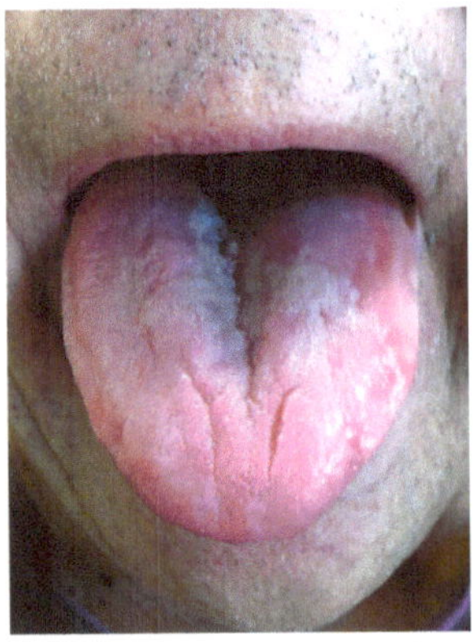
A crack in a wasting and thirsting patient (diabetes)

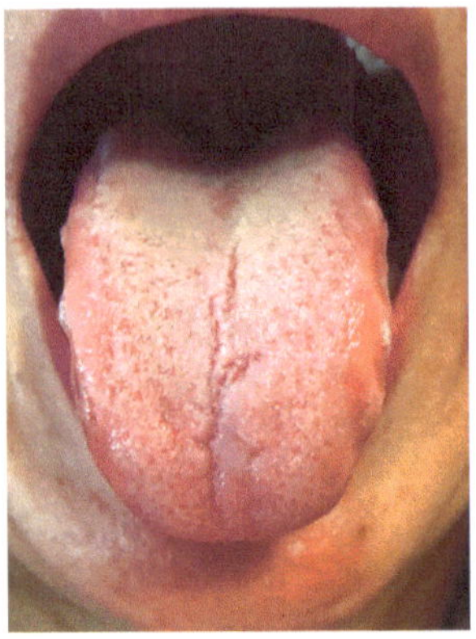
A crack in a patient suffering depression and smoking

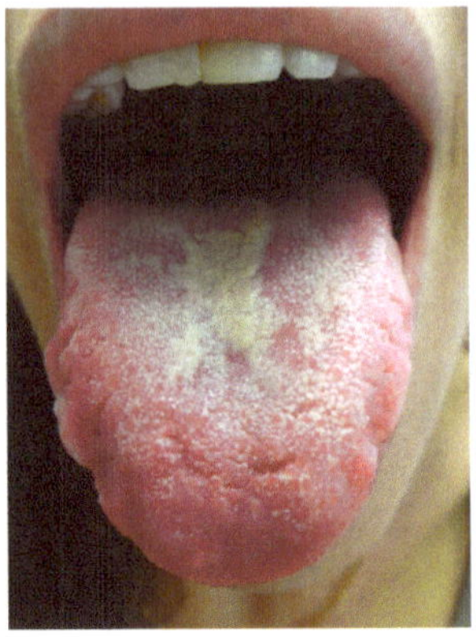
Frustration or anger

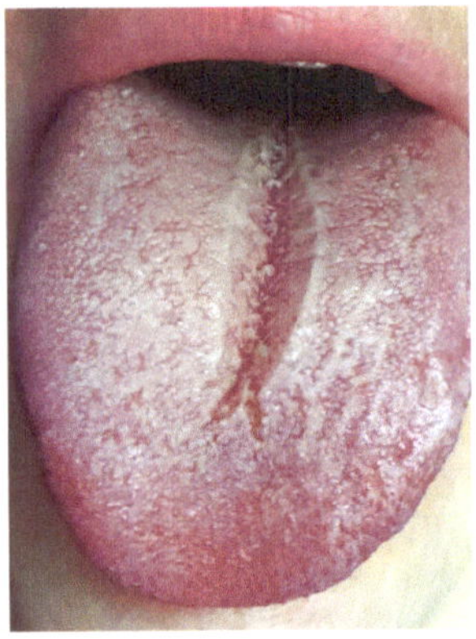
Worry cracks the midline.

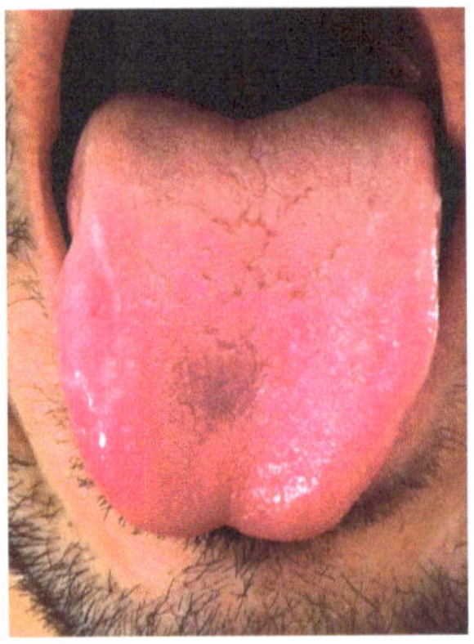
Withdrawing from relationship

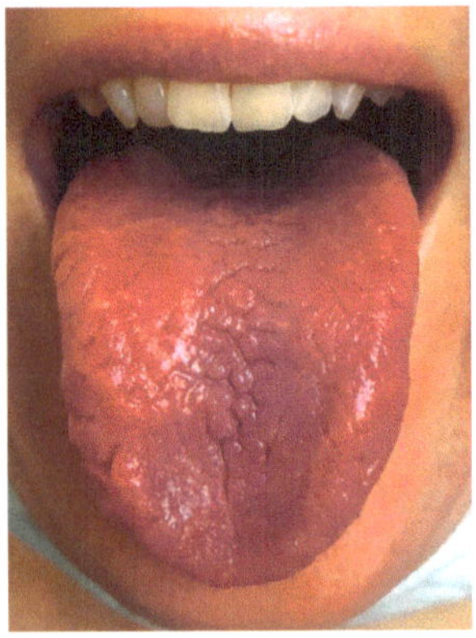
Long-term inflammation eczema

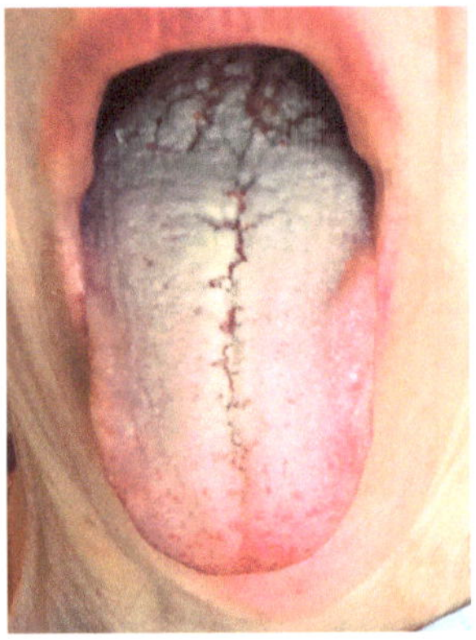
Hormone replacement therapy affecting the Jing.

Cracks can creep over time, as untended emotional issues worsen.

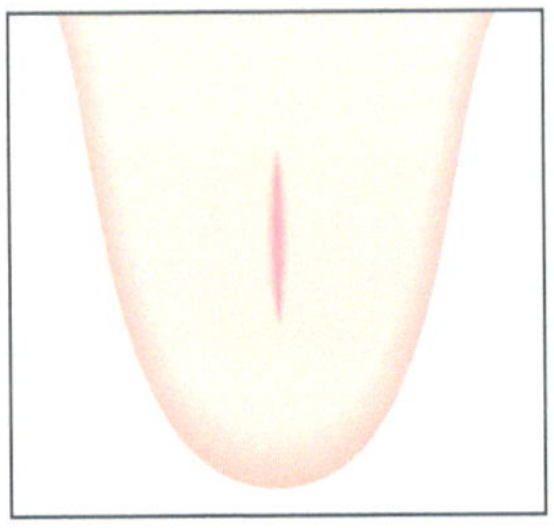
Thinking and worry damage the Spleen.

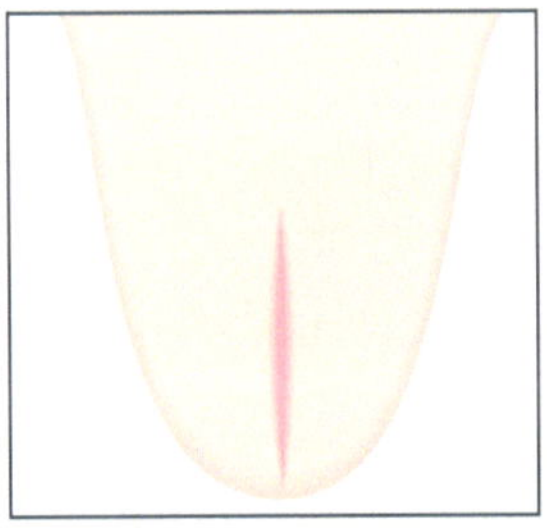
Long-term overthinking and worry can transform into anxiety.

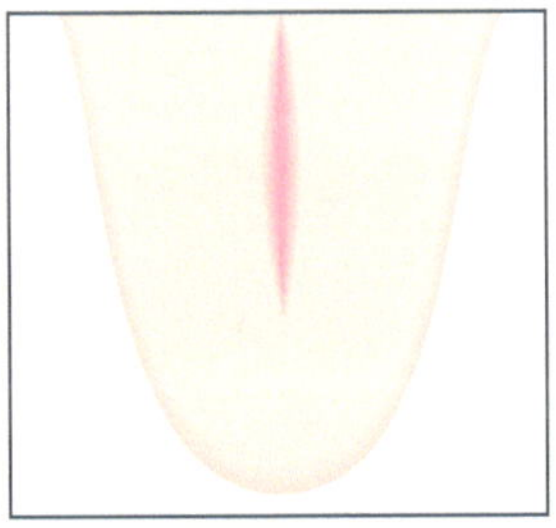
Long-term overthinking and worry can develop into fear.

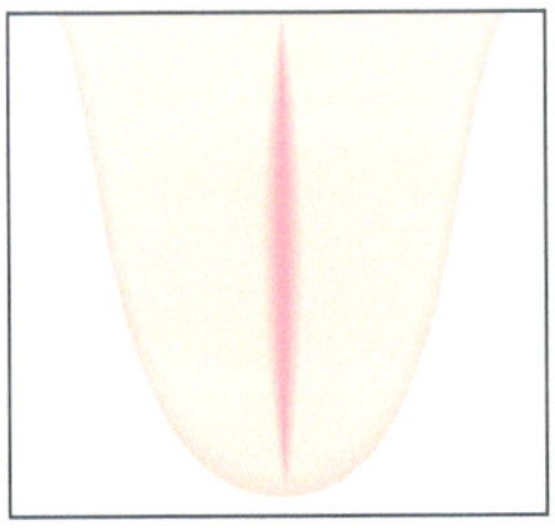
Long-term anxiety develops into fear.

The Orientation of Cracks

Cracks can be categorized as vertical or horizontal. Of course, nearly always there is a mixture, but we're interested first in which predominate, and then why that type predominates.

Transverse (Yin) Cracks

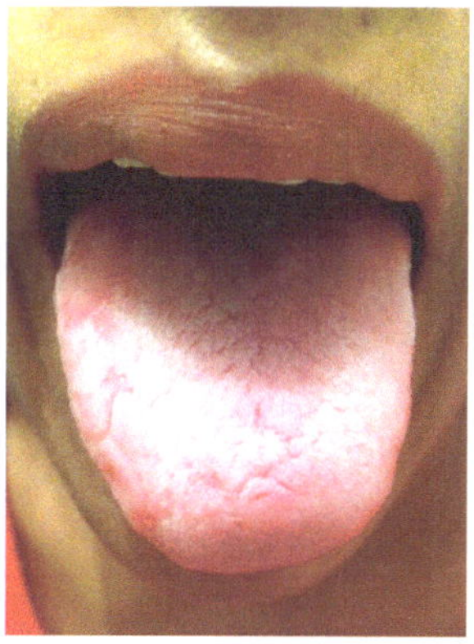

Transverse cracks show dryness. The patient is dehydrated.

The treatment principle is to moisten dryness to generate fluids.

If there are transverse cracks with Dampness—if the tongue is very swollen—Damp should be cleared as you generate Fluids. But there must be Qi present to carry out that Damp clearing. If the tongue is pale, there is insufficient Qi to clear the Dampness. In those cases, tonify Qi before you ask the body to generate Fluids.

Generally, transverse cracks tend to localize, to be concentrated in one area. Cracks can migrate as the Heat resulting from dryness looks for alternative locations to vent. This shows as cracks that develop Y-shaped junctions, new cracks that branch off from other cracks, and jagged turns. Over time, increasingly depleted resources (deficiency of mediumship) leads to the arising of Wind. The Wind shows in lengthening of the cracks. If the cracks extend all the way to the sides of the tongue, the Liver has become extremely dry.

Dryness

Left untreated, Heat leads to full-blown Dryness. The term Dryness refers to dehydration that has become advanced enough to inflame the huge complex membrane (the peritoneum) that wraps around each organ. In the long-term, Heat is able to penetrate the actual organ and the disease becomes serious. Moisture must be returned and Heat cleared before the organs atrophy. If a patient reports that they drink much more than they urinate out, the body is retaining fluids to respond to and contain Heat (inflammation).

Early stage Dryness can show in:

- a dry coat, leaving the tongue lacking in luster or even appearing powdery
- a peeling dry coat leaving patches of coat remaining
- a completely evaporated coat
- many horizontal cracks as Heat threatens to breach the peritoneum

Late stage Dryness can manifest in:

- significant horizontal cracks in a given area indicating severe inflammatory illness in the anatomical region reflected by that part of the tongue

• cracks that are lengthening over time

• cracks extending to the sides

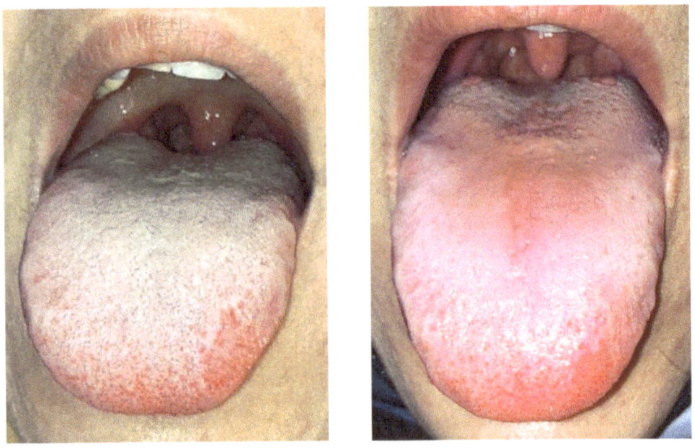

Early stage Dryness responds quickly to treatment. Dehydration caused gastrointestinal misery in this patient, leading to a blood deficiency and in turn, anxiety, insomnia, palpitations and repressed anger. In the second photo, fluids are largely restored after two treatments and dietary advice given by my colleague.

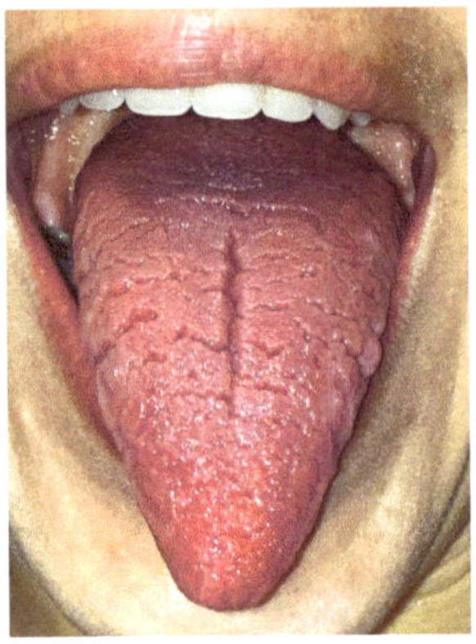

Late stage dryness has set in with this patient. Significant horizontal cracks result from long-term dehydration. The fluid deficiency is now severe and affecting the Ye-Thick Fluids, resulting in symptoms described as infertility and hypothyroidism. Significant and consistent changes in diet and lifestyle in addition to treatment are required for healing this stage.

Very often the patient is not helping because they avoid water. Such a patient will often say they "don't like water" and dehydrate themselves by drinking fluids that are actively dehydrating—coffee, all teas, anything carbonated. All are diuretics. This becomes complicated because although water is essential and helpful, it is not the best hydrator for the digestive tract, but rather a flushing agent. True hydrators that are profoundly helpful are soups, congees, broths, porridges and stews.

Cracks as Heat Respond to Dampness

If Heat is responding to Dampness, the tongue will often be very swollen with a yellow coat. The coat becomes increasingly yellow as Heat accumulates in the effort to overcome the Dampness. If Heat is allowed to predominate, Dryness will arise.

If a tongue is swollen and yet has a lot of horizontal cracks, more Yin is needed to conduct the clearing of Dampness. Hydration is required to move and flush it out. At first, this may seem counterintuitive, but the body will only release Dampness when it receives a clear and sustained message that the required Fluids are steadily available.

Vertical (Yang) Cracks

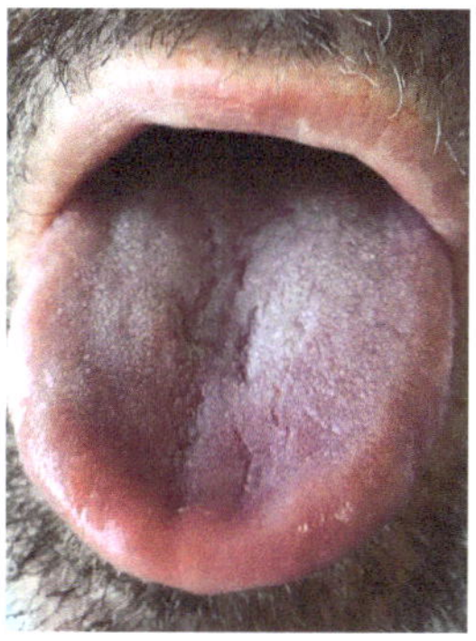

Vertical cracks indicate that Heat is damaging fluids. The treatment principle is to clear Heat.

Heat ultimately ulcerates and consumes Yin. The emotions are a common cause of this kind of pathology as they stagnate Qi. The body then creates and accumulates Heat to to try to move that Qi.

Horizontal Versus Vertical Cracks

Horizontal cracks occur when there is Dryness from dehydration. There are not enough fluids in the diet. The treatment principal is to nourish Fluids, generate Fluids, or moisten Dryness.

Vertical cracks occur when Heat—originating from the diet or from worry, stress and overthinking—is consuming Fluids and Yin. The treatment principal is to clear Heat, and/or to calm the Shen.

To be very simple, vertical cracks—particularly those down the center—are usually due to overthinking, worry, or stress. Horizontal cracks relate to physical dehydration.

Geographic Tongue

Eventually, long-term Heat radiates throughout the tongue, causing cracks all over it, resulting in the geographic tongue. Sometimes a coat (usually a partial one) complicates a geographic tongue as the body responds with Dampness, attempting to extinguish the Heat. The areas of the tongue that are missing coat altogether are said to have Dryness.

In a geographic tongue (covered in cracks):

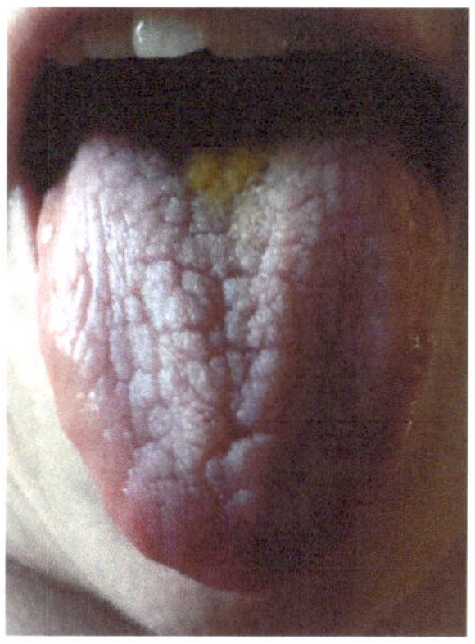

- if the sides of the tongue have no coat, there is Dryness in the Liver and Gallbladder.
- if the middle of the tongue has no coat, there is dryness in the Spleen and Stomach.
- if the front third of the tongue has no coat, there is dryness in the Lungs.
- if the rear third of the tongue has no coat, there is dryness of the Kidneys, or the Lower Jiao in general.
- if the entire tongue is littered with protrusions and cracks, heat is drying up the tongue itself.

Cracks and the Tongue Map

Cracks in Center

Heat generated by worry—circular thinking about negative possibilities—consumes digestive fluids, as digestive Qi is diverted to try to control thought. The stagnated Qi causes Heat to accumulate and damage these Fluids. In this way, worry or overthinking eventually opens a characteristic midline crack. Cracks can lengthen over time as the habit of overthinking persists.

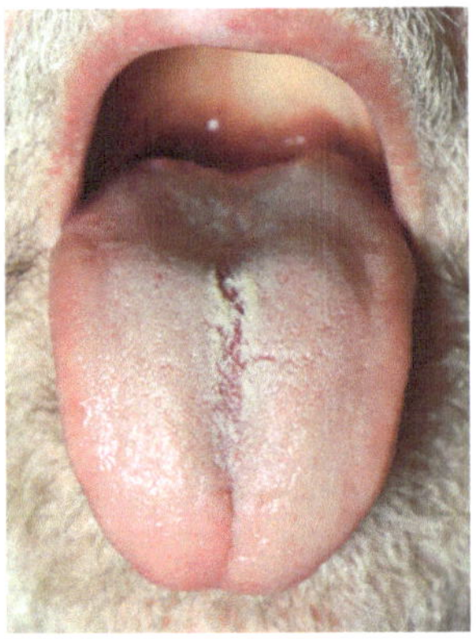

Lingering disappointment also taxes the Spleen, since it involves thoughts that persist over time. The Middle Jiao Heat caused by stagnating thoughts depletes Qi and creates a midline crack that eventually extends into the Heart region.

Heat in the digestive tract from too much Yang food—for example, too much protein—can show in the middle, but generally appears on the sides, since the Liver becomes aggravated. (See Cracks in the Sides, below.)

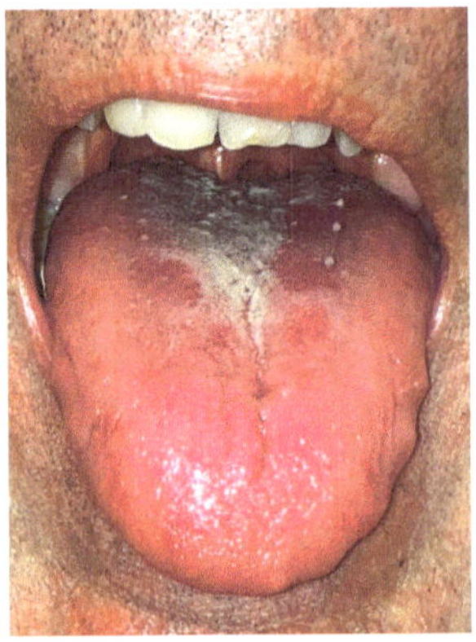

This man's digestive tract shows an enormous amount of Heat. As Heat has a tendency to move, these habits have created a systemic urgency. As a result, he speaks very quickly, is highly reactive to stimulus, is hyperactive in the gut, urgent defecation, and has seizures. A history of viral encephalitis (at age nineteen) suggests Heat is a long-term feature in his pathology. Wind resulting from the Heat has affected the Qiao Mai, resulting in serious interference with the structure, given the Western diagnosis of scoliosis. Chinese Medical diagnosis was systemic Heat generating Wind at Yang Qiao Mai.

A crack or pockets in the middle of a peeled tongue indicate Heat is not just damaging Stomach Fluids but also Stomach Yin (the Stomach lining). Remember that the coat reflects Fluid status while the tongue body reflects Yin and structure, flesh. As the crack deepens, it indicates that Heat is reaching to the material of the body, in this case, Stomach Yin (lining).

A deep crack that extends from the center toward the rear of the tongue indicates Heat is moving from the Ying level into the Yuan level. The Heat is affecting the constitution. It's rare to see a deep vertical crack extend to the rear of the tongue because the body will fiercely guard the constitution and respond with Dampness, creating a thick coat at the rear of the tongue.

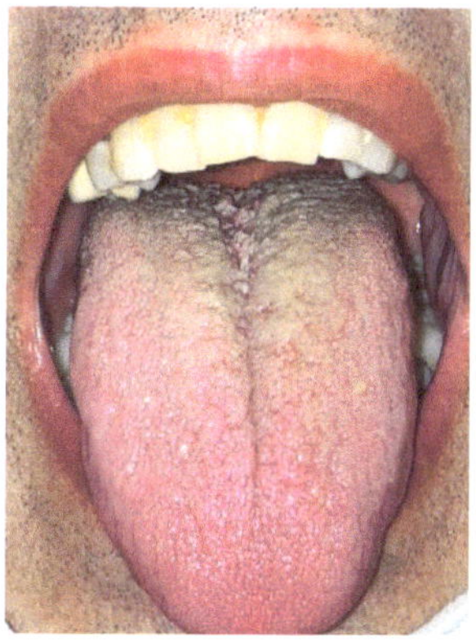

This patient's Heat sought two routes of exit, the Upper and the Lower Jiao. The Heat arose chiefly through smoking, which weakened Lung Qi, in turn stymying Wei Qi. The body responded to the Heat by producing Dampness, leading to Damp-Heat. Heat rose to the Upper Jiao, creating hypertension and anxiety. If an upward clearance of Damp-Heat is incomplete due to insufficient Wei Qi, the sensory orifices become blocked with the Damp-Heat. (This led to a reported diagnosis of rhinitis.) Next, the body tried to drain the Heat through the Lower Jiao. Again, deficient Lung Qi responsible for clearing the Lower Jiao caused the accumulation of Damp-Heat there, resulting in symptoms that led to the emergence of cysts along the paravertebral muscles, and the reported diagnoses of kidney stones, cystitis, and enlarged prostate. The weakening of the Kidneys, given their taxation, led to lower back pain. The diagnosis given by my colleague was emptiness of the Bladder Luo Channel.

Some people are born with a deep crack, indicating constitutional trauma. In children's tongues, deep cracks that were not present at birth show trauma to the constitution that likely occurred before the age of three. Chong Mai treatments will treat these issues and can ameliorate such cracks.

Cracks in the Tip

Heat generated by anxiety, worry, and disappointment causes cracks extending from the center of the tongue to the tip of the tongue.

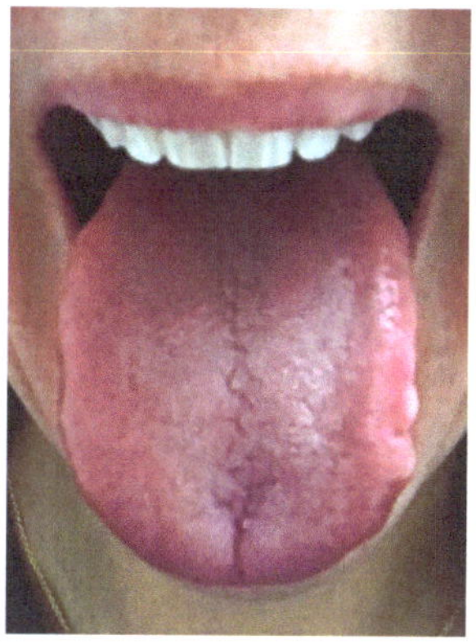

Anxiety differs from worry in that it can be about any outcome, negative or positive. One might be anxious about a second date even after the first date went wonderfully well. Anxiety eventually affects the Heart (the tip). Worry is related to negative outcomes; as, imagining an accident, one might worry about a child forgetting their skateboarding helmet. Eventually the depletion and subsequent stagnation that result from anxiety can cause in a vertical crack in the tip.

Cracks Just Behind or Lateral to the Tip

Cracks just behind or just lateral to the tip of the tongue are associated with the Pericardium. Sometimes they appear at 45 degree angles and most often they appear as folds or tight-looking grooves. As we know, the sides of the tongue reflect the Liver and the tip reflects the Heart. Heat generated by Liver constraint travels upward (showing along the sides toward the tip) and is intercepted by the Pericardium. The Heat fans out as the Pericardium disperses the Heat, buffering and protecting the Heart. If insufficiently warded off by the Pericardium, Heat rises and affects the Heart, leading to anxiety, insomnia, or angry outbursts.

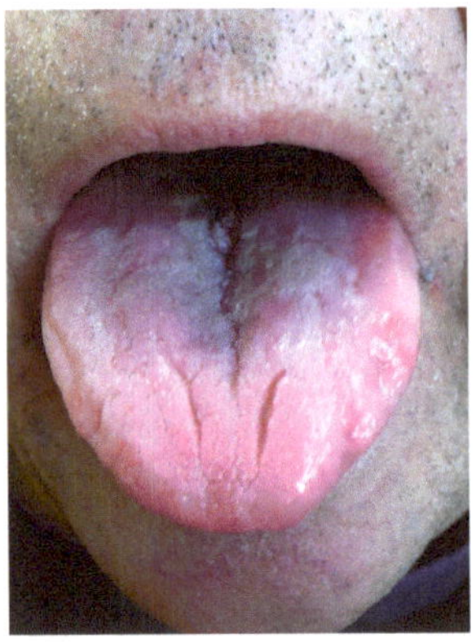
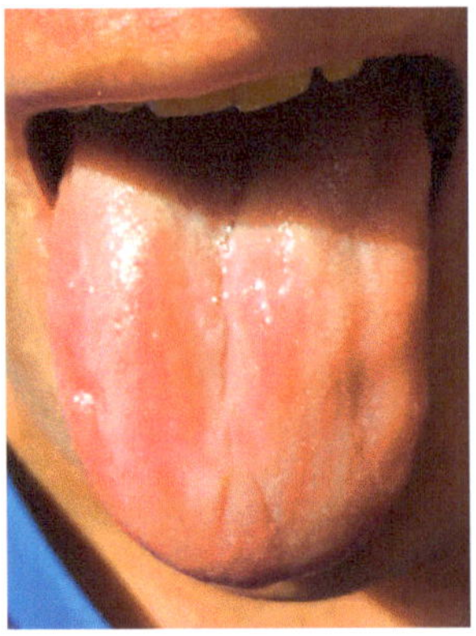

Cracks in the Lung Region

As the Heart communicates downward, it can transfer this Heat to the Kidneys. Since the Kidneys are consolidators, Heat can become trapped there.[18] The Kidneys try to vent the Heat through the Bladder.[19] Meanwhile, the Stomach or the Liver—if untreated—continues to generate Heat and the Heat continues to rise to the chest. Ultimately, the Heat accumulates in the chest and affects the Lungs. This mechanism produces cracks in the Lung area.

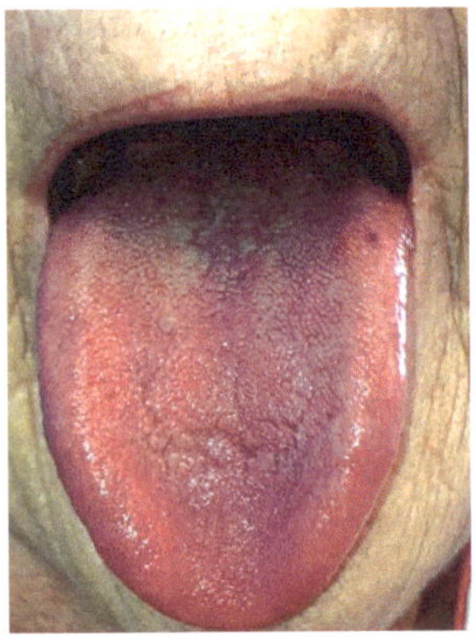

The mechanism described above is active in this patient. An overheating diet and alcohol led to excess Heat, which rose to the Lungs and was transferred to the Lower Jiao, desiccating it. Concurrently, long-term cortisone use weakened the Kidneys, leaving them unable to move the Heat through the Bladder. The Heat eventually became trapped in the Upper Jiao, where it affected the Lungs, causing Heat to move to the skin—another Lung-mediated exit— since the Lungs control the exterior and also move Blood. The Liver, constrained by the action of trying to block the Heat coming back up, is too tight to be able to store adequate blood at night to prevent nightmares, and to manage Damp-Heat. This is the cause of the current symptoms described by his Western doctor as cutaneous vasculitis and hypercholesterolemia.

Cracks only appearing in the Lung region might not relate to the progression process. If Heat is localized in the Lung area, these cracks might be signs of direct emotional stress associated with the Lungs: the experience of loss, grief, or sadness. Climatic dryness, smoking, and other pollution can also produce Dryness in the Lungs.

[18] When the Heat becomes trapped in the Kidneys, it can consume Kidney Yin, creating Steaming Bone Syndrome.
[19] This is how BL-43 (lateral to the Pericardium Bladder Shu point) works to treat Steaming Bone Syndrome and the affected Shen.

Cracks in the Sides

Again, Heat in the digestive tract arising from too much Yang food in the diet, such as protein, shows up on the sides of the tongue. The Gallbladder is stimulated to secrete alkalizing bile in response to the heightened quantity of acids needed to digest meats and fats. Overtaxation of the Liver and Gallbladder, due to excess meat in the diet, can show as cracks in the sides of the tongue.

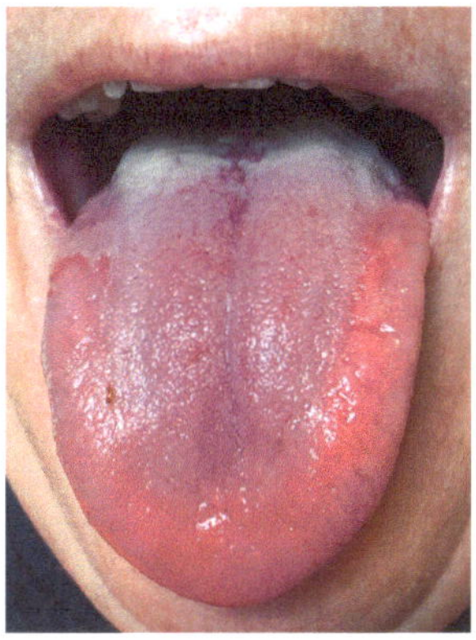

This woman craved sugar and was unable to stop eating it every time she started. Her diet was high in chicken, a particularly Yang (heating) food. A ganglion at LU-9 elicited a question about her emotional history and she reported having had a major disappointment twenty years earlier. The depression in the Lung area may reflect that. The tremendous Heat seen through the coat in the center is visibly moving to the Lower Jiao, where the body is responding with Dampness. The strain of the excess Yang animal protein and sugar has taxed the Liver and Gallbladder to the point of cracking the sides of the tongue. Since the Gallbladder is the link between the post-natal arena and the prenatal arena, the Heat gained entree to the Jing-Essence, showing as cracking in the Lower Jiao. On its way, Dai Mai attempted to contain the Heat, showing as added redness across the Dai Mai region. She arrived at my colleague's office following a diagnosis of breast cancer (left breast) and radiation treatment. Her treatments are focused in the clearing of Heat and the Triple Heater Divergent Channel.

Cracks at the Rear

Heat in the Kidneys cracks the rear of the tongue. A crack extending from the rear of the tongue to the center can indicate a constitutional weakness, since there is insufficient constitutional Yin for the digestive tract to acquire.

Deep roughness or cracks with dampness inside them can appear in the Lower Jiao area if the Liver is struggling in its attempt to control Heat, Damp, or Wind. This happens as Liver Qi becomes constrained by continually pushing downward, reversing its natural flow, to prevent Heat becoming rampant. As the condition worsens, the Lower Jiao area of the tongue becomes rough or cracked with a thickening coat. This type of constraint would manifest as headaches, abdominal signs, and Wind signs.

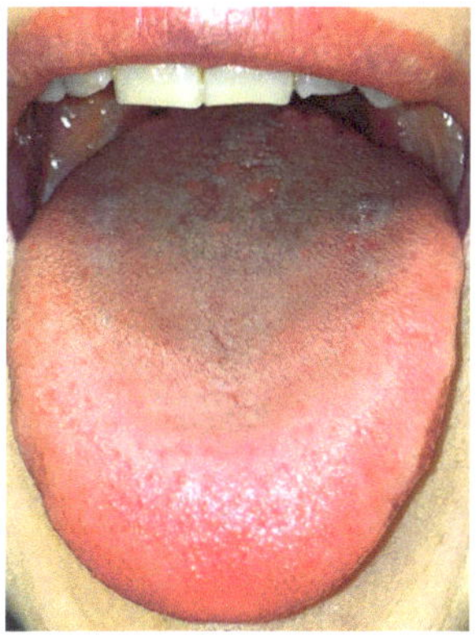

This patient experiences frustration as her own needs are unmet and unexpressed while she tends only others. Heat originated in the Middle Jiao, where it resulted in two intestinal surgeries and an appendectomy. The Heat has been shifted from the Middle to the Lower Jiao, cracking the Lower Jiao region of the tongue and causing kidney stones, urgency in the bowels, and spontaneous abortions.

Cracks in a Pale Tongue

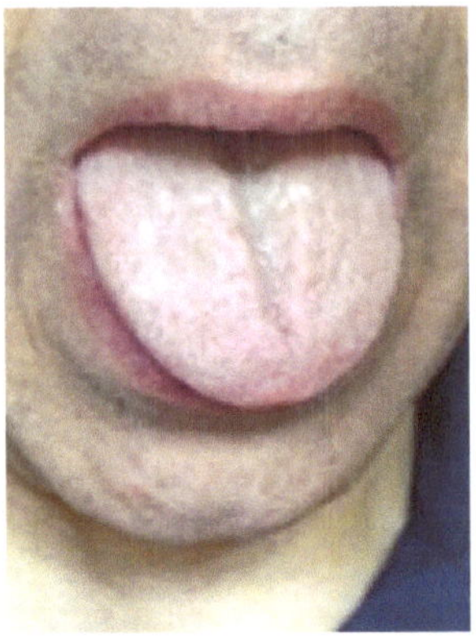

In cases of excess Stomach Fire, as long-term Heat damages Fluids, the tongue can crack open. Stomach Fire can arise as the body intentionally generates Heat in response to pathology. Often Stomach Fire results from the chronic dehydration left in the wake of eating very Yang foods and processed foods, especially sugar, hot spices, garlic, and alcohol. But generally, midline Stomach cracks are due to overthinking, from mentally generated Stomach Fire. Most people in our culture have overactive minds due to lack of calm, unstructured time. Thinking stresses the Spleen, stagnating Qi in the Middle Jiao, causing Heat to accumulate in the digestive tract. Excess fire burns and depletes the Spleen, damaging the mechanism of transformation. This is the mechanism of worry contributing to Stomach ulcers. Over time, Qi is consumed by Heat and the tongue is left pale and often swollen with a deep midline crack.

Severe chronic internal Cold can also crack the tongue open. But the tongue will be purplish or bluish.

Reading the Response to Pathology

We might expect the tongue to be dry when it is cracked, but the body tries to reduce the adverse effects of Heat by responding with Dampness. If there is a sticky coat within the cracks, Dampness is controlling the Heat. Sometimes Dampness looks as though it is actually trying to glue the tongue back together. Sometimes you'll see patches of a sticky phlegm-like coat over divots, crevices, areas of missing flesh, and tongue ulcers. This is all a response to Heat pathology. This Dampness is not pathological and should not be cleared. It's vital in controlling the Heat, buying you and the patient time. Clear the actual stimulus behind the creation of the Dampness, that is, clear the Heat. If you try to rid the Dampness, you are telling the body it is reacting inappropriately; you're sedating the immune system instead of supporting it. Symptoms will always worsen if you treat the response instead of the actual pathology.

II

Protrusions and Froth

Eruptions, Varicosities, and Thorns

Protrusions, including eruptions, varicosities, and bumps known as thorns, reflect the body's unsuccessful attempts to push a pathogenic factor out to the exterior. When Qi is deficient and therefore unable to clear pathology, the body stagnates Qi to prevent its further loss. The pathogen then sits in the body, unresolved. To create change, Qi must be replenished, the bowels must be moving daily, and the diet must shift to become one of food-based hydration (soups, stews, congees).

If Qi is very weak, and eradication is still difficult, food-based hydration remains essential because the pathogenic factor must be able to go into latency so as not to be a systemic loose cannon.

Protrusions vary in size from tiny petechiae to giant thorns (bumps) at the rear. Protrusions in small quantities are common along the sides and especially at the rear of the tongue. Markedly elevated or plentiful protrusions are less common.

Tiny protrusions often occur in clusters in the distal two thirds of the tongue, showing Qi gathering in the Middle or Upper Jiaos. Qi trapped in the Upper Jiao causes the body to respond with Heat as it tries to move the stagnant Qi, causing the tip to become red. The protrusions shift to the tip and cluster together. Minor protrusions at the rear of the tongue may indicate inflammation of the mucous membranes of the uterus or bladder.

Large protrusions at the back of the tongue can indicate the stagnation of fecal matter, intestinal polyps, masses in the Lower Jiao, or an advanced disease state. If the tongue is rough (very uneven) with protrusion and cracks, Heat is damaging the Lower Jiao. The further back the protrusion, the more deeply affected the Lower Jiao. When significant protrusions appear at the rear of the tongue, high protein diets are contraindicated, since they produce Heat that the system can no longer tolerate.

If there are many protrusions, the body is losing its capacity to hold pathology latent. There may be an overflow of fire toxins in the Jing. The tongue may be covered in thorns, indicating the condition requires urgent treatment. The tongue can concurrently become pale even though there is rampant Heat, as Heat consumes Qi, Yin, and Blood. It might become shiny, indicating that Qi has been consumed.

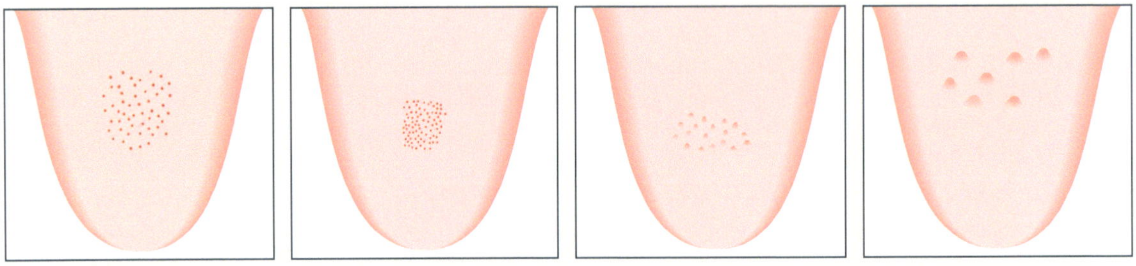

Petechiae that are spread out indicate that the body is trying to vent Heat.	Petechiae close together indicate trapped Heat.	Little abscesses (thorns) or little sores indicate trapped Heat. The resulting inflammation has damaged tissues and Damp is responding.	Large thorns indicate that fire toxins (free radicals) are present. If at the rear, Dai Mai is attempting to hold them away from the viscera.

Protrusion Color

Protrusions are generally red, purple, or white. They can also present as the same color as the tongue as Heat consumes mediumship.

- Red protrusions indicate Heat (inflammation), either from Heat itself or from Heat responding to stagnation.
- Purple protrusions show stagnation.
- White protrusions often indicate fire toxins—the Heat is so systemic and so prolonged that the redness has reached another level, transforming to white, like ash in a fireplace.
- Protrusions that are the same or a color similar to the tongue itself are either in their early stage, or Blood or Yang has been consumed leaving them pale.

Note: Petechiae, though sometimes slightly raised, are not considered bona fide protrusions. Petechiae are dots of discoloration and usually congregate. Protrusions are literally emerging from the tongue, are raised above the surface of the tongue, and are scattered.

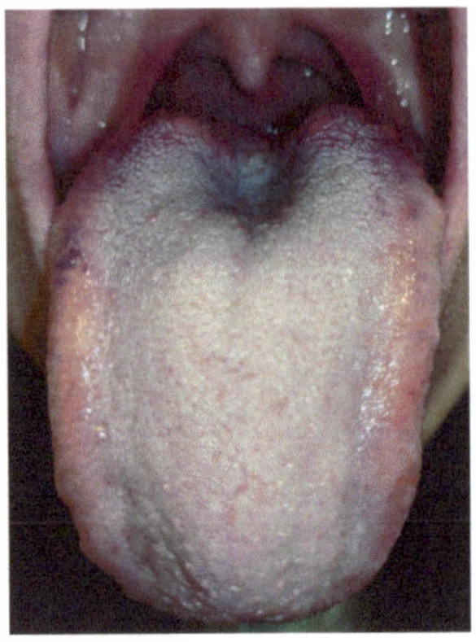

In this case, Blood was unable to deal with a pathogenic factor, leaving Blood depleted and the sides of the tongue very pale. The Gallbladder Channel and the Liver exerted effort to stagnate Blood in order to conserve it, as seen in the tension on the left side of the tongue and the coagulation of Blood on the right side of the tongue by the lip. The dearth of mediumship and the tension in the Gallbladder Channel, affecting in turn Dai Mai, resulted in the Lower Jiao being unable to release the pathogenic factor through the bowels. The toxins accrued in the intestines, as shown in the presence of many thorns in that region. The patient presented for acupuncture following a Western diagnosis of ulcerative colitis.

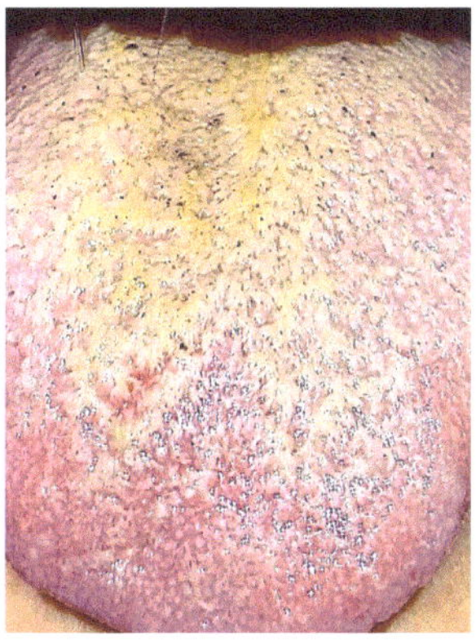

This tongue is covered in tiny white thorns, indicating a rampant spreading of fire toxins. This tongue appears on page 148. The patient sought treatment after a Western diagnosis of fourth stage cancer.

This patient's first visit was days after her Western diagnosis of fourth stage cancer of the Stomach, metastasizing to the Liver and bones, with poor prognosis. She had gone to the doctor to investigate her black stool. It's clear from the photo on the left that extreme Heat developed into fire toxins, reflected on the tongue as white ash. The Heat from the Stomach spread to the Liver, while the Gallbladder fought to lock the diaphragm down to prevent metastasis to the Lungs. The presence of white protrusions in the Upper Jiao demonstrates the exhaustion of that effort.

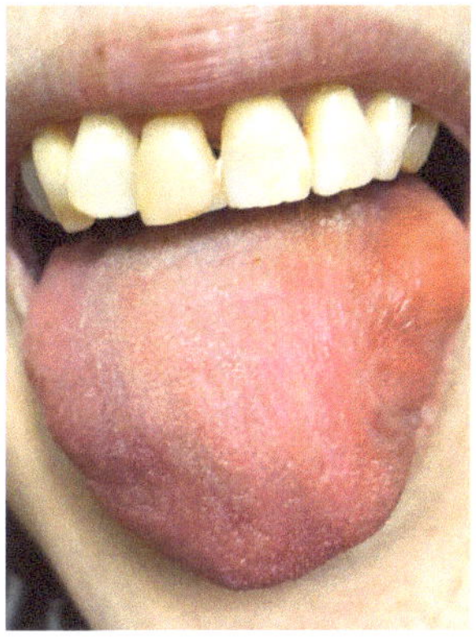

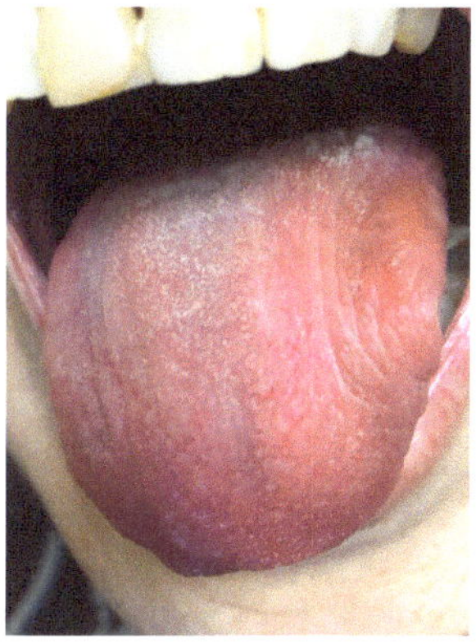

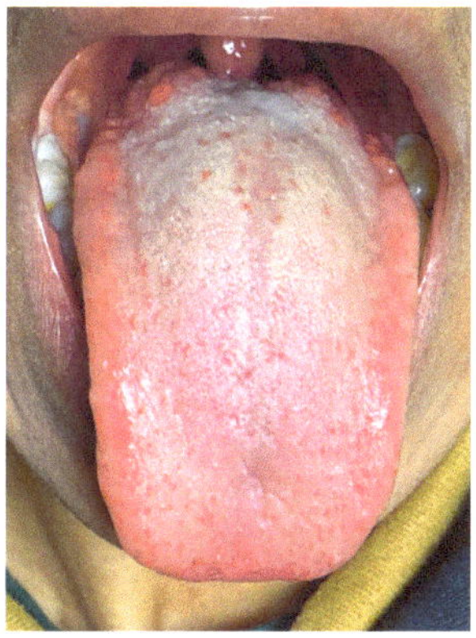

This person healed themselves of Wind-Phlegm (Western diagnosis was multiple sclerosis) but still has fibroids and digestive issues due to a current adherence to salad eating which weakens the Spleen, making it difficult to resolve Phlegm. She has fibroids because the Lower Jiao is holding pathology due to long-term insufficiency of Lung Qi. Lung Qi is derived from Spleen Qi and is responsible for descending or evacuating the contents of the Lower Jiao.

An electric shock deeply affected Wei Qi, which flows in the exterior and in the nerves, and is controlled by the Lungs and Liver. Heat intensified in the Lungs (shown in the increased size of the protrusion in the Lung area) and in the Liver (shown in the deep cracks), and consumed mediumship and Yang Qi. The patient's Lungs were already particularly sensitive and he has a history of depression (a Lung insult) and anger, which taxes the Liver, meaning there may have already been an underlying Blood deficiency. The Heat-consuming Yang leaves the tongue tending to pale. Yang Qi originates in the Kidneys. The patient presented after a Western diagnosis of kidney failure."

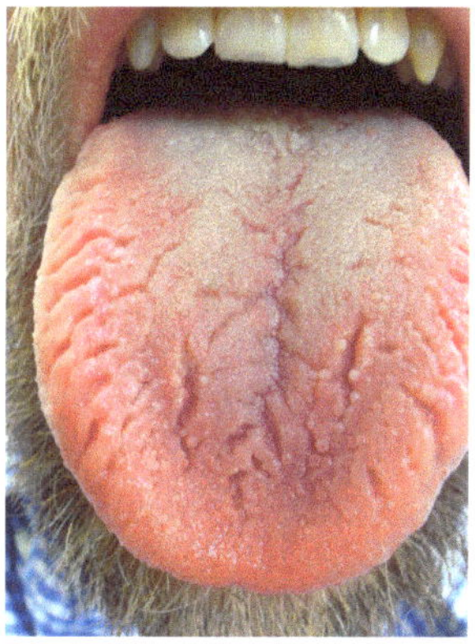

Froth

Froth indicates that the body is having difficulty moving one medium (Blood, Fluids, or Yin) to support a different medium. The most common cause of froth is persistent emotions in a person trying but unable to change. Since the emotions are held in the Blood, and persistent emotions create tremendous Heat, Blood is consumed. The Liver becomes constrained as it tries to hold on to more Blood. Yin is stirred up both by the fire created by the emotions, and also as the body reaches more deeply for resources. It strives to move one medium to support another, constraining Qi to reduce consumption of those resources. Meanwhile, the body is trying to compensate for the lack of a medium by holding on to pathological Fluids (Damp). The stirring of Yin and pathological Damp can develop into Wind-Phlegm and rise to the sensory orifices, creating tics and tremors, or at worst, epileptic seizures where the Wind-Phlegm presents as foaming at the mouth. Deep crying and violent outbursts can erupt as further expression of this rebellious Qi. The patient is unable to cultivate calm as they seek but resist the change they need.[20] The seizures will persist until the mind is able to resolve the emotions.

If the froth is near the tip of the tongue, Liver constraint is insulting Lung Yin. The Liver must be regulated. Froth at the sides of the tongue indicate the effort of moving Blood to support Yin. If the Liver is constrained, this is difficult and the stirring of resources creates froth over the Liver and Gallbladder areas. Froth at the back of the tongue indicates Kidney Yin is deficient and both Lung Yin and Liver Blood are moving down to support the Kidneys with urgency. The rushed movement creates the frothing. If Yang is floating, the Kidneys move Lung fluids back up again, and the rear of the tongue becomes frothy. The treatment principle is to separate pure and turbid Fluids in the Lungs (CV-9 and CV-12 work beautifully), then nourish the deficient medium.

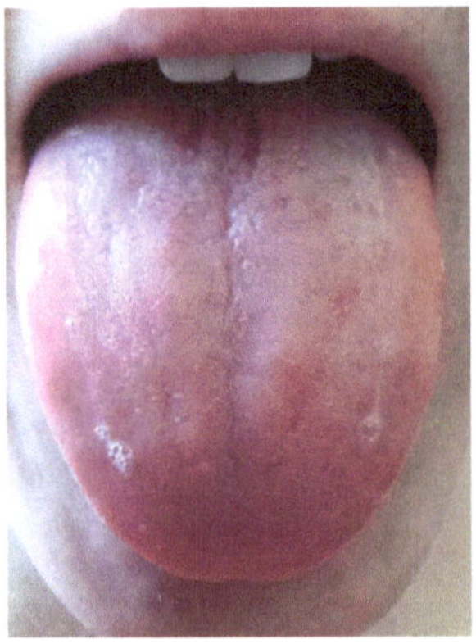

Froth in a patient with Wind-Phlegm (Western diagnosis of epilepsy)

[20] These processes are described elegantly by the Divergent Channels mechanism; as one medium is sequestered to hold pathology away from the organs, another medium is moved to compensate.

Sometimes froth is combined with strings as Dampness is responding to Wind.

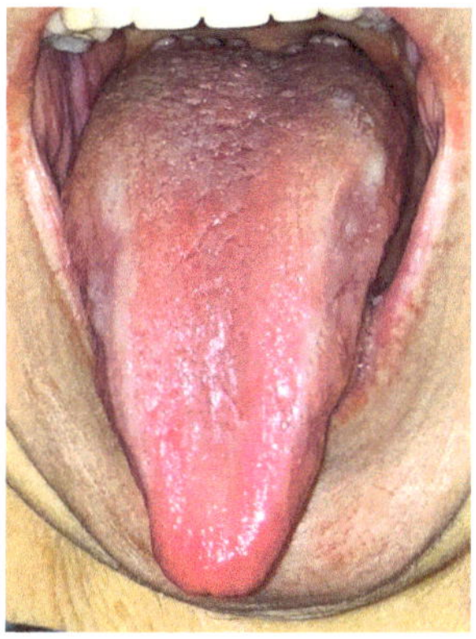

Froth over the Liver and Gallbladder regions of the tongue in a patient unable to be in present time and unable to sit still, since Blood and Wei Qi are never relaxed due to long term stagnation. The patient presented after a Western diagnosis of breast cancer, constipation and obesity. Note the fire toxins manifesting as white thorns in the rear of the tongue.

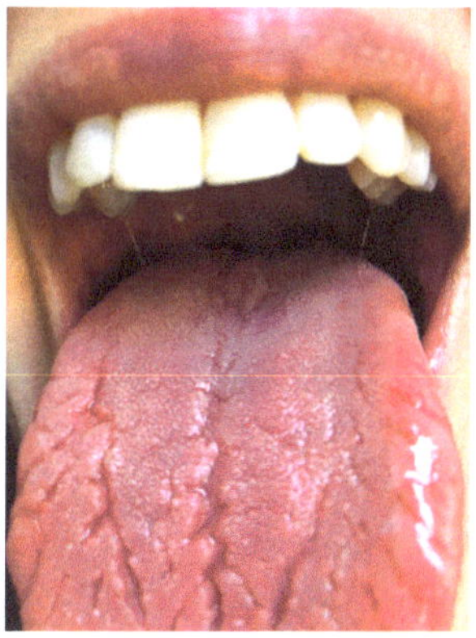

Strings in a patient with obsessive fear as Yang is stirred and Damp responds.

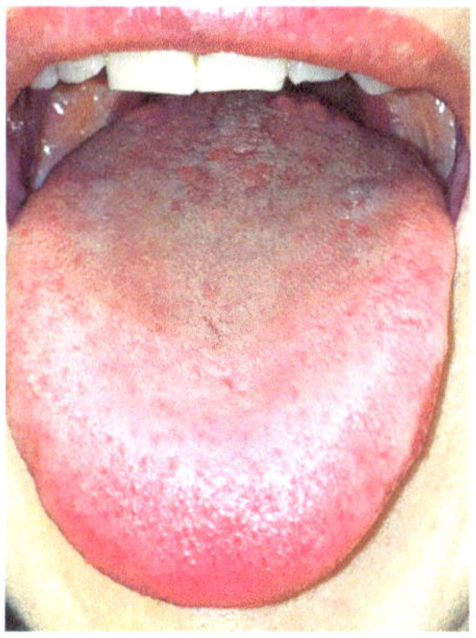

Froth in an anxious patient with escaping Yang due to a Yin deficiency. The Lower Jiao is sluggish due to a diaphragmatic blockage preventing communication between Upper and Lower Jiaos. Dampness has accumulated in the Lower Jiao in response to the Yin deficiency, further complicating the lack of movement. The body tries to move Qi in the Lower Jiao to reestablish communication with the Upper Jiao, stirring froth as it does so.

12

Tongue Diagnosis and the Complement Channels

To assess the status of the Eight Extraordinary Channels using tongue diagnosis, look for features that demonstrate the principal signs of each channel.

The Eight Extraordinary Channels and Tongue Diagnosis

The Chong Mai Tongue

Chong Mai contains the blueprint of our individual existence. It governs the way our bodies develop and sets the curriculum for one's lifetime. Living to one's full potential requires the confidence to form, embrace, and nurture relationships. When Chong Mai has not been nurtured both in utero and during the first two years of life, that is, if basic physiological and psychological needs have not been met (such as loving touch, protection, soothing, feeding), a reaction brews in the abdominal muscles. A hardened, raised muscular tension in the abdominal muscles on either side of the midline will emerge. This is known as chopstick Qi or the hidden beams, a protective mechanism, armoring both against being shunned and against further trauma to the Chong Channel. The patient will unwittingly withdraw from or block themselves from forming close relationships.

The corresponding tongue has the same two hidden beams of defense showing, usually in the anterior two thirds of the tongue. Generally, the tongue can appear purple or pale purple due to the restraint of Qi. Any combination of Chong Mai signs and symptoms may be present. If Chong pathology is advanced, you may see the hidden beams appear on the rear of the tongue, indicating that a weak Spleen has forced Jing-Essence to break down to support Blood. Regardless of the location of the beams, you'll find that the degree the Spleen is ascending is not balanced by the Stomach's descending Qi, leaving the patient with a sense of never feeling fully in balance. The distribution of Qi to the five limbs is compromised by tightness in the abdomen. SP-4 is a principal point for the harmonization of Stomach and Spleen; if needled with strong intention, it can release the rails in the abdomen and therefore in the tongue, restoring free movement of Qi in the Middle Jiao.

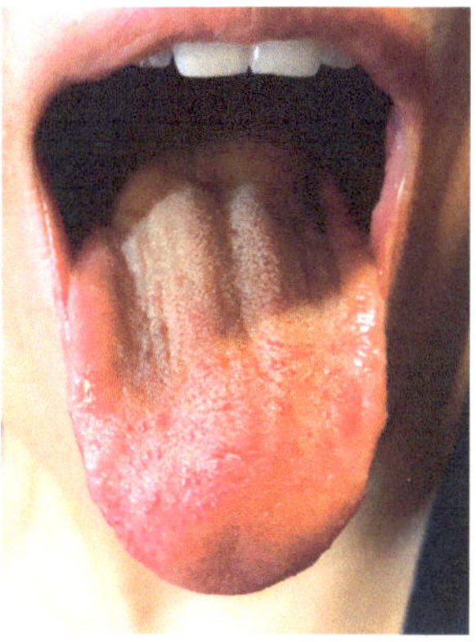

Chong Mai first trajectory.

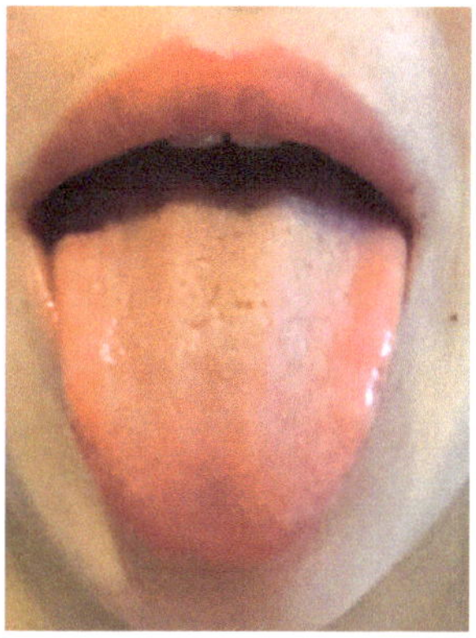

Chong Mai first and second trajectory.

The Ren Mai Tongue

Ren Mai is the Sea of Yin; it provides the resources the body requires to create, build, and repair itself. Also, as the channel propelling the need to bond for survival (initially to the mother), it generates the feeling of belonging.

If Yin is depleted, Ren Mai senses that it cannot perform these functions and stagnates Yin in response. Therefore the Ren Mai tongue will show evidence of both Yin stasis and Yin deficiency. The tongue will be swollen in places, perhaps with protrusions (bumps) as the accumulation of Yin becomes increasingly pathological and will be peeled in patches. It may be retracted, unable to fully extend outward. Looking underneath the tongue, one sees that the tonicity of the frenulum may be noticeably altered, causing it to look tight or flaccid. The frenulum, which reflects more Du Mai, will look looser than normal if Ren Mai is overactive.

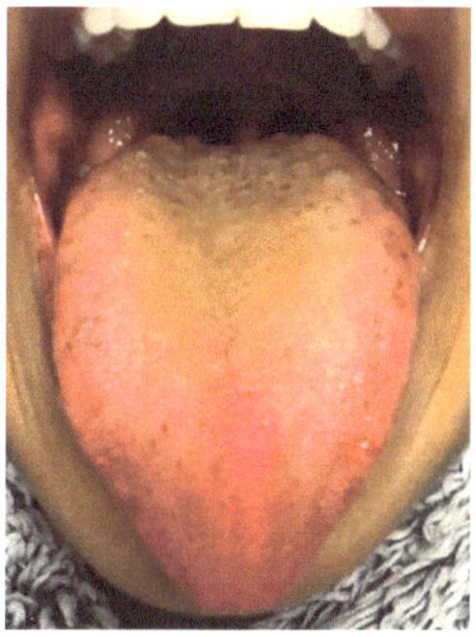

This tongue shows a Yin deficiency in that the tongue is thin and shows Yin stasis in the reactive accumulation of Yin (bumps) in the rear of the tongue. The body is stagnating Blood and directing it to the Lower Jiao where it will break down to replenish Yin.

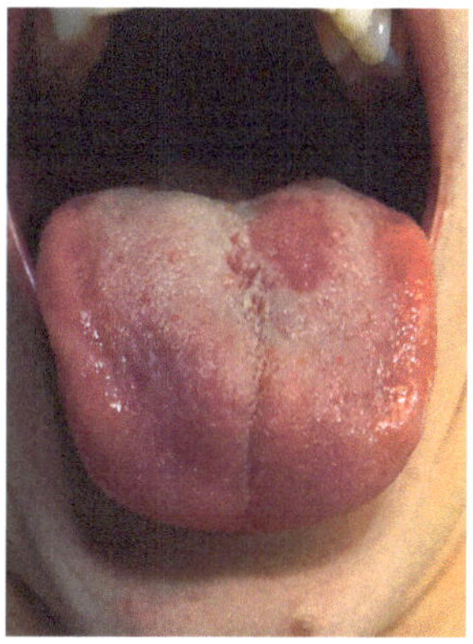

This is a more classic Ren Mai tongue. The coat is peeling off in patches while the body works to gather pathological Yin, reflected in the thickening yellow coat.

The Du Mai Tongue

Du Mai is the Sea of Yang, the origin of all Yang, source of the Qi that warms the digestive tract and therefore is responsible for the derivation of post-natal Qi from food. It supplies the Yang Qi needed for all movement, all immune function, and creates upward actions including the development of the upright stance. Du Mai governs independence, individuality, animation, and the quest to know the world. When Du Mai is out of balance, the patient will not be comfortable moving forward in life. This can go in two directions: either there will be overdependence on others, with an unwillingness to learn about the world, or there will be rebellion against that outside world, accompanied by hyperactivity.

If Du Mai is in a state of excess, meaning it is expressing too much Yang—creating, for example, headaches, seizures, dizziness, or numbness—the tongue will dart out, be quite red, and possibly shaky (the shaking means the Kidney Channel is also affected). There will be an accumulation of Heat in the Upper Jiao region of the tongue. When Du Mai is in a state of deficiency, the tongue may be flaccid and droop. In advanced states, the rear of the tongue may collapse and the tongue may be pale and damp as there is insufficient Yang to support the Spleen.

The tonicity of the frenulum reflects the status of Du Mai; when the frenulum is very tight, Du Mai is overactive. Pathologies included in this presentation include exuberant Yang, internal Wind, and exacerbated rebellious Qi. If Du Mai is in a state of deficiency, you might see that the frenulum is flaccid.

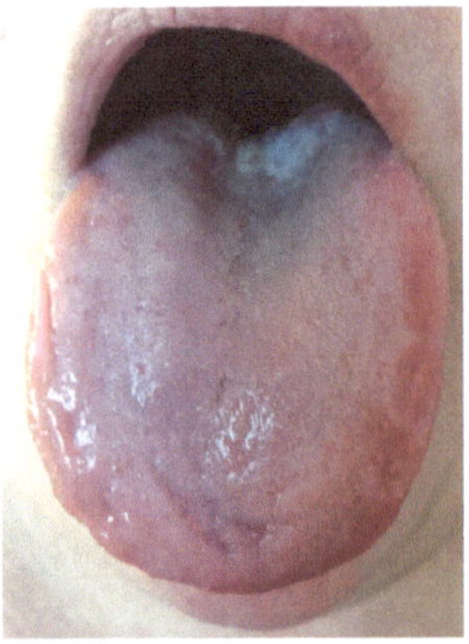

Du Mai is in a state of deficiency here. The tongue shows a history of Du Mai being overactive in remnants of a red perimeter. This person overworked and worried, exhausting their Yang. The concave rear and the floppy nature of the tongue show the eventual collapse of Yang and the consequent weakness of Spleen Qi, which led to swelling and Dampness.

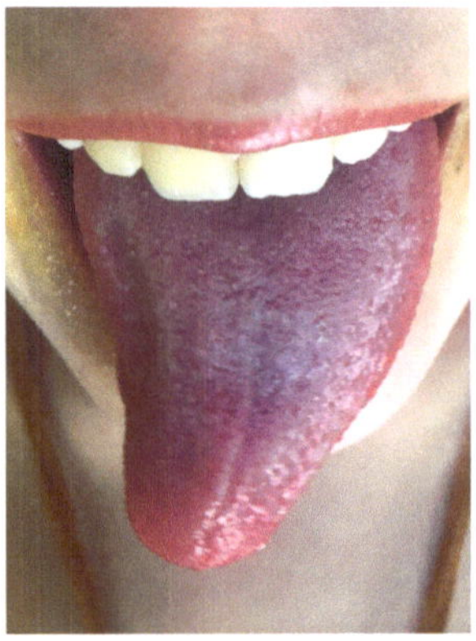

This tongue is very red, darts out, and dances around.

The Yin Wei Mai Tongue

Yin Wei Mai is the record keeper. It preserves an individual's history in its structure. This is how a depressed person develops a stooped posture, or how a fearful person develops a slightly concave chest. Yin Wei Mai also recycles Yin, preserving the origin of the structure of the body by constantly bringing excess Yin back to its origin, Ren Mai, at CV-22 and 23.

When Yin Wei Mai is out of balance, the patient is unable to let go of the past. They focus on the past and miss the opportunity to re-create and refresh themselves. The habit of reminiscence, longing for the past, or dwelling on feelings—positive or negative—about those in the past, hurts the Heart. Blood—the residence of the emotions—becomes depleted. As always, when the body recognizes that it is deficient in a medium, it will stagnate that medium to prevent further loss. And since Yin Wei Mai is producing this stagnating action, its charges, Blood and Yin, also stagnate, resulting in Shen disturbance and pain respectively.

The Yin Wei Mai tongue is characterized by tension in the Upper Jiao. The anterior third of the tongue will often be elevated and/or red, either at the Pericardium or the Heart areas. Sometimes the sides will be visibly tight, pushing Qi forward and creating a tight band in the Lung area, indicating mounting frustration affecting the Lungs. You might notice the patient revealing envy or resentment, and commonly, an inability to release the past. Sometimes, though, the sides are very tight and the tip of the tongue is elevated. In these cases, frustration has affected the Heart, resulting in jealousy or even rage.

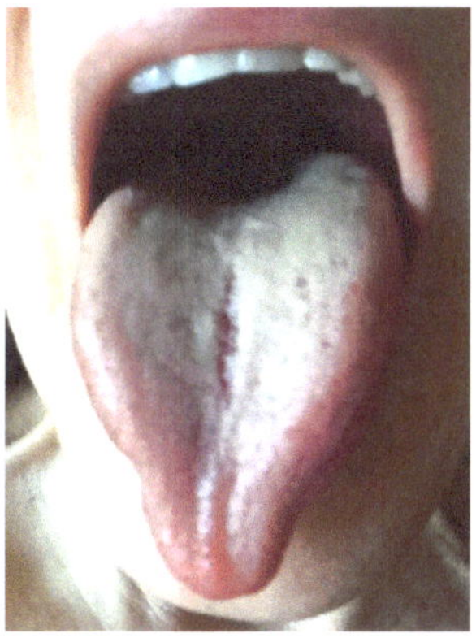

A Yin Wei Mai type tongue in a patient with childhood trauma dating from infancy.

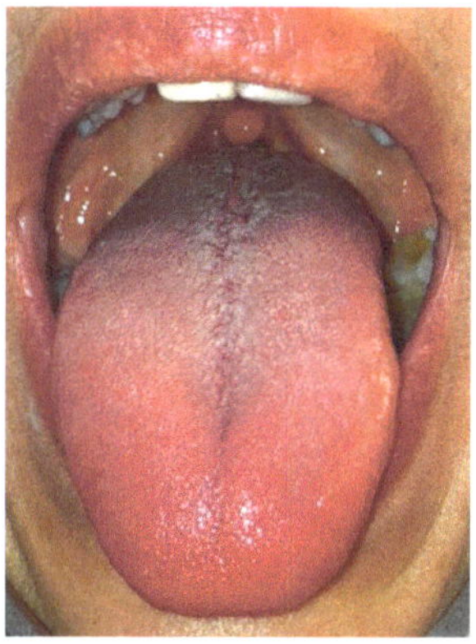

This patient presented with insomnia, anxiety, restlessness, joint pain and back pain.

The Yang Wei Mai Tongue

Yang Wei Mai creates a balance of Yang between its origin (Du Mai) and the exterior of the body. It recycles excess Yang back to the Yang's origin, Du Mai. In regulating the exchange of Yang between interior and exterior, it plays a key role in the conduct of immune responses.

It's also a record keeper, but it records the memory of actions. It records repetitive skills, such as riding a bike or driving a car, and even social skills. Life's major events, its stages, turning points, disappointments, and major achievements are all recorded as memorable landmarks onto the brain by Yang Wei Mai. Difficulty assimilating these landmarks into the fabric of one's life creates imbalances in Yang Wei Mai. The imbalances can create trepidation in making choices about how we will interact with the world going forward. Are we in or out? When Yang Wei Mai is out of balance, there is indecision, Shao Yang (Damp-Heat) conditions emerge, and there is fear of, or obsession about, the future.

If you find symptoms of Yang Wei Mai or if you find the Yang Wei Mai pulse, the tongue will often be swollen and have a thick coat (white or yellow) as Dampness responds to restrain unregulated Yang. As the conditions progress, Yang Qi (Wei Qi in particular) becomes deficient, causing the tongue to become quite flaccid, especially around its perimeter. If there is Wei Atrophy Syndrome where Yang is trapped in the exterior and has consumed Wei-Defensive Qi, the tongue may be crimson.

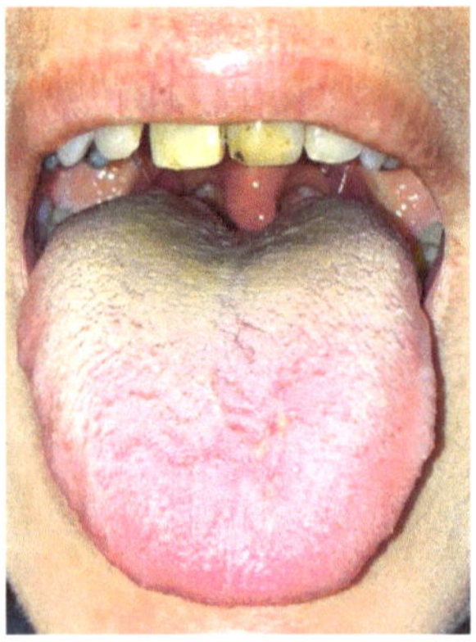

This patient shows unregulated Yang Qi, which she experiences in the form of mania, palpitations, overall tension, and a lack of coordination.
This was exacerbated by extreme anxiety. The Dampness that responded to contain Yang resulted in Phlegm affecting the Mind, resulting in the arising of suicidal tendencies. She presented after a Western diagnosis of bipolar disorder.

The Yin Qiao Mai Tongue

The principal function of Yin Qiao Mai is cultivation of one's identity, appreciation for oneself, and the ability to reside peacefully in the present moment, with structure in alignment. In the absence of love for oneself, the Yin Qiao Mai Channel stagnates and accumulates Yin and Dampness. Wind may develop. The Yin Qiao Mai tongue tends to be short, swollen, and pale purple.

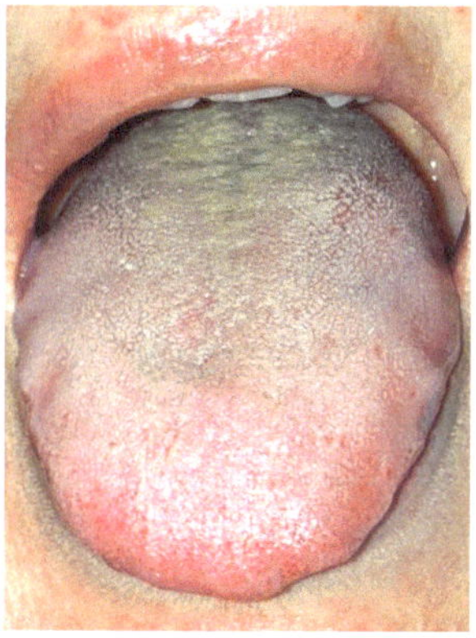

A patient with Bell's palsy.

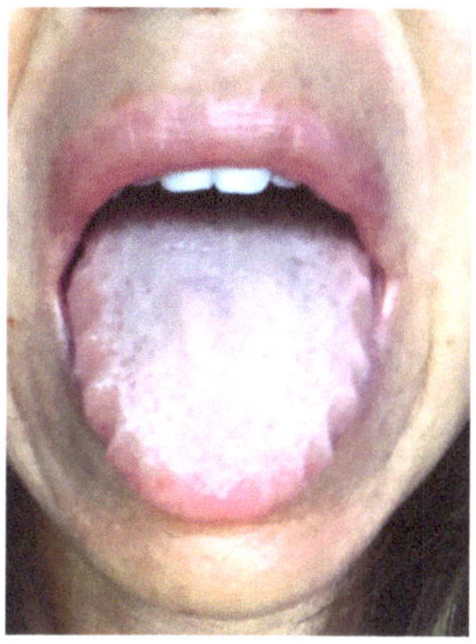

Dampness, rebellious Qi and sinus infections.

The Yang Qiao Mai Tongue

Yang Qiao Mai brings Yang Qi from Du Mai to govern our gait and alignment, keeping us in balance. When Yang Qiao Mai is tight or loose, there are musculoskeletal issues related to the alignment of the physical structure. From an emotional point of view, when Yang Qiao Mai is out of balance, the patient is never happy in the present moment, always wishing they were somewhere else, or with someone else, or doing something else. Often they feel the world is not on their side, that the world is aggressive toward them. They cannot reside happily in the moment where they are. If the patient presents with signs and symptoms of Yang Qiao Mai, or if you find a Yang Qiao Mai pulse, you might find that the tongue shows tightness down the sides, since the channel itself travels along the lateral exterior. The tension in the sides of the Yang Qiao Mai tongue causes it to be very long and red.

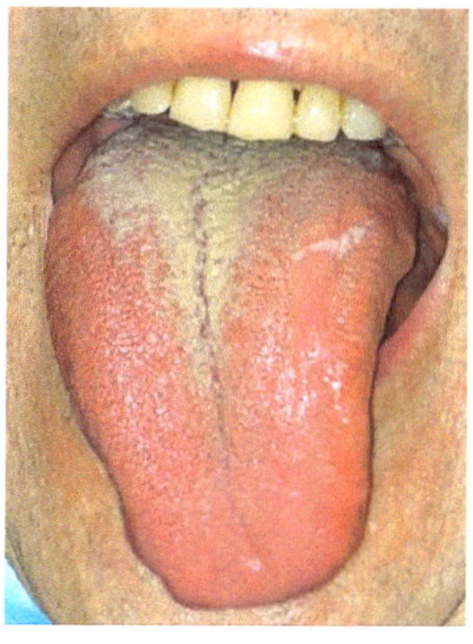

This patient presented after an injury from a fall that occurred after losing consciousness (Wind). He experiences pain in the shoulder, Wind in the legs (sciatica) and occiput, eye pressure issues, high blood pressure, and diabetes. The Wind is visible in the contortion of the tongue body.

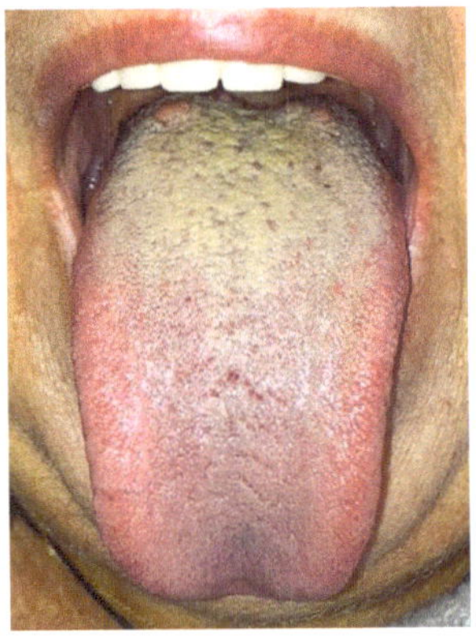

The person could do well with treatment of Yang Qiao Mai, but Yang Wei Mai would function well due to the Damp-Heat showing. She presented after a diagnosis of high cholesterol, fatty liver disease, and hypertension, and experiences headaches, a neuroma, palpitations, and obsessive fear. The cholesterol (Dampness) is being manufactured in response to the rampant Heat evident throughout the tongue. This Heat is exacerbated by dehydration and overeating poorly chosen food.

The Dai Mai Tongue

The function of Dai Mai is to use the pelvis as a receptacle for excesses. These excesses may be waste or toxins the body can't dispose of, but Dai Mai can also store Dampness that it will use to absorb unprocessed memories or emotions. Since Dai Mai is in the realm of the Jing-Essence, and since emotions reside in the Blood, the emotions contained in Dai Mai are truly repressed. When Dai Mai functions this way, the body is weighed down and there is depletion of Qi as it is diverted to fund the containment. The resulting compounding stagnation, including fluids and masses, can affect fertility, the routes of elimination, and optimism.

The Dai Mai tongue is swollen, especially in the posterior portion of the middle, and at the rear. There may be a line of constraint across the tongue behind the Middle Jiao. There may be thorns (bumps) and deposits and a thick coat in the rear of the Middle Jiao area and all through the Lower Jiao area.

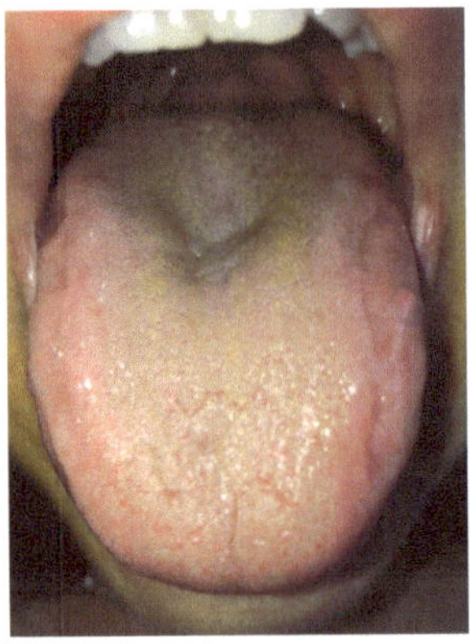

Collapse of Spleen Qi led to an accumulation of Dampness in Dai Mai, and, ultimately, its collapse.

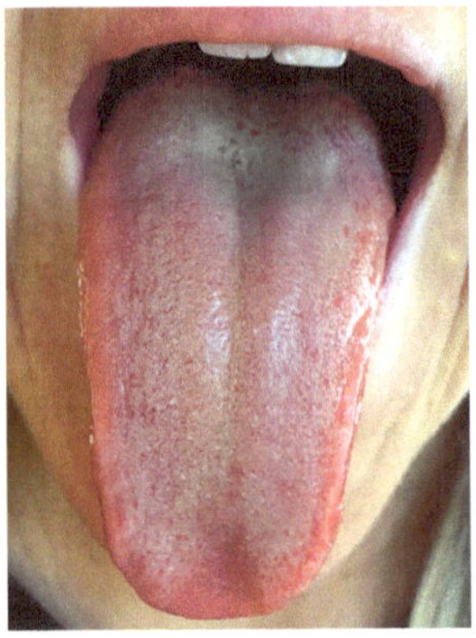

This patient presented after a Western diagnosis of reflux. She had a chronic taste of bile in her mouth. The golden rule—for the Stomach to be full, the Large Intestine must be empty—was broken. The bowels must move every day. Treatment involves Dai Mai rather than using antacids to suffocate the Stomach's clear message.

The Luo Channels and Tongue Diagnosis

The Luo Channels are created by the body to contain blood-borne pathogenic factors ranging from toxins to unresolved or unexpressed emotions. They keep these away from the organs using Blood. Luo vessels manifest as spider veins, varicosities, swellings, and later, they elicit nodules. The Luo vessels can hold pathology for hours or decades, depending on toxicity of the pathology and also depending on the amount of mediumship—Blood and Fluids—available to hold that pathology latent.

When the Luo Channels are functioning successfully—keeping the pathogen out of circulation and away from the organs—the tongue might not show pathology at all. Remember, the tongue is an instrument of expression and will not give clues about successful suppression (latency) when pathology is hidden. But when the Luos begin to fail—when they can no longer fully contain pathology—signs of Blood taxation will appear. Blood may have been consumed in the process of maintaining the Luo vessels, causing the sides of the tongue to appear slightly translucent, pale, or pale purple. If the body has stagnated Blood to try to conserve Blood, the sides of the tongue may be purple or pinched.

Small protrusions (small thorns) or roughness can indicate that the Luo Channel corresponding to that area is beginning to lose latency of a pathogen. If you suspect this is the case, look for spider veins or nodules along the relevant Luo pathways and treat the Luo Channels.

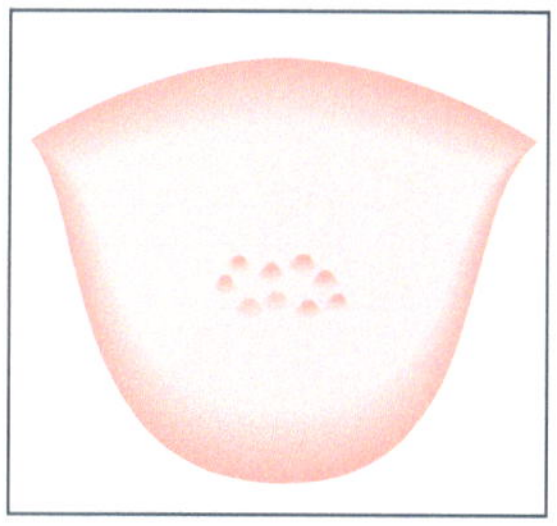

The Stomach Luo
has lost latency.

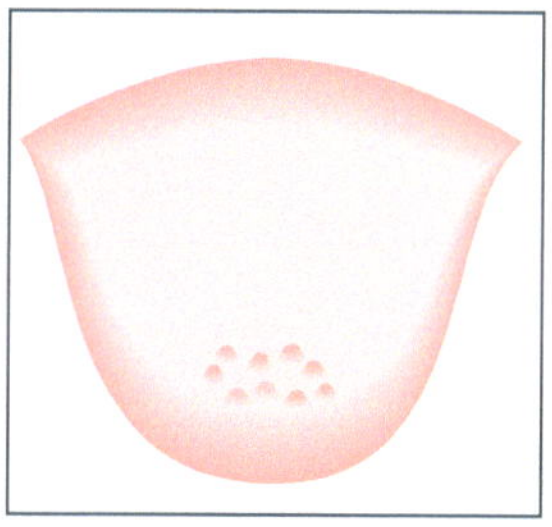

The Lung Luo
has lost latency.

When the pathology overwhelms the body and the Luo vessels can no longer contain it, the pathology comes "out of latency," emptying out into the Primary Channel. The Primary Channel tries to contain the pathology using another medium, Fluids. It creates cysts and nodules in the channel to try to arrest the pathogenic factor's progress to the precious organ. When it can sustain the delay no longer, the pathology moves to the Transverse Luo.

When pathology deepens and moves on to the Transverse Luo, the tongue becomes very interesting. The Transverse Luo is in two sections. The first connects the Luo point to the Source point of the Yin-Yang related pair. The Source point itself has the capacity to hold pathology in the relatively short term; the tongue may still not show pathology other than Blood deficiency or stagnation.

The second section of the Transverse Luos—identical to the internal branches of the Primary Channels—are like exit ramps off the highway of pathology containment; they lead pathology to a head-on collision with the Source level and, therefore, the organs. It is the action of the Transverse Luos—not the Longitudinal Luos—that is visible. Once the pathology has reached this point, the body musters as much Yang Qi as it can, sometimes creating an explosion of Heat in a last-ditch attempt to either combust the pathogenic factor, to oust it to the exterior, or at least move it away from the organ. There will be a dramatic display of Heat in the body of the tongue; it will become very red, even crimson.

As the pathology reaches and affects the organs, the underside of the tongue and the sublingual area—the reflection of the Yuan-Source level—will show unmistakable signs of toxicity breeching the Yuan-Source arena. The area becomes dark and distended, even purple or blackened. The disease is serious.

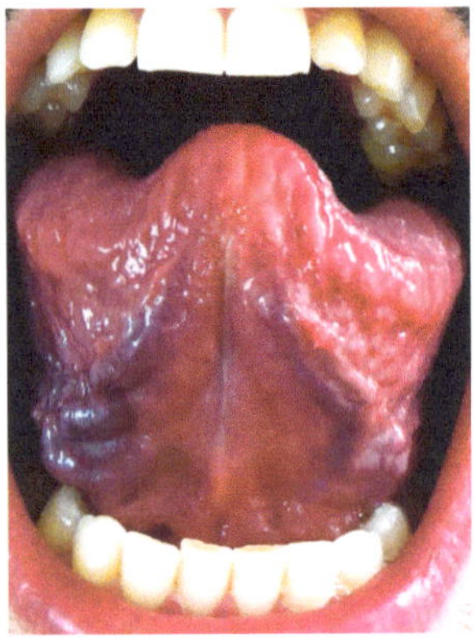

The Divergent Channels

If the Luo Channels fail, and there are sufficient alternate resources, the Divergent Channels may capture the pathogen and move it to the joints—another area of latency. The Divergent Channels can contain a pathogen for hours or decades, depending on the strength of the pathogen. They attain latency by lassoing the pathogenic factor in a sequence of brilliant moves as mediumship becomes depleted. They command first Jing, then Blood, then Jin-Thin Fluids, the Ye-Thick Fluids, then Qi, and finally Yang to ensure or strive for preservation of the organs.

When the Divergents are holding a pathogen in latency, there will be no signs and symptoms in the body related to that pathology. As resources are consumed over time, latency may become lost—the pathogenic factor can come out of hiding—and the tongue will show evidence of the body's response to the depletion of those resources. Signs can include swellings, pallor, and wasting.

Eventually, when the body cannot maintain latency, the pathogenic factor is released and evidence of the pathogen itself will show on the tongue as great Heat, or protrusions. Since the Divergents move pathology from one side of the body to the other, the tongue may become deviated, or the two halves of the tongue may become noticeably different. In some cases the tongue may point to one side.

The rear of the tongue is important, because the Divergents can only hold pathology if Fluids or Yin are sufficient. Divergent Channels will fail to hold pathology away from the organs if Yin is scarce. If the rear of the tongue is particularly cracked, dry, shriveled, or wasting, the Divergent Channels have failed or are on the brink of failing.

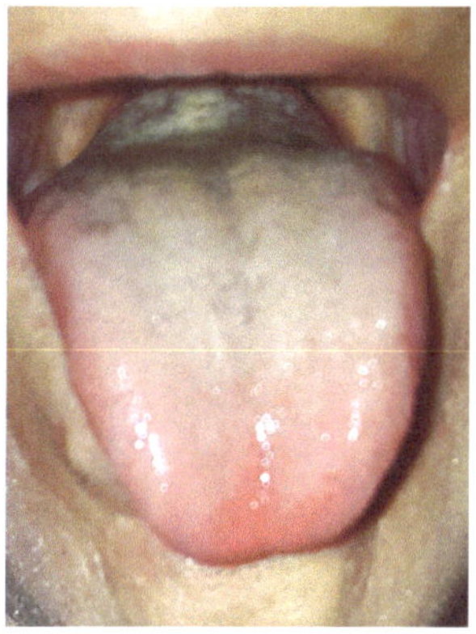

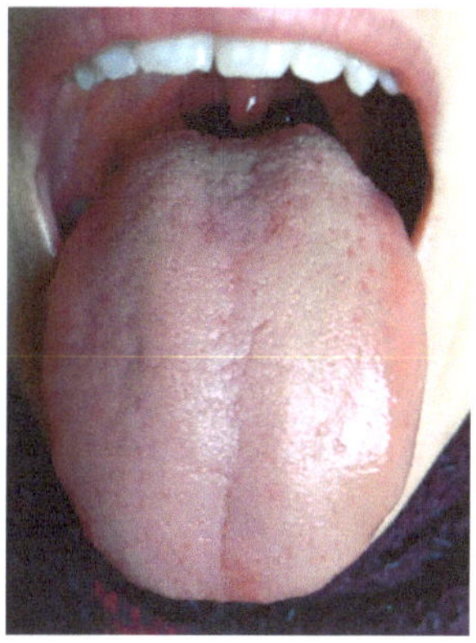

The Sinew Channels

The Sinew Channels conduct Wei Qi over the entire surface of the body, creating warmth and defense, and allowing movement of the exterior anatomy. They also control the Wei Qi that resides in the smooth muscle: in the lungs, heart, gut and uterus. Wei Qi is formed by Kidney Yang and Stomach Fluids. It is spread evenly by the Liver and brought fully to the exterior by the dispersing action of the Lungs. When the body wishes to expel a pathogenic factor, Wei Qi acts to initiate sneezing, sweating, coughing, vomiting, urination, and defecation, moving the pathogen to the exterior and out of the body. When Wei Qi is engaged in this process, the outer rim of the tongue often becomes red. This is because the Liver is active in moving the Wei Qi, trying to get the pathogen to exit, first through the upper Jiao. A more primitive map of the tongue is best used to see the evidence of the response of Wei Qi.

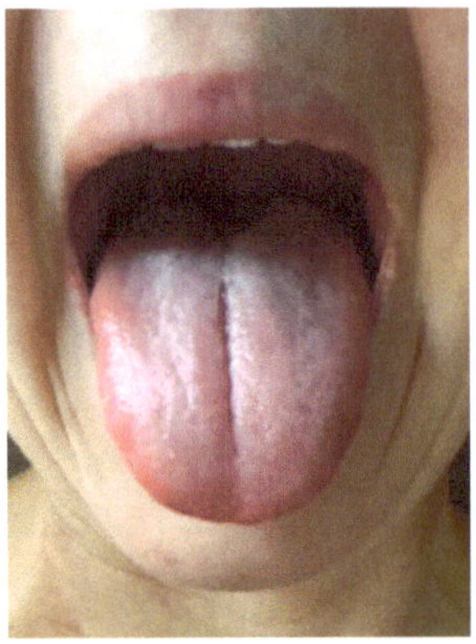

This photo shows Wei Qi trapped at the exterior. The patient has chronic, itching, weeping rashes all over her body.

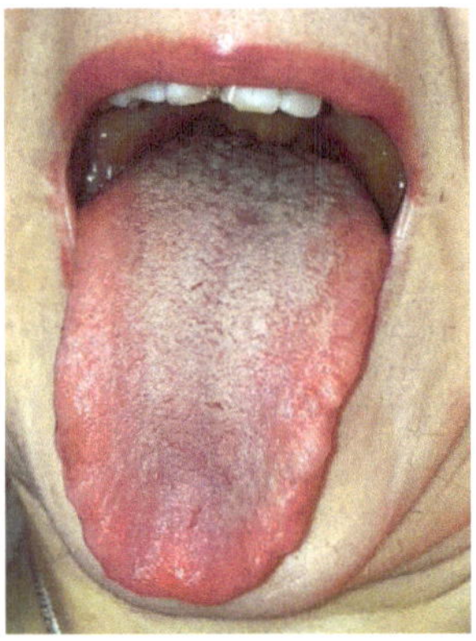

This patient presented with eczema. Wei Qi is trapped in the exterior.

When Wei Qi is chronically trapped in the exterior, the accumulating Heat consumes the local anatomy. After experiencing chronic eczema for many years, this patient presented to her practitioner with a diagnosis of multiple sclerosis. The tongue shows the history of intense redness that was at the edge of the tongue but, left untreated, was able to migrate to the Ying level, where it burned the flesh. The body responded with copious amounts of Dampness, which developed into Wind-Phlegm.

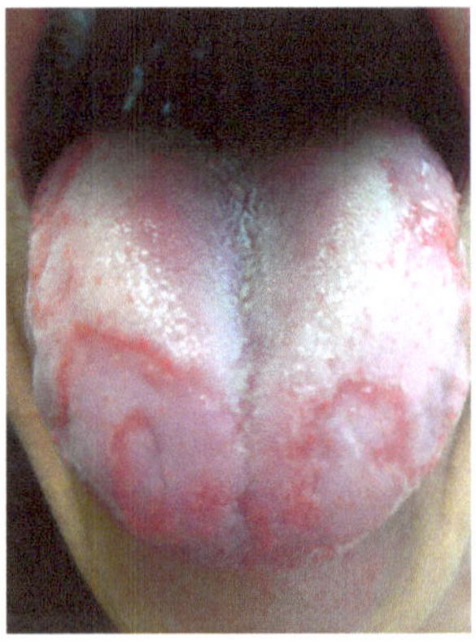

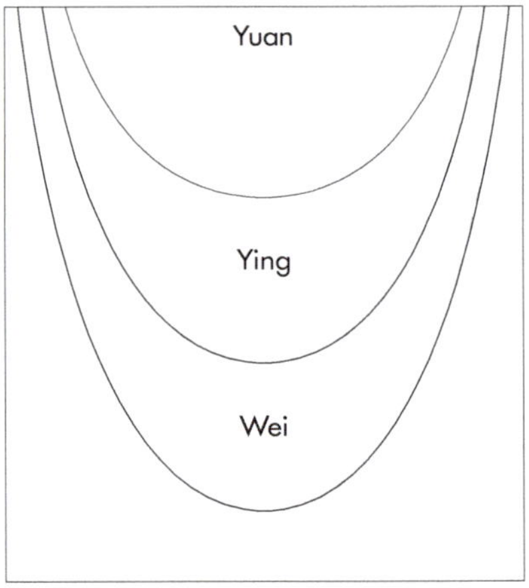

13
Wen Bing (Febrile Disease Theory) and the Tongue

When viewed through yet another lens, the tongue can show the four stages of the Wen Bing model of the Ming Dynasty, the last major tradition in Chinese Medicine. The basis of Wen Bing theory is that Heat is the originating pathogen. One can hardly blame the early Ming Dynasty practitioners for their belief that Heat must be pathological. The presentations of pestilent Qi (the Black Death) were terrifying and cruel. Pestilent Qi aside, with the advent of Wen Bing theory, a key fact disappeared from the medicine: Heat is a vital, crucial response to pathology. Most fevers are our friends, yet even today, fevers are seen as signs of impending grave illness. In the clinic, we find that it's important to differentiate between the Heat of pathology and the Heat that is clearly an appropriate response to pathology. The pulses will save the day again. If the deep and moderate pulses are rapid, it's time to clear Heat. If the pulses are only rapid at between one and six beans of pressure, it's likely Wei Qi is doing its job, acting against a pathogenic factor. Nourish Fluids and support it, then watch that it clears when healing is complete. Wen Bing theory is best used as emergency medicine for fast-progressing, highly infectious illness. The theory is divided into four stages: Heat in the Wei Level, Heat in the Qi Level, Heat in the Ying Level, and Heat in the Blood Level.

1. Heat in Wei Level

With Heat in the Wei level, the initial stage of response to so-called febrile disease, the patient experiences fevers and chills, aversion to Cold, thirst, headache, sore throat, cough, nasal congestion, and sinus inflammation. The pulses are floating and rapid.

Tongue: The tongue is red at the perimeter, all along the edges to the tip. As Wei Qi scatters to meet the invasion, a slightly yellow coat may form.

As the Wei level stage develops, complications of Dampness may arise including heaviness of the chest, nausea, and loss of appetite. Symptoms can be intermittent.

Tongue: At this point, the tongue may develop a thin, greasy coat, usually yellow but maybe white. The sides of the tongue become red.

Meanwhile, the pulse remains rapid and floating but becomes slippery.

2. Heat in Qi Level

At the Heat in Qi level stage, the pathogen has entered the interior. This would equate to Yang Ming in the channels in the Shang Han Lun tradition. Heat has become exuberant as Wei

Qi confronts the pathogen, creating fever. The patient has thirst, a bitter taste, aversion to Heat, dark urine, yellow mucus, hard stool, restlessness, diaphragmatic constraint, disturbed Shen, loud cough, rapid breathing, even wheezing or panting. They may present with a scorched odor. If the Heat is extreme enough, sweat may be absent. Not surprisingly, the pulse will be rapid and flooding, since Heat is exuberant and forceful.

Tongue: The tongue is deep red with a yellow coat, at least slightly greasy.

As the Qi level stage deepens, it becomes complicated as the body creates Dampness to stem Heat damage to tissues. This equates with the Shao Yang stage in the Shang Han Lun tradition. The patient experiences nausea, abdominal distention, difficult urination, diarrhea alternating with constipation, borborygmus, afternoon fever, chest oppression, lack of thirst, and Dampness in the chest. The pulse becomes wiry, rapid at both the moderate and deep levels.

Tongue: The tongue becomes dark red with greasy, yellow coat.

The Qi level stage can become further complicated as Heat consumes mediumship, leading to vacuity in the channels. There may be difficulty breathing, a cough with yellow phlegm, canker sores, and early internal Wind signs. The pulse becomes unpredictable, perhaps flooding and rapid or deep and rapid.

Tongue: The tongue becomes dark and quivering as Kidney Yin is consumed.

3. Heat in Ying Level

The next stage, Heat in the Ying level, is marked by fevers (high or low but worse at night). As the fevers progress, Yin is consumed and internal Wind manifests strongly as neurological signs, including seizures and tremors. There can also be insomnia, fibrosis, cough, and skin outbreaks (even necrosis). As Heat consumes Fluids and Blood and there are no resources to buffer the pathogen, fire toxins (free radicals) become rampant. The pulse is rapid and thin.

Tongue: The tongue is crimson or purple or dark red, peeled and rough-looking.

As the Heat in the Ying level stage worsens, more Damp responds to the extreme Heat. The Damp-Heat complex damages metabolic mechanisms, leading a variety of wasting scenarios including Wasting and Thirsting Syndrome (diabetes). The pulse is rough, thin, and rapid.

Tongue: The tongue body becomes dark due to damage to Fluids. The coat becomes thick, greasy, parched, sometimes brown.

4. Heat in Blood (Shen) Level

In the final stage of the Wen Bing model, Heat in the Blood or Shen level, hemorrhaging begins. Diseases such as Ebola are so rapid, so pestilent, they whip through the previous three stages and arrive in the fourth stage soon after the disease is contracted. This fourth stage has all the signs and symptoms of the third stage, but much more severe. Fevers at night are even worse, leading to severe insomnia and disturbed Shen, eruptions on the skin are now dark, bruised and purple, and there is reckless Blood (hemorrhaging). The pulse is thin, weak, rapid, rough, all due to extreme depletion of Yin.

Tongue: The tongue is dark purple, bruised-looking, bright and shiny, since the Qi that was managing Blood is seriously depleted. Yin is so depleted, there is no coat and the tongue can take on a luminescence as Yang escapes. The tongue may also be stiff, and protrusions can erupt all over the tongue.

As the Heat in the Blood level stage worsens, and both Yin and Yang are lost, Wind signs become extreme and deep depression sets in. If the body is able to create more Damp, depression can deepen to manic-depression. The pulse becomes rough and irregular. At this point, the disease is considered terminal.

Tongue: Ultimately, the tongue becomes pale and flaccid as Yang is consumed.

14
Step-by-Step Diagnosis

Make thorough observations before turning attention to diagnosis.

Observations on the Fly

If you're running short on time and you want to ensure the effectiveness of a brief treatment, focus on the moisture on the tongue. This is more important than the color of the coat or body, protrusions, the map, size, shape and posture. If the tongue is dry, moistening will be a chief strategy. If there is clumping of the coat, as you nourish Fluids, ensure their movement and ensure that the bowels are moving.

As a Chinese Medical practitioner, you are treating the individual, not the disease label. We're making a unique diagnosis for that individual. No two patients diagnosed with cancer, no two patients diagnosed with arthritis, no two patients diagnosed with hormone imbalances, no two patients with skin rashes are the same; the root cause is a unique combination of the factors you are analyzing in the tongue or the pulses. For one single Western diagnosis, the causes, when viewed through the lens of Chinese Medicine, could be any combination of countless of factors. This is what makes Chinese Medical diagnosis special—the absence of labels, seeing behind the symptoms, and deducing root causes. All diseases originate in a state of dehydration, not necessarily of water, but of wet food and fats. Tongue diagnosis focuses on tracking that dehydration, and the resulting Heat and Dampness. Your diagnosis, therefore, should focus on fluids first. Remember not to be seduced by the tongue map!

Below are step-by-step protocols arranged from very quick to more in-depth. Naturally, you'll treat according to your own training.

Step-by-Step Observations (Very Simple)

1. Does the tongue seems to have good Qi? Does it come out of the mouth and have good posture, or is it either floppy and overextended, or stiff and retracted?

2. Is the tongue moist?

Treatment: If retracted or flaccid, tonify Spleen Qi. If not moist, nourish Fluids.

3. Does the tongue stick out too far?

4. Is the tongue body red or purple?

Treatment: Clear Heat and nourish Fluids.

This very simple approach is not comprehensive but can be a starting point, since Spleen Qi and adequate Fluids are the cornerstone of health.

Step-by-Step Observations (Simple)

1. Note how far the tongue protrudes.
2. Note the posture of the tongue (how it sits).
3. Note the:
   a. moisture of the tongue coat
   b. color of the tongue coat
4. Note the:
   a. moisture of the tongue body
   b. color of the tongue body
5. Note the locations of:
   a. cracks
   b. coat
   c. color
   d. spots
   e. accumulations
   f. protrusions
6. Note the color and state of the sublingual veins.

Step-by-Step Observations (Complex)

Note:

1. Distance: how far and how quickly does the tongue move out? Does it:

    a. come out a long way?

    b. barely exit the mouth?

    c. stay within the confines of the mouth?

    d. dart out?

    e. emerge slowly?

2. Posture of the tongue (how it sits). Is it:

    a. turned under?

    b. turned up?

    c. stiff?

    d. flaccid?

    e. pointed sideways? Left or right?

3. Shape. Is it:

    a. narrow in general?

    b. narrowing anywhere across the tongue?

    c. narrow at the rear of the tongue?

    d. pointed at the tip?

    e. squared off at the tip?

    f. thickened anywhere?

4. Coat. Note the location of any of these qualities. Is the coat:

    a. moist?

    b. dry?

    c. thick?

d. patchy?

e. powdery?

f. absent?

g. color noteworthy? (white, yellow, brown, black, etc)

5. Body. Note the location of any of these qualities. Is the body:

    a. moist?

    b. dry?

    c. withered or atrophied?

    d. swollen?

    e. color noteworthy? (pink, red, translucent, purple, crimson, etc.)

    f. shape in general noteworthy?

6. Profile. When turned sideways, is it:

    a. swollen in the Upper Jiao?

    b. compressed in the Upper Jiao?

    c. swollen in the Middle Jiao?

    d. compressed in the Middle Jiao?

7. Note the location and depth of:

    a. vertical cracks

    b. horizontal cracks

8. Note the location of:

    a. spots

    b. accumulations

    c. petechiae, protrusions, thorns

    d. erosions, divots, missing flesh, pockets

9. Note the state and color of the sublingual veins. Are they:

a. swollen, protruded, sunken, or not visible?

b. red, purple, blue, pale, black, and so on?

10. Note locations of froth:

a. sides, front?

b. sticky, clinging to the palate?

Example of Observations

1. Unremarkable (Distance)
2. Very flaccid (Posture)
3. Narrow at rear (Shape)
4. Thick, greasy, dark yellow coat at rear, no coat on sides of tongue, thin yellow coat elsewhere (Coat)
5. Thin, pale purple, wet body, swollen in the middle (Body)
6. Compressed Upper Jiao in profile (Profile)
7. Very small horizontal cracks in the center (Cracks)
8. Petechiae (red) are present in the area between the Spleen and Liver areas (Spots)
9. Sublingual veins are slightly swollen (Sublingual veins)
10. No froth (Froth)

Example of the Related Diagnostic Thought Process

Note: The following considerations are best made in conjunction with pulse findings. If you feel you are not very skilled in pulse taking, or feel bewildered by them, please know it really is a skill you can acquire. The mythology about the difficulty of becoming confident and accurate in pulse reading is overstated and has no place in our profession. (See *The Art of Pulse Diagnosis.*) Additional note: I'm completing this book during the COVID-19 period and as mentioned in the first chapter, the tongue is holding up beautifully without pulses being available.

1. Unremarkable.
2. Very flaccid. *Is there a Yang deficiency? Qi Deficiency?*

3. Narrow at rear. *Are these deficiencies constitutional? Is there also a Yin deficiency? Is there a Dai Mai blockage? Are Qi and mediumship in the Middle Jiao being shared with the Lower Jiao? Is there profound dehydration affecting the intestines?*

4. Thick greasy yellow coat at rear, no coat on sides of tongue, simply wet elsewhere. *Is Damp-Heat accumulating in the Lower Jiao? Is it a response to the deficiency of Yin (and/or Blood)? Is the Yang deficiency disabling the movement of Fluids in the Lower Jiao? Is there a Liver Yin Deficiency resulting in no coat appearing on the sides of the tongue? Is there systemic Dampness leaving the tongue wet?*

5. Thin, pale purple, wet body, swollen in the middle. *Again, is the swelling and the wetness revealing systemic Damp that has accumulated due to a deficiency of Yang, since the tongue is pale and flaccid?*

6. Compressed Upper Jiao in profile. Is there a diaphragm blockage? *Is there Qi constraint in the Upper Jiao?*

7. Very small horizontal cracks in the center. *Is there dehydration? Are there insufficient Fluids in the Middle Jiao?*

8. Petechiae (red) are present between the Spleen and Liver areas. *Is there disharmony between Spleen and Liver? Is the Liver trying to support the Spleen because the Spleen has been weakened?*

9. Sublingual veins are slightly swollen. *Is Dampness beginning to affect the Yuan level?*

10. No froth. *The pathology has not yet resulted in enough depletion to cause internal Wind.*

Treatment Principles

Integrate your observations of the tongue with your pulses readings. Then integrate that combination with your clinical knowledge and intention.

Remember, one of the most important principles in Chinese Medicine is that the body does not make errors. In its ingenious way, the body keeps rearranging its resources, trying to hold on to these resources to ensure that pathology cannot reach the organs. The organs are the deepest level of the interior, precious gems that govern and preserve life. So most of what we see is simply a response to pathology; sorting out the difference is key to a successful treatment. Be sure you're positively treating (nourishing or tonifying) what the tongue is telling you is missing. Sometimes, of course, what you see is actual pathology. If the patient is eating a quart of ice cream in front of the television every night, and you see a thick cheesy coat and the pulses are slow and slippery, probably you are looking at pathological Damp. But if the patient is eating a quart of ice cream every night and the pulses are rapid at the deep level, they might be craving it simply to counter Heat at the Yuan level. The tongue in both cases might have a thick coat but there will be a deep red body in the second case. If you begin by clearing Damp in the first case, the treatment may be successful, but if you begin by clearing Damp in the second case, the Heat may become rampant and the condition will worsen. Steer clear of blind protocols. Take pulses carefully and really examine and think about what you see. If you are working remotely and cannot access pulses, it's okay as long as you look at all the parameters of the tongue. Allow enough time to take yourself through the diagnostic protocols above. Perhaps ask for a photograph in advance.

- If the cracks are transverse, the treatment principles must include moistening Dryness. Nourish Fluids.
- If there are swellings and cracks at the same time, moisten dryness and also nourish Yin so that the body stops accumulating Dampness (pathological fluid) in an attempt to hydrate itself.
- If the cracks are vertical, the treatment principles must include clearing Heat.
- If the tongue has many transverse (horizontal) cracks and there are also swellings, one must promote Yin to moisten Dryness and generate fluids so the body will clear Dampness. The patient must have ample Qi to accomplish this. If the tongue is pale, it can't be done. Tonify Qi if that's the case.
- If there is a coat, the practitioner can purge if needed. If there is no coat, purging is not possible. There must be available Yin to create a purge.
- If the pulses are floating in the Kidney positions, do not try to eliminate Dampness. If you do, the Heat will gain dominance since it would be unchecked, and Fluids would be further consumed. The Dampness is there as a perfect response to Heat. Clear the Heat but leave the Dampness response mechanism undisturbed. It will correct itself in most cases, once the body recognizes that the Heat to which it was responding has been cleared.
- If a patient enters a healing crisis—a situation where the body is trying to offload pathology—and there are insufficient Fluids to fund a purge (to take them all the way out to the exterior for eradication), the patient can enter into a state of serious autointoxication as the toxins are released from latency. The patient must have sufficient Fluids to sweat, urinate or defecate (or vomit). If these functions are not enabled, the patient's illness can deepen. Keep the routes of elimination freed; the bowels must be moving.
- If fire toxins (thorns) are present on the tongue, ensure there is not too much protein in the diet. A high protein diet will add enough Heat (Yang) to spread and add to the pathology.

15
Tongue Diagnosis and Dietary Therapy

By Andrew Sterman, author of *Welcoming Food: Diet as Medicine for the Home Cook and Other Healers* (Classical Wellness Press, 2020)

Diagnosis is the art of discerning from apparent signs what is happening hidden from view. Further, diagnosis is an application of what we know about how things work when functioning well, along with a familiarity with how things go awry. In other words, we diagnose through our working lens, or paradigm, while always aware that other perspectives are possible.

For example, a patient arrives (in person or remotely over video) and we investigate the tongue. We want to see not only which systems are strong and which are in disharmony, we also want to be able to see a history of dietary habits. Then we want to be able to recommend shifts in diet, small or large, either as a single presentation of recommendations or as a beginning of a series of supportive dietary changes.

The tongue is very responsive to internal changes. If the tongue presentation is consistent, or a patient reports, "My tongue always looks like that, it has for years," then we have to consider that the habitual diet and lifestyle is actively holding this individual in place. So often we eat to affirm and establish our character in the stance where we are comfortable, and that includes holding our pathologies in place through our dietary habits. In simple terms, our diet effectively locks us into the results of how that diet interacts with our health status as individuals.

There are nearly infinite details of tongue presentation to be considered with an eye for recommending dietary change for health improvement. It is very common that clinicians will view a tongue and quickly point to a few specific features, without assessing overall health status as it relates to diet. This is the common clinical approach. It can be much more helpful (and satisfying for both clinician and patient) to first assess overall health before placing details into the picture. This overview sets the stage for a more complete health and lifestyle picture (not simply "what is wrong"), and creates a more meaningful context for the dietary recommendations to come. In order to assess this big picture, the clinician will want to know how the patient's current diet is working for them, specifically regarding the three macronutrients: grains (carbohydrates, including sweets and sugar products), proteins (including animal foods, dairy, and beans), and oils (lipids, including dairy, nuts, cooking oils, and animal fats). To do this we look at the tongue body shape, tongue body color, and coat, respectively.

Tongue Body Shape

Assessing the size/shape of the tongue body gives us an overview of how an individual's digestion is handling grains and other carbohydrates. Although the Stomach and Pancreas-Spleen areas of the tongue are located in the central region of the tongue body, the overall size and shape of the tongue is meaningful in terms of how the individual is assimilating carbs from the diet. Can this person handle the carbs they are eating? Is this person assimilating enough from the diet to maintain fullness of flesh and fluids? Things to look for: swelling of the tongue body, thinness of the tongue body, scalloping of the sides of the tongue (imprints from the teeth).

Tongue Body Color

Assessing the color of the tongue body gives us an overview of how an individual is regulating Heat, especially heat or cold in the digestion. Redness all over can indicate that Heat has entered the blood level. Noticeable paleness shows that Blood is deficient, perhaps because digestive fire is insufficient to transform foods and assimilate blood building elements (including dietary iron). Cold in digestion (or elsewhere) can also have a pale appearance but more reliably appears as slightly dark areas, possibly hinting at blue.

Tongue Coat

Assessing the tongue's coat (or lack of coat) gives us an overview of how an individual is handling oils or fats in the diet. This requires actively applying theoretical understanding of how health changes over time. What we're seeing is in progress. Signs move and change as the body handles pathology. Resist the temptation to assign set treatments for symptoms in an absolutist way, outside of the profound awareness of change embodied in the fabric of classical Chinese Medicine. Looking at the tongue coat is important for assessing the individual's history of pathology.

Tongue and Diet Considerations

What follows below are a series of door-openings for finding meaningful associations between tongue presentations and digestion, with a basic guide to appropriate dietary recommendations. Often, what a patient should avoid is more important than what he or she should add. Remember, we may recommend foods, but people eat meals (and snacks). Our recommendations should include meal planning and even cooking tips. At the very least, we should be including advice on selecting grains (advising on carbs), vegetables, proteins, oils, and spices. Advice on snacking is also important, in order to be practical and address how our patients really live, offering changes they can willingly and successfully make.

Every acupuncture or herbal session should include dietary recommendations. Sometimes they are absolutely necessary for survival, other times they simply support the treatment and help ensure success of the healing strategy employed. And that's the point: our dietary recommendations should be fully integrated with our other therapies. It is possible to match specific strategies in diet to strategies being used in acupuncture, herbal medicine, or any other modality, rather than performing a sophisticated treatment only to offer dietary advice based on other paradigms altogether.

As with any series of "door-openings," take these recommendations as starting places to be explored in your own practice. And remember, food touches all levels of a person's life. Apply with a sensitive eye for ancestral background, current habits, emotional tenor, cooking skill, economic context, and, of course, accurate diagnosis, supported by tongue presentation.

Finding: Swollen tongue body

Interpretation: Spleen Qi is not successfully transforming carbs in the diet, causing stagnation. Location of swellings can add information on focus of stagnation.

Recommendations to Consider:

- Eliminate glutinous grains (wheat, barley, rye, but especially modernized wheat)
- Increase non-glutinous whole grains to move and clear stagnation (e.g., millet, brown rices, buckwheat, oats)
- Regular inclusion of spices that aid in digestion of grains (rosemary, oregano, fennel seed, cumin, caraway, coriander seed, cardamom, nigella, etc.) as well as spices to warm digestion (fresh ginger, turmeric, cinnamon, etc.)
- Look honestly at sugar consumption. Deliberate or hidden sugar consumption can significantly disrupt digestion of otherwise healthy grains. Abstaining from all grains may be necessary for a time.
- Assess for SIBO. If present, abstain from all sugar and most grains while rebuilding microbiota through gradual introduction of varied fiber foods, fermented foods, and if desired, pre-and probiotics.
- Assess alcohol use (alcohol is fermented from sugar and functions similarly to concentrated sugar in the system).

Finding: Narrow tongue body

Interpretation: Spleen and Stomach not able to digest and assimilate substance from diet. Inability to absorb and assimilate Yin.

Recommendations to Consider:

- Assess what factors in diet and lifestyle are draining Yin and/or over-firing Yang.
- Build Yin (slowly) with nuts, seeds, shellfish (clams, mussels, scallops, abalone, those which do not turn red when cooked as do lobster, shrimp, crab, which should be avoided).
- Homemade nut/seed milks are excellent to build Yin.
- Grains also build Yin, especially as congee and porridges.
- Soups, stews, wet-cooked dishes. Wet-cooked foods are easier to digest and assimilate.
- Add digestive spices and kitchen herbs to solve specific problems of digestion. The narrow tongue is usually indicative of problems assimilating carbs; add spices into various dishes to aid carb digestion: fennel seed, cumin, nigella seed, caraway seed, cardamom, coriander seed, star anise, rosemary, oregano, basil, dill, shiso, mint, and more. Sprouts of all types also strongly aid digestion of carbohydrates.

Finding: Thinness at the back. Ideally, tongues remain full all the way back.

Interpretation: Indicates Yin deficiency in the lower burner, including gonadal hormones.

Recommendations to Consider:

- Foods with healthy oils: avocado, coconut, oily fish (salmon, sardines, mackerel, herring, black cod, and other cold water fish).
- Healthy kitchen oils: olive oil, butter, nut/seed oils. Avoid overly processed commercial oils.
- Include eggs, nuts, seeds.

Finding: Tongue Body shows red color

Interpretation: Heat in the blood is showing in the tongue. Uneven locations of brighter redness indicate greater specificity of where heat is located (usually toward the tip; how that appears is significant).

Recommendations to Consider:

- Reduce meat consumption.
- Reduce stimulants that raise heat: coffee, alcohol, chocolate, hot spices, garlic, onion, and nightshades.
- Use more stable oils such as olive oil, butter, and saturated fat, rather than the more reactive polyunsaturated fats.
- More green vegetables will strongly help clear excess heat.
- Add more Yin-building foods (congee, porridges, soups, stews, rice, millet, amaranth, barley, clams, mussels, mushrooms, seaweeds).
- Add more bitter vegetables, as the bitter taste strongly cools and drains ascending fire (dandelion greens, radicchio, endive, chicory greens, escarole, broccoli rabe, etc.)
- Sprouts strongly help cool excess heat.
- Root vegetables help bring down heat.
- Mint tea opens the exterior that can help vent heat to relax the Heart, useful if redness appears more at the tip.

Finding: Pale tongue body

Interpretation: Blood Deficiency casts a pale color into the tongue body.

Recommendations to Consider:

- Stomach Fire may be too low; add more warming spices (cinnamon, nutmeg, ginger, turmeric, rosemary, oregano, cumin, mustard seed, cardamom, etc. Avoid hot spices, although black pepper may be used.)
- Cooking with vinegars can raise Stomach Fire (sufficient stomach fire is necessary for assimilation of dietary iron and the building of rich blood.)
- Gradually increasing red meats can help build blood.
- Vegetarian Blood-building foods include beets (beetroot), blueberries, raspberries, black berries, goji berries, black beans, adzuki beans, red lentils, and dark leafy greens.

Finding: Dry tongue

Interpretation: Thin fluids are not available from Stomach, or not being ascended by Pancreas-Spleen Yang Qi.

Recommendations to Consider:

Water is essential, but too often water passes quickly through the body. What we need is to slow hydration to increase assimilation of fluids. With this in mind, wet-cooked foods can be more beneficial for hydration than water alone.

- Congee, porridges, oatmeal (cooked somewhat wetter than most do), polenta/grits (without cheese or hot spices). All grains can make excellent porridges for breakfast, late night eating, or through convalescence.
- Soups, stews. The water cooked into stews and soups is released gradually during digestion.
- Steamed rice, millet, etc. These grains are moistening; steaming is the cooking method that best supports stomach and pancreas-spleen, together the distribution hub for fluids.
- Healthy oils are essential as part of overall hydration: olive oil, butter, nut oils, seed oils (all good quality if at all possible), avocado, coconut, eggs, gently cooked fish and meats. Shellfish and cold-water oily fish are particular good sources of dietary oils from the animal food side.

Finding: Midline crack

Interpretation: The midline crack indicates an overheating of Stomach and digestion, either from overly spicy foods, or, more commonly, from excess worrying and thinking.

Recommendations to Consider

- Consider reducing meats.
- Reduce or eliminate foods that stoke stomach fire, including: garlic, onion, chili peppers, coffee, chocolate, nightshades, and alcohol.
- Add or increase foods that clear heat: green vegetables, root vegetables, well-cooked grains, small beans, sprouts of all types, mushrooms, seaweeds, fish and seafood (avoiding seafood that turns red when cooked such as shrimp, crab,

lobster).

- Add Yin-building foods such as congee, soups, stews.

Finding: Horizontal Cracks

Interpretation: Horizontal cracks are usually signs of dehydration.

Recommendations to Consider:

- Develop a water practice; warm water first thing in morning and regularly through the day.
- Include porridges, congee, etc.
- Include steamed rice, millet, oats, polenta.
- Include more soups and stews.
- Avoid foods that stoke stomach fire and consume stomach fluids: garlic, onion, chili peppers, coffee, chocolate, nightshades, and alcohol.
- Rely on plain water and wet-cooked foods rather than non-hydrating drinks such as tea, coffee, alcohol, herbal tea, carbonated water or drinks, etc.

Finding: Wet or Sticky tongue

Interpretation: Sugars or oils are not being digested/transformed well enough.

Note: A wet or sticky tongue, or even a thick coat, can appear to increase or appear where there was none when a person starts a cleansing diet or healing protocol. As dampness clears internally, a new or thickened coat often enough appears on the tongue. Don't be surprised; continue through the healing process.

Recommendations to Consider:

Sugar is such a concentrated simple carb that the tongue coat quickly shows a response indicating something from within, usually as a wetness, sometimes glistening, and sometimes sticky.

- Have sugar-free days, saving the sweet taste for several times a week only, or less.
- Have sweets or desserts only after meals digest at least for a good duration,

between 30 minutes and 2 hours.

- Add sprouts to your diet to aid digestion of sugar.
- Be honest about snack sugar and hidden sugar, even in "healthy" foods, especially store-bought things.

Excess oils can also bring a presentation of shiny or oily tongue. Through experience and hearing a patient's story it is usually possible to discern the role of sugar and oils, knowing where to focus (it may be a combination).

- Avoid fried foods; instead, add a drizzle of olive oil (or other healthy fat) on vegetables, grains, or animal foods when serving. Too much heat denatures oils.
- Add spices that aid digestive success with oils and fatty foods in order to gain the benefits of healthy oils without their potential drawbacks: fresh dill, cilantro, parsley, fermented foods, radishes, seed spices such as mustard seed, cumin, coriander, cardamom (especially black cardamom), and more.

Finding: Thick coat, white or yellow

Interpretation: Response to heat or Yin-deficiency is causing the internal body to gather pathological Yin. If the tongue coat is yellow, long-standing heat has been present along with dampness.

Recommendations to Consider:

- Before enacting clearing strategies, satisfy the body's need to gather Yin by providing Yin-nourishing foods, as listed above (grains, greens, seaweeds, nuts, seeds, mushrooms, eggs, shellfish, porridges, etc.)
- Once satisfied, clear pathological Yin through avoiding dairy, sugar, and gluten. Also avoid irritating foods that elicit a protective response within: onions, garlic, hot spices, alcohol, coffee, chocolate, nightshades. Avoid personal allergens or irritants.
- Consider separating proteins from carbs, to create clear meals that digest better and avoid internal fermentation.
- Gradually and steadily add more fiber to rebuild the microbiome and clear food stagnation (bitter greens help here, too).
- Add more fermented foods to aid digestion and gain control of the microbiome.

Finding: White or yellow coat gathering in the front or the back, or along the center line, or bumpiness growing on the back.

Interpretation: Locations of stagnation are being identified. Bumpiness in the back indicates sluggish and insufficient clearing of toxins from the lower belly, perhaps along with hormonal deficiency.

Recommendations to Consider:

- Congestion in the upper burner indicates more need of green vegetables such as bok choy, collard, kale, and Napa cabbage.
- Cook with fresh ginger and scallions to help clear lungs and lymphatic system (bok choy sautéed with slivered ginger is a strong example dish for clearing the lymphatic system).
- Aromatic spices help clear stickiness and phlegm from the upper burner: mint, shiso, tarragon, sage, dill, parsley, cilantro, cumin, coriander, cardamom, black cardamom, etc.)

Finding: Bumpiness or thorns in the back of the tongue

Interpretation: Problems of toxins in the Lower Jiao. Improve the microbiome, resolve food stagnation, clear constipation, and attend to conglomerations in lower burner.

Recommendations to Consider:

- Follow advice listed previously for clearing stagnation and congestion with vegetables and aromatic spices.
- Strongly reduce sugar, irritants, and dairy, while also increasing fiber and root vegetables to aid clearing.

Finding: Lack of coat (naked "raw meat" appearance)

Interpretation: Spleen Yang Qi isn't bringing enough Yin upward to the chest; this is reflected on the tongue by profound lack of normal protective coat.

Recommendations to Consider:

First, hydrate and nourish Yin, then support ascension. Diet will vary based on further specifics of diagnosis.

- Warming spices help transportation of nourishment: cinnamon, ginger, turmeric, cumin, clove, nutmeg, rosemary, oregano, mustard seed, more.
- Sprouts and spring greens (eaten any time of year) stimulate ascension, e.g., asparagus, pea shoots, cooked bean sprouts.
- Steaming supports Spleen, but more ascension is needed here. Pair steamed grains with sautéed asparagus or other vegetables, with warming spices.

Finding: Abnormal sublingual veins

Interpretation: Swollen sublingual veins indicate stagnation of blood circulation. Causes can include Spleen Yang Qi deficiency resulting in insufficient blood transport, Liver Qi stagnation and Heat, Heart Heat and Luo Channel issues.

The sublingual veins also offer another look at the status of Yuan Qi; the sublingual veins and the back of the tongue offer two glimpses of the lower burner, providing insight into progression of conditions.

Recommendations to Consider:

To work with conditions of the Lower Jiao, be aware of nourishing Yin before clearing conglomerations and accumulations.

- Congee and porridges are important for ease of digestion and the contribution of fluids. Be sure to include healthy oils (toasted sesame oil, eggs, etc.)
- Whole grains help clear accumulations from the bowels. Cook brown rice, oats, wild rice, bulgur wheat, and others, with plenty of olive oil or other healthy oil.
- Nuts and seeds nourish the Lower Jiao while also clearing accumulations through their oils and fiber. Add pumpkin and sunflower seeds to grain dishes, and include walnuts (best served after soaking over night then drying in the oven set to lowest possible temperature for an hour or two).
- Mushrooms drain dampness and strengthen the lower burner.
- Seaweeds resonate at the Lower Jiao level and also help clear accumulations and conglomerations.
- Root vegetables are important for clearing the lower intestines and improving energy there.
- Shellfish can powerfully nourish the Kidneys and the Lower Jiao. For Kidney

Yin, have clams, mussels, oysters, abalone: the shellfish that does not turn red when cooked. For Kidney Yang, first nourish Kidney Yin, then judiciously add the shellfish that do turn red when cooked: shrimp/prawns, crab, and lobster.

- Spices are very important to help uplift Spleen Yang Qi that is suffering from lack of contribution from Kidney Yang Qi and the Lower Jiao (rosemary, oregano, tarragon, sage, chive, scallion, fresh ginger, etc.) Spices used well (and not overused) are also very important for freeing the circulation of stagnated blood (important for clearing conglomerations) including turmeric, ginger, cumin, cardamom, star anise, cinnamon, saffron, and vanilla.

From this brief guide, the clinician can extrapolate dietary recommendations for all the varied tongue presentations in this book, and in the clinic. The main point here is that dietary change is essential for real and sustained systemic change.

16
Cases

Case 1

I'm presenting this tongue as an example of the life-preserving mechanism of accumulation of pathological Dampness in a last-ditch attempt to buffer a pathogen. This woman's Western diagnosis was fourth stage liver cancer metastasized to the lungs, breast, large intestine, brain, and bone. The pulses suggested that the initial pathogen might in fact have been in the Lungs, however, and that it had metastasized to the breast and Large Intestine, then Liver, then Gallbladder and the rest of the Curious Organs because the Lung pulse was at 14 beats per breath and the others' significantly slower. It's hard to say. Clearly, looking at the left side of her tongue, the Gallbladder was very taxed, trying to assist the Liver in its management of Blood and eradication of toxicity. Regardless of the chronology of the disease, her body was trying to gather any Fluid and Phlegm it could, to buffer the pathogen (fire toxins) since the Divergent mechanism was exhausted through the complete consumption of Yin, Yin it would normally call upon to contain the pathogen. It was essential, therefore, not to drain any of this Dampness. Her brief to me was to relieve pain and a wish to have a painless death. As you can see (it's not just the light), the tongue is very shiny. This is a sign of Yang escaping, which it will do if there is no Yin to anchor Yang down. There are also Chong rails evident here since the constitution is deeply affected. While the Eight Extra channels can be used in the treatment of fire toxins, her treatment involved Triple Heater Divergent Channel to ask the digestive tract to generate more Fluids so that Fluids could be spared to nourish the Sinews to relieve pain. After that was achieved, I did a scar treatment on several major scars up to fourteen inches long crisscrossing her abdomen. She did get her wish for a painless death soon after this photograph was taken.

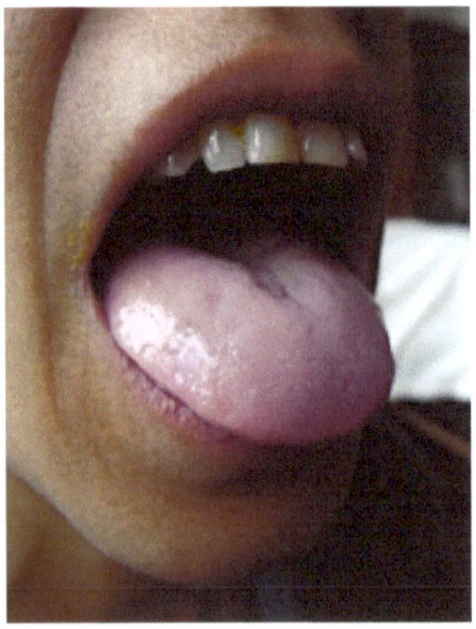

Case 2

This patient presented with Western diagnoses of eczema, psoriasis, and also complained of excessive thinking and an inability to sit still. His regular diet included onion, garlic, chicken, and, for many years, daily cold smoothies. The tongue shows consumption of Qi by Heat and the resulting weakness of Spleen Qi. The narrowing of the rear of the tongue shows depletion of constitutional Qi. Thorns in the Lower Jiao are either accumulations of indigestible dietary matter or they're pathological accumulations of Dampness gathered to lessen the impact of Heat on the Jing-Essence. The Spleen is very depressed, possibly due to the cold smoothies. Yet the entire tongue is deep red, showing systemic inflammation due to Heat further complicated by garlic, onion, and too much chicken. The digestive tract is unable to process the food due to the extinguished Stomach Fire. This creates inflammation in the digestive tract as Wei Qi identifies material in the gut that is not absorbable. The inability to sit still is resulting from an accumulation of this Wei Qi Heat; Wei Qi is always ready to move. Constraint arises as the Liver seeks to bolster the Spleen, rendering the Liver unable to relax the diaphragm, causing a visible swelling in the anterior third of the tongue. The region of the Small Intestine shows an inability to separate pure from impure and difficulty with elimination. The rear of the tongue is dramatically narrowed as Heat is affecting the constitution.

The second photo, taken after one treatment shows much less swelling, with a strengthened Spleen. The resulting lessening of turbidity shows in the Small Intestine region at the rear of the tongue. The width of the rear of the tongue will take much longer to shift.

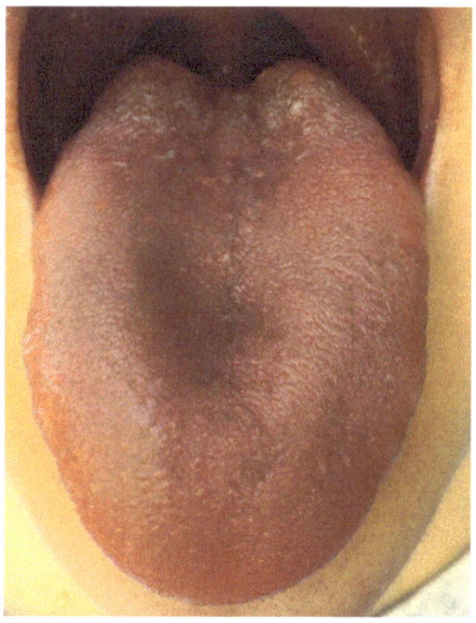

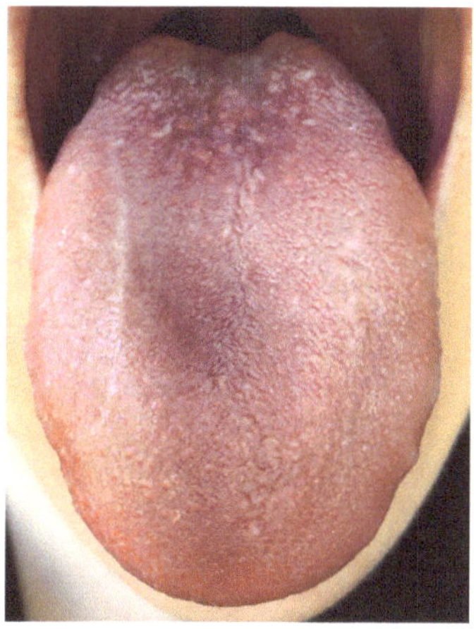

Case 3

This tongue is a good example of consumption and exhaustion of Yang Qi due to Heat resulting in a very pale and blue tongue. The patient has exhausted his Blood through alcoholism, especially the consumption of hard liquor, also known as "fire water." Whatever he was trying to avoid using alcohol is no longer suppressible, since Blood is exhausted. Blood normally provides a buffer for the emotions but this has been eroded hence this patient experiences extreme anger and rage.

This scenario has put pressure on Fluids, making the patient profoundly dehydrated, as seen in the wrinkles at the medial border of the Lung and Gallbladder regions. The Liver, constantly strained with daily intoxication, has been unable to store Blood. The tongue would have appeared much tighter along the edges at one point, but now, as Yang is depleted, the ability to astringe Blood is waning and the accumulation of Damp in lieu of Blood is swelling the sides of the tongue. This creates the illusion of plentitude, but is simply a response to the deficit.

The main complaint is "painful reflux." The tongue is discernibly blue. Remember that in tongue diagnosis, we're thinking about Yang exhaustion, resulting in Cold, rather than the introduction of Cold itself. I would argue that the hard liquor that he only drank "on ice" was a contributor to the Cold. Cold draws into the center, and in this tongue we can see the Qi gathered into a large region, pushing the center of the tongue up. A large bulging tightness at the rear of the tongue reveals defense of the Lower Jiao against further cold invasion, since Cold naturally wants to sink. The result is that Qi is pushing upward in reflux. The fact that the Liver is tight from alcohol abuse compounds this reflux since Wei Qi (controlled by the Liver) is unable to move downward in the gut. The Stomach is unable to descend due to the compounding constraint of Cold. The constriction itself is painful, but so is Cold. There is also an echo of tightness in the Upper Jiao, showing as pale petechiae. Moxa was a feature of the treatments to tonify Yang. Then the belt channel relaxed and his symptoms disappeared, all within the few weeks of treatment during which he stopped alcohol consumption and adopted a warm diet.

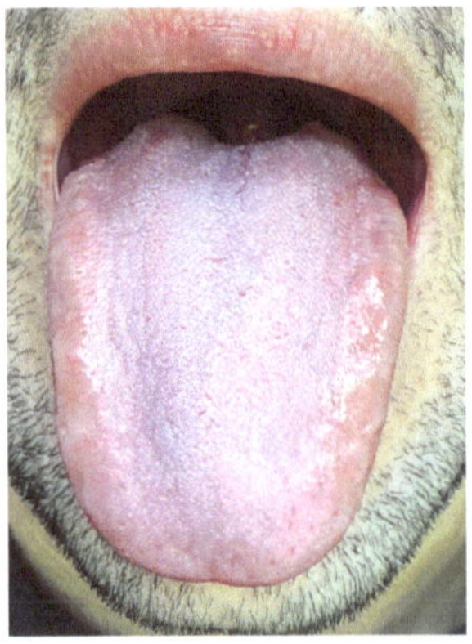

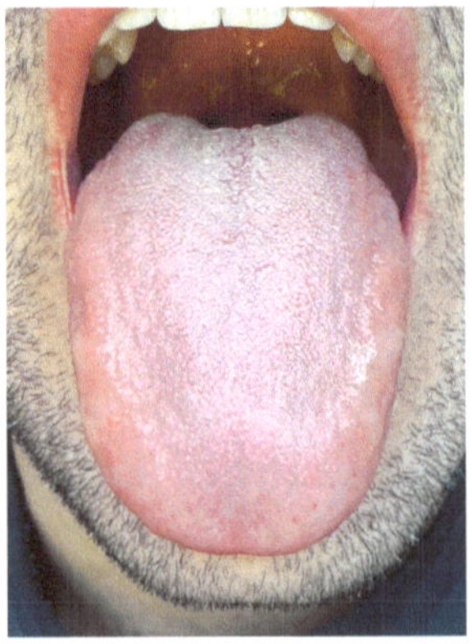

Case 4

This person suffers depression, deep fatigue, Cold, and a sense of the world being unsalvageable. This tongue reveals a tendency to extreme privacy in that it is very short. The Lower Jiao cannot be revealed, as the mouth cannot be enticed to open, although the tongue protrudes a little further as the patient engages in trust. Tension in the Pericardium region is evident in the impression of a horseshoe-shaped depression. The cracks in the Lung region are diagonal, indicating both dehydration through Heat and through loss or erosion of Yin. Sadness shows, since the focus of these cracks is at the meeting of the Lung and Heart regions. The patient reports that she is disenchanted with the world, feels things with great intensity, and always "takes things to heart." She then suffers from the effects of overreacting. The dramatically collapsed sublingual area indicates collapse of Kidney Yang. This in turn has taxed Spleen Qi, leading to pain following meals and poor digestion.

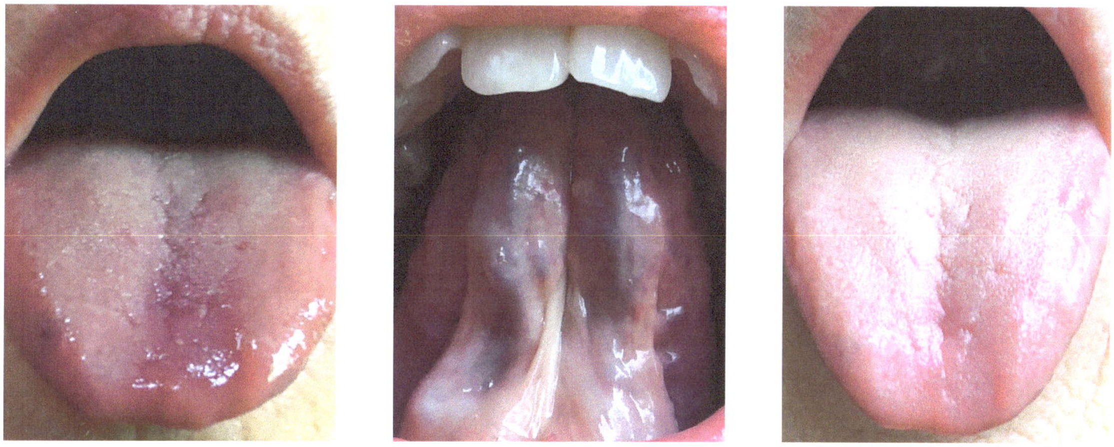

Case 5

This tongue shows the expression of extreme long term Heat manifesting as rage. The rear of the tongue—ideally the widest part of the tongue, is very narrow. In this case, this shows extreme consumption of Jing as a result of a twenty-year pornography addiction, now resolved. Loss of Jing resulted in Yang escaping, causing rage. Yang is expressing in the digestive tract, in the Lungs, and as dermatitis via the Lungs. The cracks in the Lung region show damage to the Lungs due to dehydration. Compensation for the loss of Yin is seen as an accumulation of pathological Yin (Phlegm) in the Lower Jiao.

It's difficult to see in the photo, but the tongue points to the right and the jaw is also torqued to the right. The patient was treated once with Yang Qiao Mai, and the face and tongue shifted dramatically and became aligned. The Gallbladder and Liver regions are inflamed and constrained, tensing the diaphragm, forcing Heat to accumulate in the Middle Jiao. The sides are also moist, indicating Damp-Heat in the Liver and Gallbladder. This may be due to alcohol or fried food consumption. The Heat, trapped in the Middle Jiao and unable to rise, seeks alternative vents in the Lower Jiao, showing as a fork in the crack as the crack enters the Lower Jiao. The initial treatment of Yang Qiao Mai created much relief, released and realigned the jaw, and dissipated the rage.

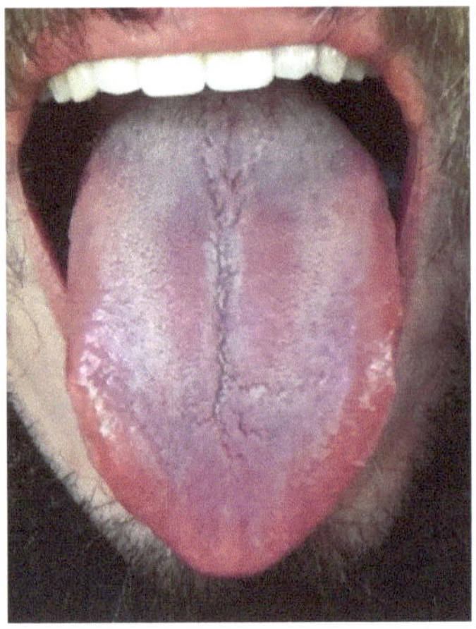

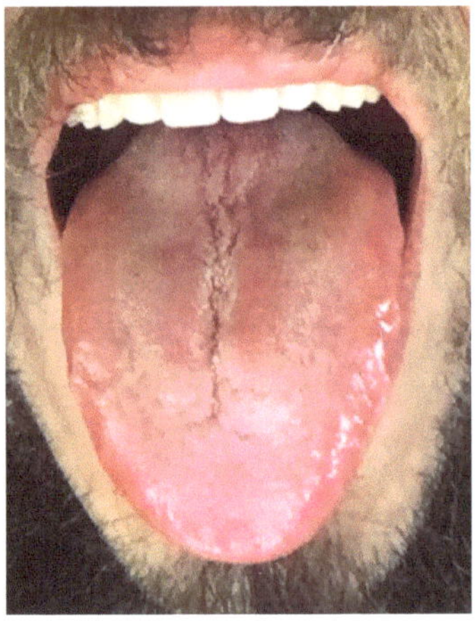

Case 6

This tongue belongs to a young woman with bleeding sigmoid colon and rectum, which began with the taking of medications for upset stomach. Prior to treatment, the bleeding would be copious, daily. The photo is not an illusion; the midline of the tongue is curved and sits in a long, wide channel. I interpret this as a Chong Channel tongue. Long-term sexual abuse, the trauma of which was compounded by the inaction of those around her, has distorted Chong Mai. The rails we might expect to see in a Chong tongue are visible in the front third of the tongue, but separated more than we usually see, because Chong is in a challenged state as it tries to buffer the chronic insult to the constitution. Anger, causing a crimping in the sides of the midsection of the tongue, is being suppressed by the Mind—as can be seen in the Spleen region, where the curve is most dramatic. Where the tongue is crimped, it also has a translucent quality, since Blood is very deficient. The entire tongue is very small and is about half the width of the mouth from corner to corner, echoing the dramatic Blood deficiency due to loss and emotional strain. Stomach Divergent treatments stopped the bleeding within three weeks, before we moved onto Yin Wei Mai to treat the trauma.

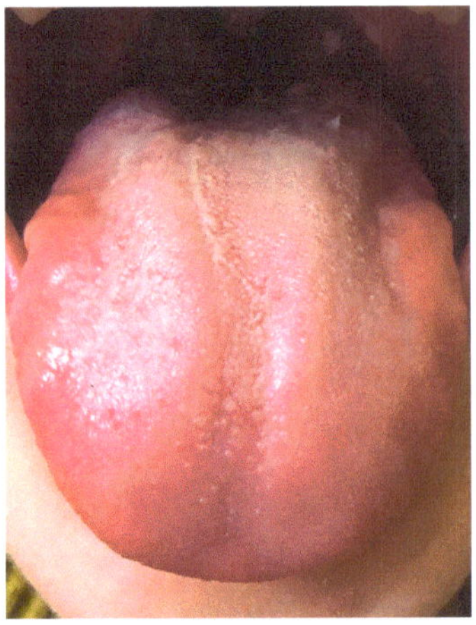

Case 7

The patient experienced a spontaneous pneumothorax soon after the unexpected break-up of a relationship. The surgery intended to repair the injury was unnecessarily invasive, involved malpractice, and caused further damage. The patient's main complaint is great tightness in the solar plexus, at the lower ribs, and at GB-22. All these areas show as compromised on the tongue. Inflammation is evident in redness and swelling in the areas reflecting the Lungs, the sides of the chest, and the solar plexus at the junction of the Spleen and Lung regions. The strings of petechiae between the Spleen and Liver regions indicate their disharmony. Petechiae in the Heart region suggests inflammation is trapped in the Upper Jiao. Some tongue flesh is actually missing in the Lung region. The tightness in the diaphragm is graphically reflected at the diaphragm regions of the sides of the tongue. The body is trying to push the inflammation from the surgery up and out. At the same time, the patient is questioning his decisions, causing more disruption in the smooth flow of Qi in the Liver and Gallbladder Channels.

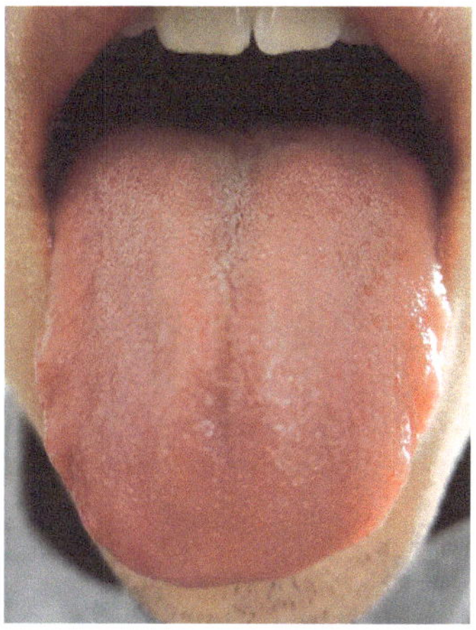

Case 8

This patient presented with a thirty-year history of opiate use for chronic low back pain. Opiates dehydrate and even desiccate the gut, slowing it down, resulting in constipation, gas, and indigestion. In the center of the tongue we see exactly that: the area is gathered and pursed and dry, as the Spleen, Pancreas, and Stomach struggle to acquire Fluids. The tongue is shrunken, not meeting the width of the mouth; the capacity to create mediumship in the Middle Jiao is severely compromised. His blood pressure was very high due to the inability to anchor Yang down to the Lower Jiao which clearly is depleted since it narrows toward the rear. Hence Heat has not just accumulated in the Upper Jiao (seen in the red petechiae), it is trapped there by the Cold in the Middle Jiao, showing as a pale area where the Upper and Middle Jiaos meet. (A daily ice cream habit, recently ceased, and beer and fried food were reduced.) Treatment focused on acquiring and assimilating fluids.

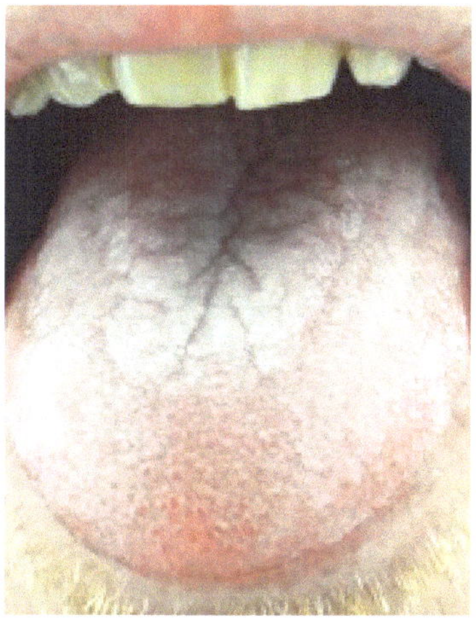

Case 9

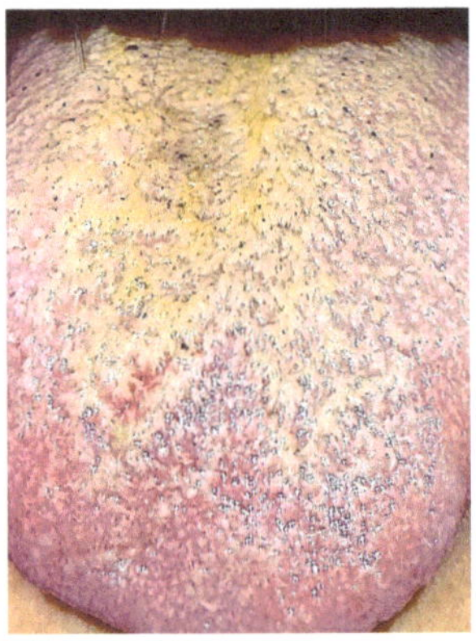

Fire toxins, (known in Western medicine as pre-cancer or cancer) often show on the tongue as white thorns or white exudation. These pictures show extreme fire which has damaged the constitution. I was asked to help this patient remotely, but in the end she declined treatment as she elected not to speak any more. Remember that the sublingual area not only reflects the constitutional level, but also what was overtaxing the organs. In other words, ultimately, pathology that cannot be contained in arenas of latency can then penetrate the Yuan-Source (constitutional) level where it can corrupt essence (including DNA). The photograph of the top of the tongue shows extreme Heat. The body responded to this Heat with Dampness, creating Damp-Heat. This created tremendous strain on the Liver. Although I didn't receive much information about the patient, it seems clear to me that the tongue cancer originated in the Liver, since the lesion on the tongue is directly under the Liver region. The spread of pathology can be seen in many ways on the tongue. First, the sublingual area is affected, even to the floor of the mouth where the Spleen Channel, the Kidney Channel, and the Heart Luo all attach. But more dramatic is the prevalence of tiny white thorns peeking through the yellow dampness. White thorns (fire toxins) peeking through all over the tongue is a reflection of complete cancer metastasis. In treatment we would be looking at the fifth confluence of the Divergent Channels to try to reestablish latency. The diet would have to change radically. Later I heard that the patient did indeed have a long history of eating the major inflamers: garlic, onion, sugar, hot spices, chocolate, caffeine, hard liquor. Perhaps she also consumed nightshades to excess, including tobacco.

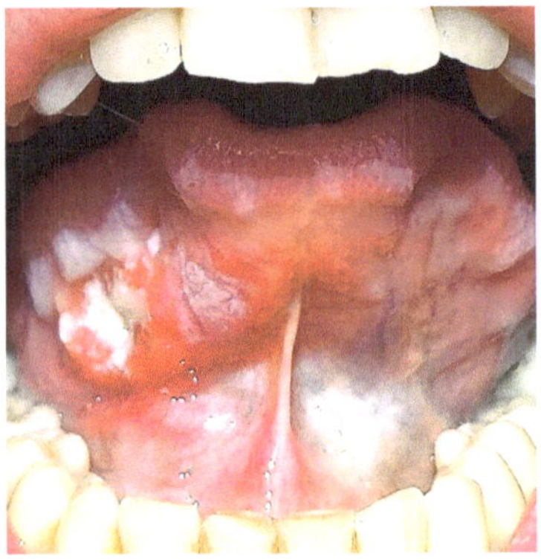

Case 10

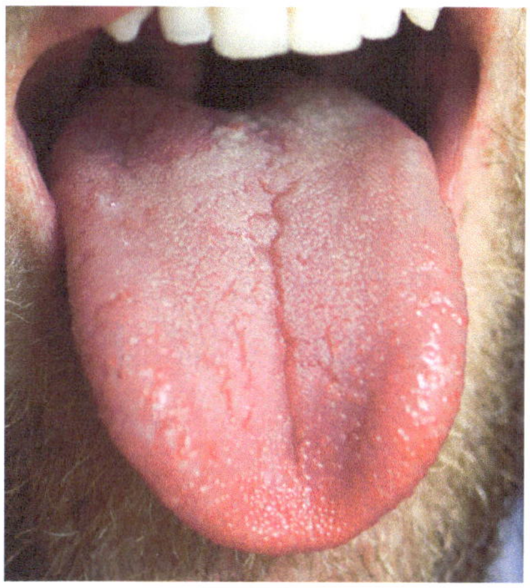

This twenty-nine year-old male patient of a student had debilitating, chronic allergies, obsessive-compulsive issues, depression, and injured self-esteem. The tongue shows great inflammation in the Upper Jiao and a compression of the Heart region—the tip is pinched flat. The edge of the tongue is redder than anywhere else, showing that Wei Qi is overactive on the exterior. The substantial midline crack extends all the way to the Heart as worry affects the Upper Jiao. Heart and Kidneys each show a depression and, given the Heat accumulated in the Upper Jiao, are likely not communicating, causing anxiety. The center of the tongue is very dry; the Middle Jiao is unable to produce adequate fluids. Hence, the Lungs in turn are drying out. Pulses showed no ascension from Spleen to Lungs, a Yin Qiao Mai pulse on the right and a Dai Mai pulse on the left. Treatment involved ascending the Spleen, bleeding ST-40 to release Heat, and consolidating Dai Mai for stabilization. The allergies improved dramatically.

Case 11

This ten year-old boy suffered from stuttering. His tongue was withdrawn when I asked him to show it, and when I asked him to extend it, it appeared stiff and with very defined curves at the diaphragm and at Dai Mai. Liver constraint had trapped Heat in the Upper Jiao, causing anxiety and compromised confidence.

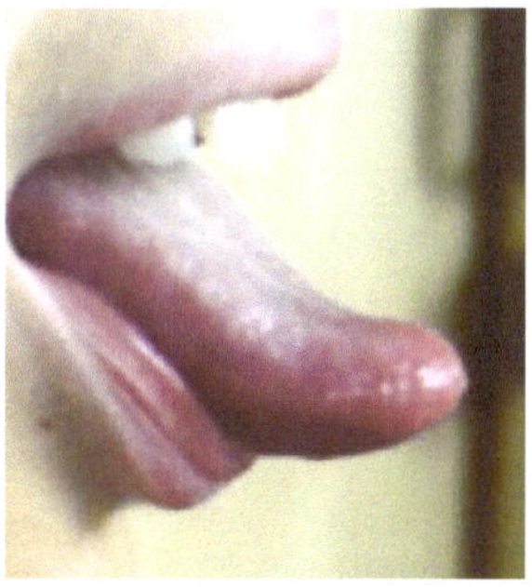

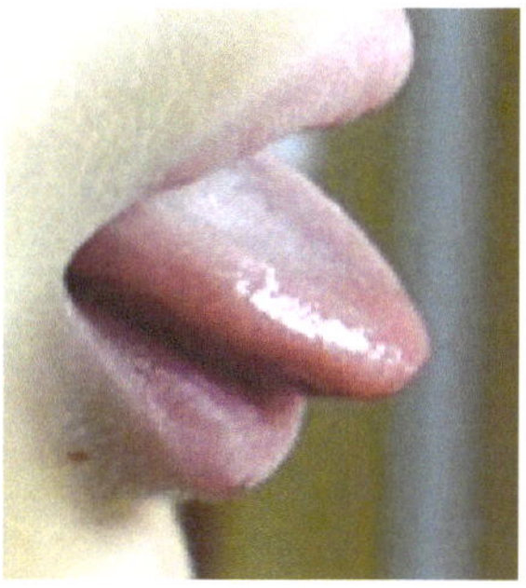

The second photo, taken twenty minutes later, shows the tongue relaxed after bleeding and moxaing HT-5 during a Luo treatment for stuttering and other speech issues.

Case 12

This patient arrived in considerable pain in the hip (the tongue is pulled to one side), vertigo (the tongue is frothy), overthinking (substantial midline crack), and with compromised self-esteem from missing out on an important job he wanted (the tongue is withdrawn).

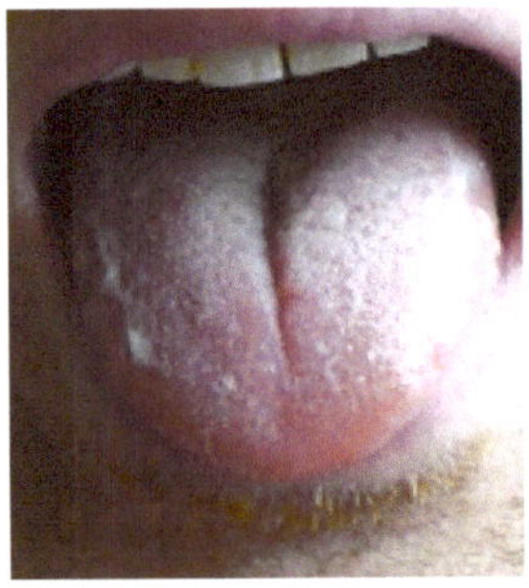

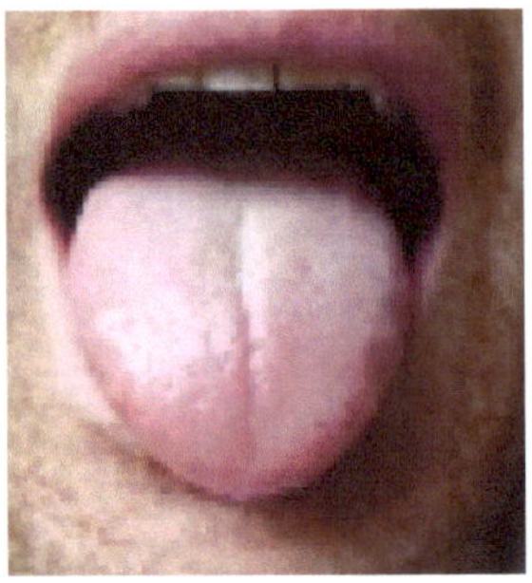

The second photo, taken forty-five minutes later after a Yin Qiao Mai treatment, shows the tongue returned to its natural length, the tongue crack relaxed and the froth cleared.

Case 13

This patient has a cholesterol reading of 455. Cholesterol-lowering drugs bring it down to about 300 and severely impact her memory. Excess cholesterol manifests as Damp-Heat, and this shows in the thick, slimy tongue coat. The pallor of the tongue shows a chronic Blood deficiency. The severe tightness, especially at the right side, shows the Liver constraint as it tries valiantly to accrue Blood while being given a signal from the drug not to create cholesterol. The patient wakes at three a.m., since the Liver is unable to satisfactorily connect with LU-1, showing as stress in the Lung region. The Jue Yin pair of the Liver—the Pericardium—is constrained, causing the tongue to curl upward at the tip. The strain and Heat evident in the Gallbladder pushes the tongue far forward, stretching it out, so much so that there is a convergence (cross-eyed) issue in the eyes. All symptoms were alleviated with Gallbladder and Liver Divergent courses with deep-superficial-deep needling technique. The convergence issue cleared completely from the eyes with the first treatment.

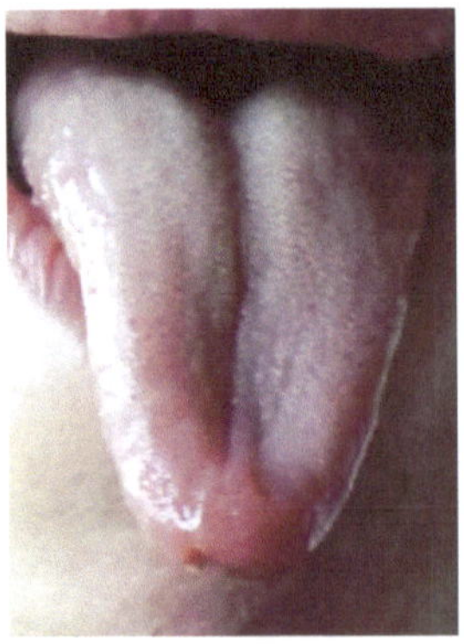

Case 14

This patient tried for ten years to become pregnant having "tried everything," including many IVF attempts. She came for acupuncture as a "last resort." The unfortunate thing about fertility patients is that they come as a last resort after having spent so much time chasing fertility while cultivating infertility at every meal. When we first meet these women and ask about their diet in general terms, they invariably report something along the lines of having a "very healthy diet, no sugar, all organic, and lots of raw vegetables and juices." For this patient, breakfast was a cold smoothie made from raw vegetables and frozen fruit, lunch was skinless chicken on a large salad, and dinner was another juice and large salad with tuna, beans, or a different protein. This diet—nearly all raw, cold, and devoid of grains—instructs the body to become Cold and to engage in daily purging of Fluids, Yin, and warmth. The net effect is great depletion of the very resources needed to cultivate fertility.

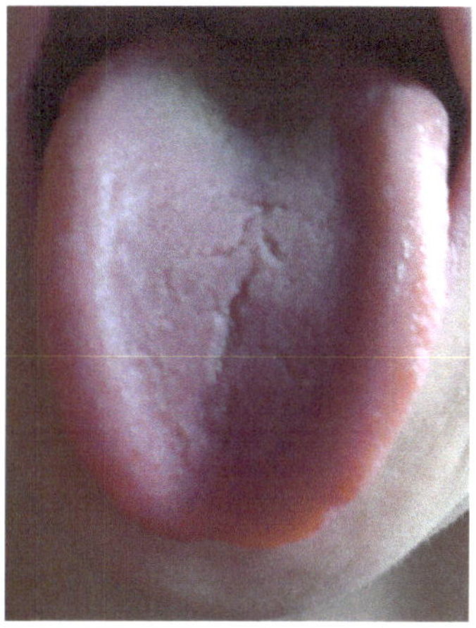

In the first photo (first visit), we see the result of a deeply dehydrating diet where every meal sent a message to the body to evacuate, since this is the function of cold and raw. The resulting deep cracks in the tongue are a mixture of dehydration (lateral cracks) from the clearing diet, and heat (vertical cracks) from the coffee and garlic supplements.

Initially, the suggestion was to adopt a diet of only cooked food served warm or hot, to add gluten-free grains to every meal (rice or millet especially), and a strong suggestion to vastly reduce coffee consumption. (Information about this kind of food knowledge can be found in Andrew Sterman's *Welcoming Food*.)

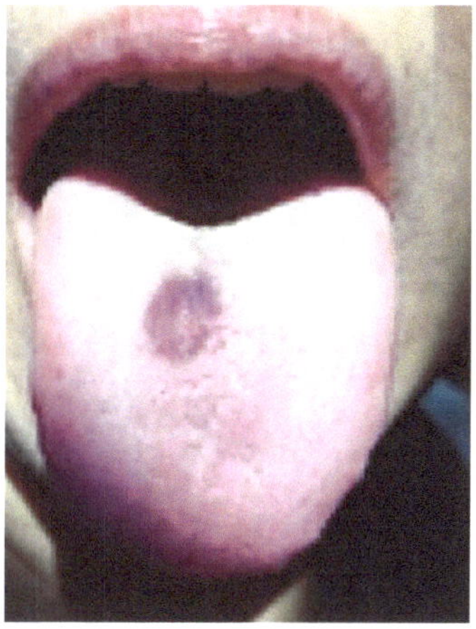

We spent a few sessions doing a great deal of moxa over the Middle Jiao and Lower Jiao to scatter the Cold. At the end of one of these treatments, a clear blue ring emerged in the Spleen region. This was a reflection of the cold breaking up and moving to the exterior. Cold consolidates, and as it breaks up and comes to the surface, it scatters and spreads out. The patient began to feel the cold emerging, then felt it move through the Sinews and exit through the hands and feet before disappearing. The blue ring vanished that night. The following week we embarked on a short course of Chong Mai treatments. She became pregnant about six weeks after the day of the second photograph.

Case 15

This patient came for treatment after receiving a Western diagnosis of SIBO (Small Intestine Bacterial Overgrowth). She complained of debilitating abdominal pain, anxiety, insomnia, and skin issues. It was clear that she engaged in overthinking, since she supplied me with copious lists including a detailed food diary, a long list of medications and supplements, a list of sleep hours, and a twelve page bulleted history of her life. She believed the world was against her and that every effort made to move forward was met with resistance and aggression. Stress was a feature of every day. She had a daily popcorn habit and believed it was good for her since it was organic. The same applied with coffee. She had a long history of scheduled fasting, eating salads every day all year, and took garlic capsules daily. All these habits resulted in extreme heat showing in the long, deep red tongue.

The sides stand up, indicating tension in both Gallbladder and Liver due to extreme tension and frustration combined with toxicity due to drugs and extreme heat due to popcorn and garlic capsules. There is a discernible swelling in Dai Mai. The Gallbladder is more swollen than the Liver, creating a Dai Mai bulge on the left as it strains to contain the toxicity evident in the thorns at the rear and on the sublingual area. The back of the tongue is narrow, concave, and set in a V-shape, indicating contraction due to the steady strain on Kidney Yang.

The tip of the tongue is retracted and the Pericardium is active guarding the Heart. The stream of Heat emanating from the Middle Jiao to the Upper Jiao for venting is evident in the tongue body as a continuous redness emanating from the Middle to the Upper Jiao. The perimeter of the tongue is red in the Upper Jiao, indicating Wei Qi is congested at the exterior, hence, the patient has skin rashes, especially on the face. However, the sides of the tongue are paler than the rest of the tongue, indicating a deficiency of Blood in the Liver since Heat has consumed Blood (and the diet is unfortunately overly constricted). Concurrently, the Gallbladder Channel cannot find enough Blood to gather back to the Liver and it, too, is comparatively pale.

The coat is accumulated in the vertical cracks as the body seeks to contain Heat using Dampness. The coat is thicker in the rear of the Middle Jiao and the entire Lower Jiao, but the sides and tip are without coat. The coat appears to be thicker in the region of the Small Intestine. The sides of the tongue are wet, as Dampness accumulates in the Liver and Gallbladder to quell the Heat. The coat is slightly yellow as the body responds to Heat with Dampness, but it only succeeds in smothering it (the slightly yellow tint indicates this process has been sustained for some time). The cracks are vertical, indicating Heat has consumed fluids. There is a double crack extending from the Middle to the Upper Jiao as Heat seeks alternative routes for venting upward. This Heat is not releasing all the way out, however, since petechiae show all the way around the perimeter of the front portion of the tongue.

In short, Heat has consumed Blood and Fluids, resulting in constraint in the Liver and Pericardium. Gallbladder is tight as it tries to draw Blood back to the Liver. Heat has accumulated in the Upper Jiao, causing, anxiety, depression, obsession, and rashes. Overthinking and daily cold and raw food weakened the Spleen and daily popcorn and coffee desiccated the gut, resulting in crippling abdominal pain. After the cessation of causative habits, treatment involved relaxation of the Liver and Gallbladder, clearing of Heat, strengthening of the Spleen and nourishment of Blood and Fluids. The abdominal pain subsided during the first week of treatment.

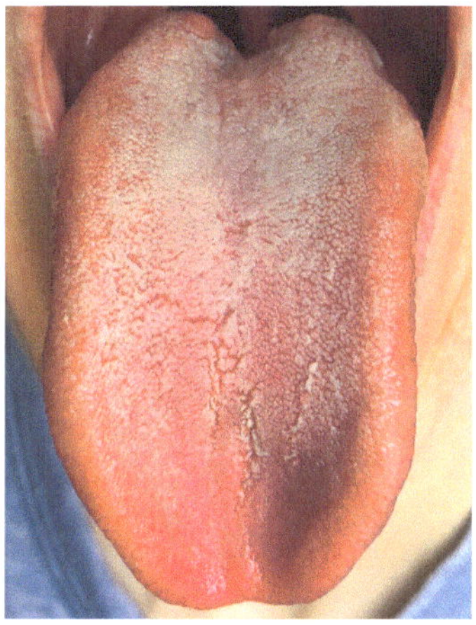
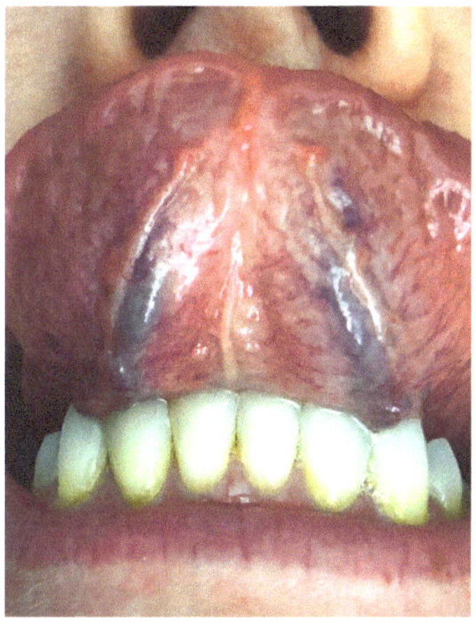
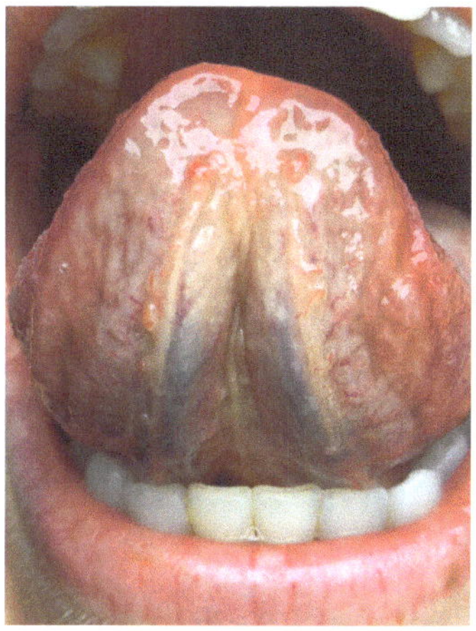
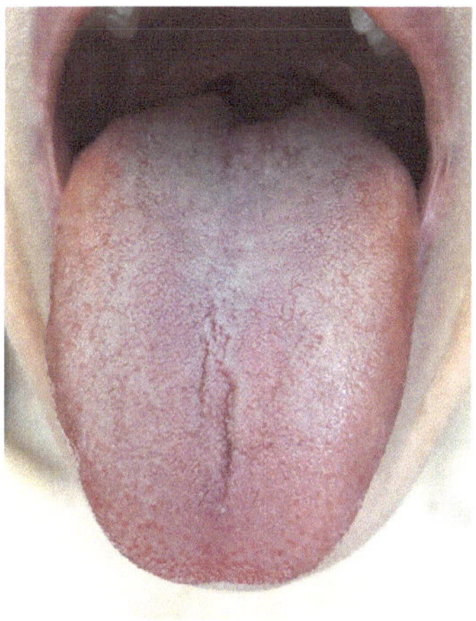
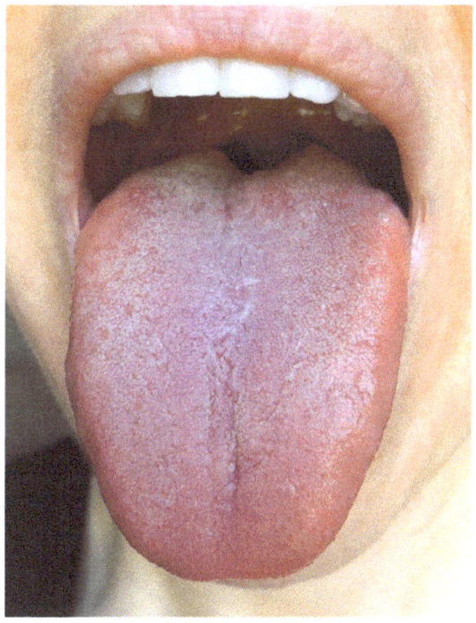
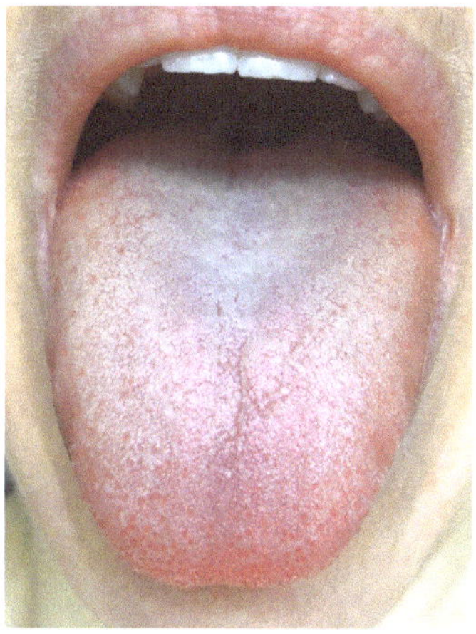

Case 16

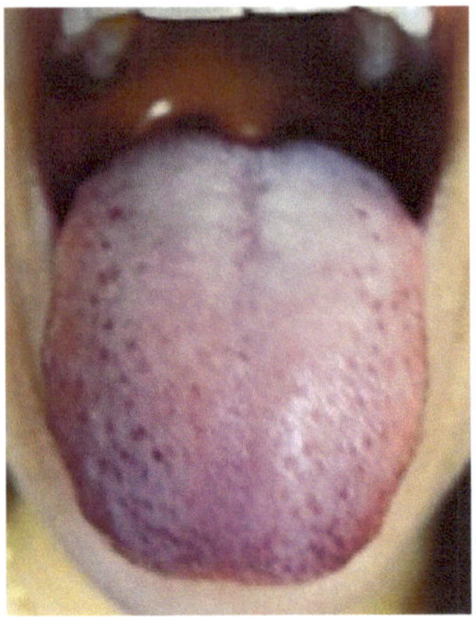

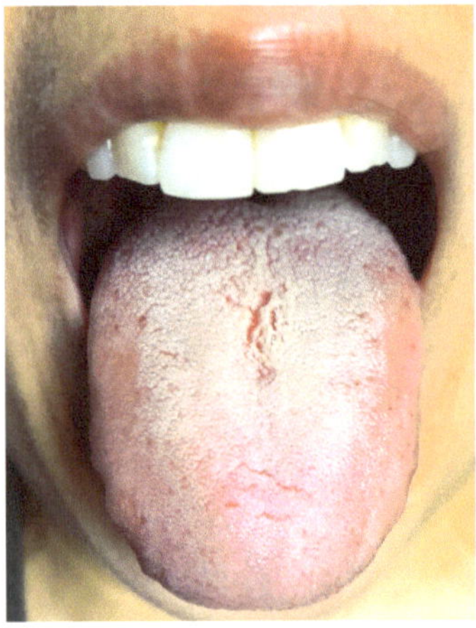

These two photos are taken pre-pregnancy and then postpartum while breastfeeding. The first photo shows the purple hue and blueness associated with the accumulation of Cold and the resulting Blood and Qi stagnation. The patient had patches of discoloration on the Stomach and Gallbladder Channels on the legs due to Blood stagnation. The etiology was fear and withdrawal due to significant childhood trauma; all the treatments focused on the Eight Extraordinary Channels. After the scattering of the Cold the patient moved far away, found her partner, married, and had a baby, all in a short period, and became genuinely content (allowing for the natural ups and downs of life). Although the Pericardium is still slightly guarded (dark petechiae in the right, lateral to the tip) the Cold is largely gone. Now we see the challenge of reconstituting Fluids postpartum while breast-feeding since that requires a combination of Stomach fluids and Blood from the Liver. The sides are pale and there are cracks in the Lung and Stomach regions. A mild Damp accumulation compensates in the Middle Jiao. This tongue is also an example of how emotional change (and also pregnancy, for that matter) moves Blood.

Case 17

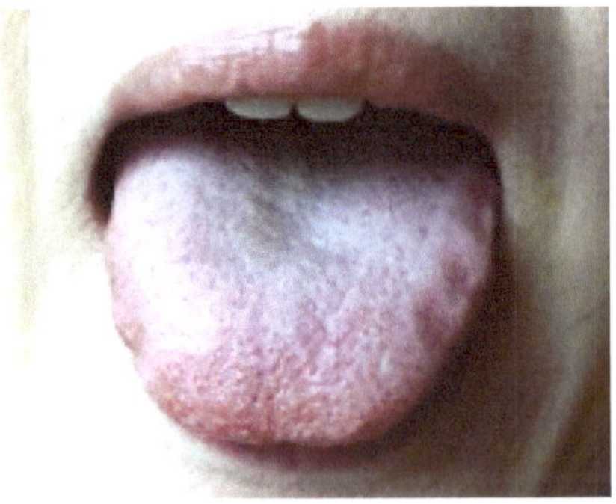

This woman, habitually consumed by obsessive thinking, has a depleted Spleen, showing in the central depression in the tongue. Overthinking results in the accumulation of Heat in the Middle Jiao, which then affects neighboring organs, especially Lungs and Liver. Turbidity in the Stomach shows in the same region, since the Spleen is unable to transform and transport fluids. The Gallbladder (left side) shows crimping or scalloping, as it must try harder to move the Liver Blood. This results in Gallbladder constraint, which in turn creates more frustration and then finances more overthinking. A cyclical pathology sets in. This great constraint in both the Liver and the Gallbladder inhibits the suppleness of the diaphragm. Blood, Qi, and Yin, which should have clear passage from the Upper Jiao to the Lower Jiao, are blocked at the diaphragm, trapping all these resources in the Upper Jiao. Therefore, we see petechiae and considerable redness in the tip of the tongue and a swelling in the Upper

Jiao. The treatment involved bleeding Luo points to release pent up anger, frustration and obsessive thinking, and then releasing the diaphragm and communicating Heart and Kidneys to reestablish the openness of these vital highways.

Case 18

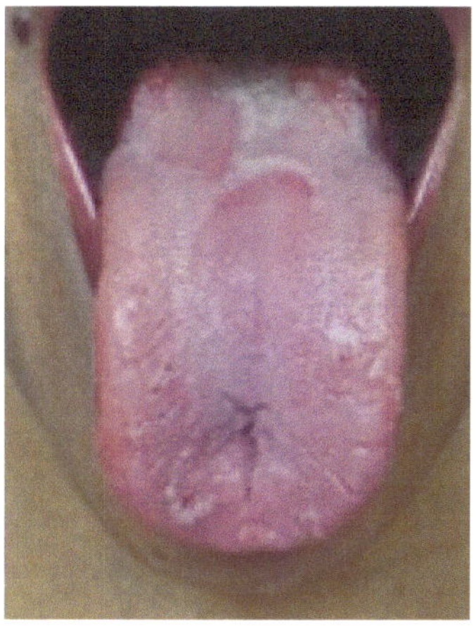

This patient presented with bleeding from the Large Intestine. (The Western diagnosis was Crohn's disease.) She had been taking steroids but stopped after they caused necrosis in both hip joints. In this photograph taken before her first session, she is post-bilateral hip replacements, but her teeth had just started cracking.

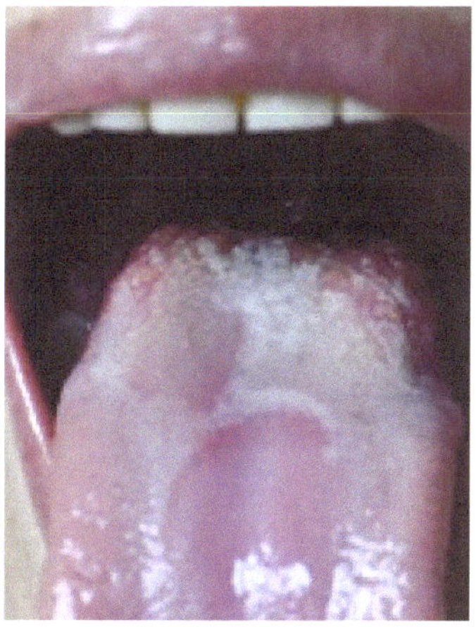

It was clear from the tongue that the damage to the Large Intestine was caused by long-term smoking, as seen in the very deep, cracked depression in the Lung region. If the Lungs are Yin deficient, they cannot bring Yin to the Large Intestine to moisten it. This results in inflammation and then bleeding in the Large Intestine. In this case, Dai Mai responded, trying to astringe Blood in the Lower Jiao, as seen in the significant "waist" toward the rear of the tongue. This resulted in the trapping of toxins in the Lower Jiao, seen in the significant thorns at the very rear of the tongue. The trapped toxins then create more inflammation, causing more bleeding, then more constraint in Dai Mai, and so it goes. The steroids, aimed at stopping the symptoms including the inflammation, affected the realm of the Curious Organs, in this case the bone—hips and teeth—both sites the body will employ to try to hold pathology latent. They also resulted in a major Yang deficiency, shown in the floppy or drooping tongue and its shininess. We also see Yin deficiency in the peeled coat and in the attempts of the body to repair the coat by accumulating Dampness.

The treatment involved relaxing Dai Mai, communicating Lungs down to the Kidneys and stopping bleeding with moxa on LR-1 and SP-1. Yin-tonifying foods replaced her highly stimulating diet. The bleeding stopped within forth-eight hours and, apart from needing some dental repair, she was symptom-free in less than a month.

Case 19

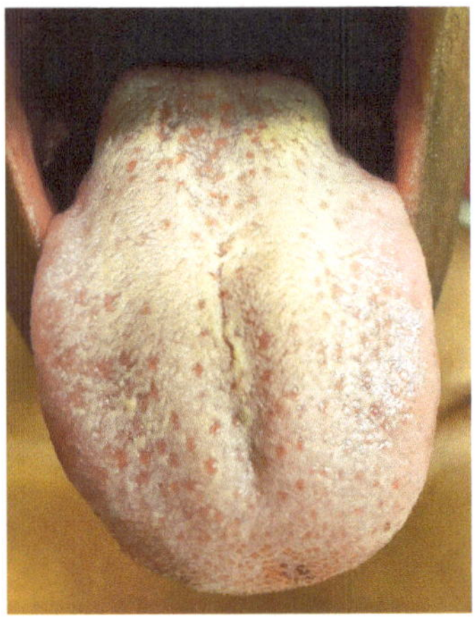

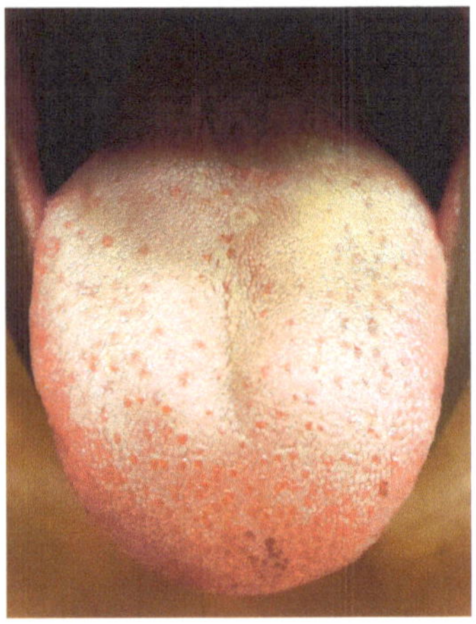

This set of pictures came from a member of my community who wanted to make sure she was on the right track.

Dear Ann, The pictures here are from 3 different weeks (consecutive and labeled). She has been drinking warm clear soup daily and achieving more hydration. She says the inner lining of the sinus passageway is "inflamed" rather than fluids getting stuck, according to her. She feels best with hot liquid and when she exercises.

She had a stomach infection in 2015 while living abroad, a longer history of asthma, was four pounds in weight at birth, wakes up hot at night, often sweaty and with an itchy nose and her period is 30 to 34 days. Her bloodwork showed mild hypothyroidism. She has a painful right knee and tight right upper arm. Her left LR-13 area is sore and she belches.

Since her treatments, her energy is better, there is no more belching, more appetite, and she wakes up less at night. She has fewer clots but more cramps this month. Pulses are not as thin anymore. Left cun and guan are still relatively thin compared to the other pulses but the right guan is wide. Left guan is no longer rapid.

She has a big knot on the upper back/neck area which she wasn't aware of. Gua sha and cupping didn't reduce the size significantly, but she felt a release of tension.

The treatment was Stomach Divergent Channel deep-superficial-deep:

(BL-1, ST-30, CV-12, LI-20. Even though it was DSD, I added very light ST-45 for exit just in case.) Left BL-1 and ST-45 came out on their own.

This tongue shows tremendous systemic stagnation. As mediumship and pathology fail to move, the body creates Heat to try to produce movement. That Heat then becomes stagnated. The asthma predates the "stomach infection" and so we know that there was stagnation already entrenched before 2015, since the Lungs were unable to communicate with the Lower Jiao back then. The Lower Jiao became depleted, as shown in the dramatic narrowing of the rear of the tongue. The stomach issue was not cleared due to a Yang deficiency (perhaps constitutional as she was born tiny), showing in the drooping of the tongue. The Stomach Divergent Channel became active, employing the sinus cavities as an area of latency, causing them to swell. A Stomach Divergent treatment will dramatically move stagnation, treating the clots, cramps, blockages, even the asthma and hypothyroidism (via CV-22, 23 and ST-9), and bring the pathology out after it generates Fluids to flush the pathology through the sensory orifices. She wakes up hot and sweaty, with an itchy nose in the Yin part of the day as the Divergent channel makes an attempt to use the Fluids to move the pathology, but still, there is too much stagnation to enact that fully. The period is long, since Blood is stagnated in the Lower Jiao. The painful right knee is also a Divergent sign as the body is trying to shift the pathology. Gua sha on the Yang Ming zone will release the knot and the upper arm. The very dark petechiae in the tongue indicating disappointment or heartbreak may underly the entire picture. Ultimately, the treatments will have to focus there, or the practitioner will needle CV-17 on the Stomach Divergent trajectory with specific intention to free the Heart.

Case 20

This woman presented for treatment after unsuccessful attempts at conceiving a baby through IVF protocols. Lung Qi is the principal factor in maintaining fertility. If the diaphragm is locked, as it is here, there can be no descension of the egg from the ovary to the fallopian tube and also no descension of Heavenly Qi from the Lungs to the uterus. Treatment to release the diaphragm and to descend Lung Qi is indicated. The tongue is also quite pale and Blood building is necessary.

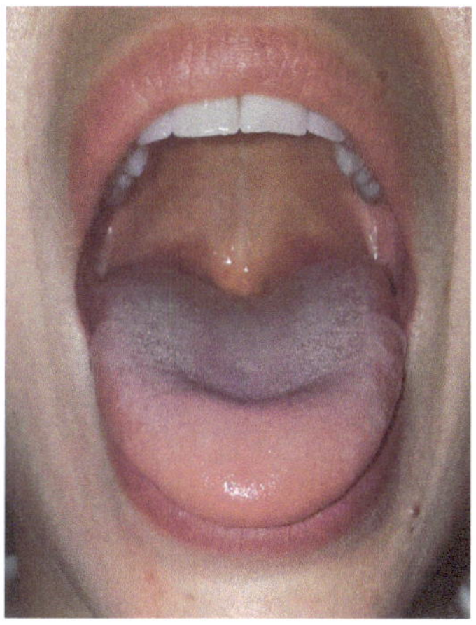

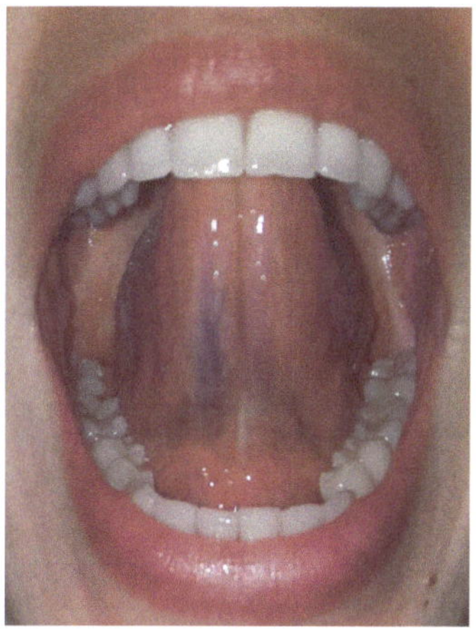

Case 21

The tongue belongs to an intensely private woman breastfeeding her fourth child presenting for remote treatment. Her life has regularly been punctuated by disappointment, as shown by the dramatic retraction of the tongue tip. This action results in outbursts of anger as the Liver and Gallbladder are in turn affected. The geographic tongue shows both chronic overthinking and deep worry, combined with the deep depletion of Fluids given the demands of continuous breastfeeding for nearly eight years. The tongue is devoid of any coat. The cracks in the Liver and Gallbladder regions arose through depletion of Blood, since breast milk is a meeting of Stomach fluids and Liver Blood. The tongue is also quite wet, indicating the body is trying to accumulate Dampness as compensation.

The second tongue photo was taken after the patient was caught in a draft while standing in a high wind talking to a relative she met on the street. Here we see a comparative pallor in the upper Jiao, delineated by a line across the diaphragm which has tightened to block the passage of Cold to the interior. The deepening of the tongue body redness shows the raising of a fever to break up and release the Cold. Wind is evident in the slight froth. The cracks have deepened as the fluids are further tied by the fever. The deep, darkened tight bands between the Spleen and Liver regions reflect the Heat being generated to combat the Wind-Cold invasion; also, the Heat is not fully articulated so that it becomes Wei Qi, and therefore interferes with the smooth flow of Qi in the Middle Jiao.

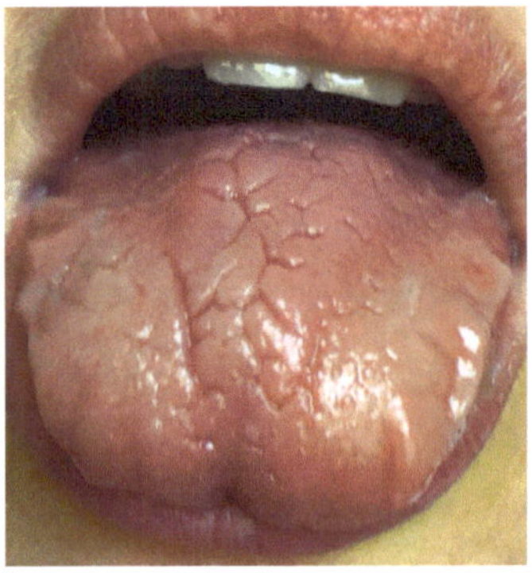

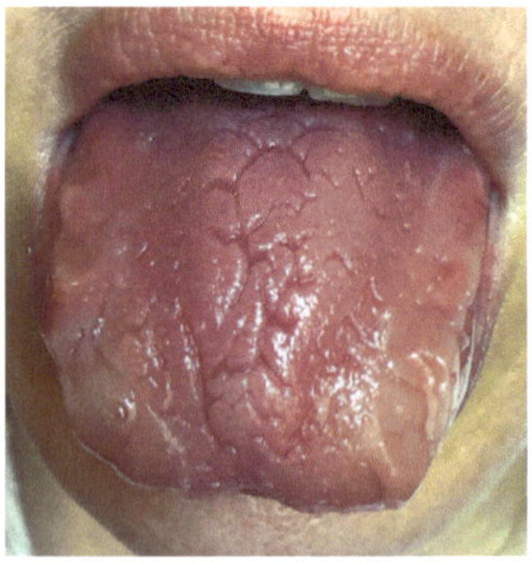

17
Questions and Discussion

General Questions

Why don't you talk about how to locate specific diseases on the tongue, like cancers of certain organs?

Chinese medicine is the art of understanding and treating the mechanism underlying illness, not the symptoms or even manifestations. Cancers (damage by fire-toxins) arise as a result of a complex chronology of deficiencies and excesses that result in an internal environment in which a disease can arise. For this reason, Chinese medicine never treats diseases, it only treats the cause of diseases, it treats the failure of mechanisms and functions that allowed that disease to present. The location of cancer signs on the tongue might be interesting, but it will not help with diagnosis. The diagnosis must be based on how those fire toxins arrived there in the first place. What happened to allow that illness to arise? And where is the pathology headed? Also, fire-toxins show up on the tongue in locations that might be quite removed from the origin of the disease. Fire-toxins might arise in the breast but have originated as Heat in the stomach, for example. Treatment focused in the Upper Jiao in a common case like that will completely miss the root. Always treat the patient, not the disease.

How can I tell if Heat is responding to Dampness or Dampness is responding to Heat?

If you're finding it difficult to work out whether Dampness is responding to Heat or Heat is responding to Dampness so that you can treat the root, ask about history and cravings. Is there a long history of Damp-related issues or Heat-related issues? Issues that arose a long time ago could be the root. Then ask about cravings. Very often, a patient will crave the response to pathology. For example, they might look forward all day to arriving home to a cold beer—Dampness is craved as a response to Heat pathology. Or maybe the patient wants to put hot sauce on everything—Heat is craved as a response to Dampness. Remember, if Dampness is responding to Heat, the Dampness must be kept in place to protect the viscera and Yin until the Heat is cleared. Don't clear Dampness when it is protecting the body from the Heat that preceded it.

Can I tell if Heat is responding to Damp or vice versa from Lower Jiao symptoms?

Generally, if Heat is responding to Damp, there will be urinary symptoms of Damp-Heat as it clears, including urinary tract infections. (Treat Bladder Divergent, perhaps, and remember the gua sha.) If Dampness is responding to Heat, there will be bowel symptoms of Damp-Heat as it clears. (Use the lower He-Sea points, perhaps.)

What message am I sending if I treat the response to pathology instead of the pathology itself?

If you clear the response to pathology instead of the cause of disease, you are sedating the immune system and deepening the disease; you're telling the body it's reacting wrongly.

My patient's tongue is very thin, like a crepe, and dry. Where should I focus?

This is often a sign of Dryness of the Stomach mucosa. Stomach Yin is insufficient to create movement and lubrication. Nourish Stomach Yin and Fluids. Pay attention to the diet; they need soups, broths, stews, and wet breakfasts.

I see a big midline crack, yet the tongue is very pale. I thought Heat causes cracks!

Yes, Heat (or dehydration) causes cracks, but over a long time, Heat consumes Qi, leaving the tongue pale. However, a big midline crack is generally present in those who cannot stop thinking.

Can I generate a purge if the tongue is pale?

No, if the tongue is pale, there is not enough Qi to mount a healing crisis. Heat has exhausted the Qi needed for a purge. Clear Heat and engender Qi to nourish Fluids.

When my very overweight patient showed me her tongue, I was amazed to see it. It was so tiny and withered and gray. How does this make sense?

The patient is likely very swollen. They may be accumulating Dampness in a desperate attempt to accumulate Yin, or perhaps in this case, since the tongue is gray, Jing-Essence. The channels that reach the tongue are so deficient in mediumship that they are not able to carry enough Qi to move Qi and Fluids to the tongue. The tongue becomes gray as the Kidneys become weaker.

My patient insists on scraping her tongue just prior to appointments. Can the appearance of the tongue coat be so changed that is it not useful in diagnosis?
Yes, but the rest of the tongue will still yield valuable information.

My patient's pulses are very rapid on the deep level, but the tongue is not red or dry at all. In fact, it looks very sticky. Why can't I see this serious Heat on the tongue?
The responses to pathology are complicated. Sometimes the body responds to Heat by retaining Dampness. If successful in this response, Dampness succeeds in controlling the Heat and keeps it suppressed; it keeps it from expressing upward and outward. You might see cracks, crevices, or ulcers, but there might be stickiness around them. These are clues that the body has felt the need to respond to Heat with Dampness. You're seeing the aftermath of the Heat (the cracks and the glue) trying to come to the surface. The pulses confirm that the Heat is very much present and must be released from the viscera or the constitution. Clear Heat.

My patient's tongue looks enormously long. Is this pathological?
It can be. A long tongue is showing you plenty of Yang, perhaps an exuberance of Yang.

My patient's tongue looks extremely lustrous and shiny and yet it is deep red.
Heat has consumed Yin. Yin is no longer able to anchor Yang Qi down and so it is escaping. Both Yang in general and Wei Qi, which is a subset of Yang Qi, are escaping. When Yang escapes, it creates a luminescence. Nourish Yin to anchor Yang.

My patient's tongue is incredibly stiff, so stiff he has trouble speaking!
Heat stiffens the tongue and blocks Stomach Yin from reaching the tongue. If there is also obstruction of the Heart's connection to the tongue, the speech will be affected. Begin by bleeding the Heart Luo point.

Why does my patient's tongue droop like a dog's?
The Spleen is unable to uphold the muscle of the tongue. Ascend Spleen Qi.

The pulses are so slippery, but the tongue is very short, not protruding at all. It looks like a ball stuck in the patient's mouth. Why?
You might be seeing turbid Phlegm. The function of separation of pure and impure is harmed. Turbidity from the Stomach and congealed Phlegm from a weakened Spleen may be sent to the Lungs for expectoration, but if there is overwhelming epigastric distention and/or diaphragmatic constriction, Qi cannot move. Free the diaphragm, separate pure and impure, tonify Spleen Qi, and nourish Fluids.

Why might my patient's tongue be curled under, as though the tip is touching the chin?
This usually manifests in a patient who has experienced long-term disappointment. Moxa KI-6, KI-2, and KI-8 (the foundation of Yin Qiao Mai) in that order, to straighten it out and to give you a clearer view of the big picture in the pulses.

Why might my patient's tongue look like a canoe when showing it?
Yin is depleted and the flesh is retracted, creating a hollowing of the tongue.

How does the appearance of the tongue relate to Wen Bing theory?
Heat in the Wei level is reflected in the coat; Heat in the Qi level is seen in the tongue body; Heat in the Ying level affects the distribution of the coat; Heat in the Blood level shows as protrusions.

You haven't spoken about Cold very much. I'm a Shang Han Lun practitioner. How can I see Cold in the tongue?
Tongue diagnosis originated in the Ming Dynasty, the time of the Wen Bing tradition. Therefore, tongue diagnosis is focused on Heat as pathology, not Cold. Tongue diagnosis was not a practice in the Han Dynasty. The tongue was merely observed briefly as a sign in itself, as a whole. You could invent a new system and try to apply it to earlier periods, but it wouldn't be classical.

My patient's tongue is floppy and covered in bleeding lesions. Where should I focus?
The Spleen is not controlling Blood and there is Heat in the Blood. Heat has consumed Qi. Focus on strengthening the Spleen. Clear Heat from the Blood by bleeding Luo points.

What does it mean if the tongue is very stiff and rigid?
This is a sign of internal Wind. It may be trembling, also, showing Kidney Yin is depleted. Do not simply release Wind, but locate the mediumship that's deficient and nourish that first. This can be done in the same session.

My patient, who is very thin, has a chief complaint of canker sores in the mouth. She doesn't appear strong, but when she sticks her tongue out I'm very surprised at how long, red, pointed, dry, and energetic it seems. How can one explain this apparent contradiction?
If the patient has canker sores you wouldn't be surprised to see a red, dry tongue. It's long and energetic because Yang is escaping. There is insufficient Yin to anchor Yang, and hence, it spills forth, giving the tongue a very Yang presentation.

After the treatment to clear Heat in the Wen Bing style, my patient's tongue became pale! What does it mean?
The Wen Bing style of treatment spends Yang and posits the idea that it is never too late to purge. (The Shang Han Lun style reveres Yang.) It may be that you cleared Yang Qi when there was a deficiency of Yang. When you examine the pulse and complexion after treatments, there should be evidence of Heat having cleared. The clearing should be immediate. If the pulse becomes thin

or the complexion pales, there was a Blood and Qi deficiency and you expended Qi that could not be afforded. Find which pulse is narrow and nourish Fluids or Blood accordingly.

Can I tell whether Dampness is responding to Heat or vice versa from looking at the tongue?
Swellings indicate Dampness. If the tongue is dry and swollen, there is more Heat than Dampness. Dampness is likely responding. If it's swollen and moist, there is more Damp than Heat. Dampness may be primary there. The pulses help tremendously with this. Also, ask the patient about what they crave. Frequently, the response is craved.

My patient has a history of treatment-resistant thrush. The tongue is coated in thick stubborn Dampness. What should I do?
Inquire about the diet. You can treat till the cows come home but these Damp conditions will not budge until there is no sugar in the diet. Refined carbohydrates should come out, too.

My patient has a strange vacant look about them. There is a thick turbid-looking coat all over the tongue.
Examine the possibility of an entitic invasion. If likely, perform a Sun Si Miao entitic treatment: needle GV-26 and moxa LU-11 and SP-1.

My patient has sciatica that is not responding to treatment for pain. The tongue is so narrow that there are large gaps between the sides of the tongue and the sides of the mouth. What might I be doing wrong?
Treatment for pain cannot be effective if a patient is so deficient in mediumship that the tongue has shrunk dramatically. Drop your treatments for pain and treat to replenish Yin, Blood, and Fluids. Give strong dietary advice: the patient needs a wet diet, rich in soups, stews, broths, porridges. Send them to sleep early. Build them back and then treat for pain. By the time you get to that point, the pain may well have disappeared.

I feel very slippery pulses, but I can't see Dampness on the tongue; I can't even see much moisture on the tongue. Why?
The Dampness might not be evident on the tongue if it is smothering deep internal Heat.

My patient's tongue is very wet. What does this mean?
This usually indicates very early stage Dampness. The chronology of Dampness can extend from very wet tongue to a thick, cheesy-looking tongue.

What does it mean if the sublingual veins are severely distended?
Remember, the sublingual veins tell you that a condition originating in the Middle Jiao is so chronic that it has begun to affect the constitution. If the veins are very swollen, there was long-term stagnation in the Middle Jiao.

My patient's tongue is unremarkable except for its dryness. How do I know where the dryness is coming from?
The moderate level of the Spleen pulse might be thin or narrow, indicating Stomach Fluids are deficient. You might find the Spleen pulse is not ascending to the Upper Jiao. Either nourish Stomach Fluids or ascend Spleen Qi. Or the Lungs are not dispersing, so Fluids are not moving. Disperse Lung Qi. Check the pulses after the needles are inserted, to make sure you're on the right track.

Why does my patient's tongue look like polished glass?
Yang is escaping. You'll find the Kidney pulses sitting up high. Nourish and anchor Yin.

Why might my patient's tongue look dull?
The tongue receives Blood from the Heart and Fluids from the Stomach. Take the pulses and find out where they are blocked.

What does a tongue that looks like a strawberry tell you?
The strawberry tongue, which can described as shaped like a strawberry and deep red with white dots on it, is showing you that there is stagnation of Qi with tremendous Heat, perhaps with spiking or unrelenting fevers, Heat in the Ying level, disturbed sleep, and possibly fire toxins. This condition can quickly become critical.

My patient's tongue is very short but has a thick turbid coat on it.
These two facts are related. If the Stomach has turbidity, the Fluids it sends up are also turbid and inherently stagnating. The tongue will have less freedom of movement and cannot be fully extended.

Questions About the Coat

Why might the coat not be evenly distributed?
The Kidneys might not be supporting Spleen Qi. Perhaps the Lungs are not distributing Wei Qi adequately.

My patient's pulses are nice and wide without being slippery; I don't see dehydration, but the tongue coat is very unevenly distributed.
The Lungs are unable to distribute Fluids to support Wei-Defensive Qi.

The tongue has no coat at all. Why?
The body is unable to produce Wei-Defensive Qi.

The tongue has a patchy coat and is geographic with a depression in the Lung region. What might be happening?

The Lungs are unable to distribute Wei-Defensive Qi. Find the broken link in Wei Qi production. Is the Spleen unable to send Fluids upward from the Middle Jiao to the Lungs? Are the Kidneys unable to provide Yang Qi to the Spleen for it to ascend to the Middle Jiao? Are there sufficient Fluids in the first place?

My patient's tongue coat looks like a layer of white powder. What does it mean?
You'll likely find the Spleen pulse very weak and thin. There are inadequate Fluids, but also Spleen Qi is unable to hold the coat to the tongue.

My patient's tongue coat looks like sandpaper.
Stomach Yin is drying.

Can there be Heat if the tongue coat is thick and white?
Yes, Heat can be so smothered by Dampness that the Heat is hidden even on the tongue. The pulse will show you the location of the Heat that has become trapped. Look on the moderate or deep level for rapid pulses. Clear or drain the Heat, leaving the Damp in place until that is achieved.

What can it mean if the tongue coat is greasy?
If there is dryness in the Middle Jiao, the Spleen can become weakened, unable to transform what Fluids there are; Dampness results. The body responds to the Dampness with Heat, and the resulting Damp-Heat combination is sent to the tongue, appearing as a greasy coat. Or the Heat pushes the Dampness to the surface in a Hot-Phlegm presentation.

My patient's tongue is covered in a thick, greasy coat. The sides are red. Why might my treatments not be clearing the coat?
Heat is trapped in the Zang Fu and the Damp is playing an important role of mediation. The body will not release the Damp until the Heat is released.

What does it mean if there is a coat only on the interior of the tongue cracks?
It means that Dampness is responding to Heat. The body is trying to use pathological Yin to glue mediumship back together.

Why is the coat of the tongue peeled in patches in patients with deficient Yin?
In cases of Yin deficiency, the body is unable to consolidate Yin. It's not able to hold it together, so the coat—an expression of substance—is unable to maintain integrity in its coverage.

My patient eats a quart of ice cream every night and has a very thick tongue coat with a red body. His pulses are very rapid at the deep level. Should I clear Dampness?
No. The patient is most likely craving the response to his pathology (internal Heat). Clear Heat first and deal with the Dampness later.

My patient's tongue is narrow but very high. I mean there are large gaps between the tongue and the sides of the mouth and yet the tongue is very thick. What causes this?
This occurs when the body is gathering Qi but not distributing it. There may be blockages in the diaphragm and in Dai Mai, preventing outward movement of Qi.

My patient's tongue is very swollen but has lots of clear fluid on it. Given the swelling, shouldn't the tongue have a sticky or turbid coat?
The Spleen is likely in an early stage of weakness; the accumulations haven't had enough time to gather.

The left side of my patient's tongue is very swollen and red and has a much thicker coat on it than on the right side. The chief complaint is brain fog and constipation.
The left side of the tongue reflects the Gallbladder. Due to stagnation, the Damp-Heat has become so advanced, it has likely gained access to the Curious Organs via the Gallbladder and entered the Brain. Move the bowels first.

Questions About Color

My patient has a history of exuberant Heat but her tongue appears very pale. Why?
A tongue can become pale as Heat consumes Blood, Fluids, Yin, and Qi, leaving the tongue reflecting expenditure of resources.

Does a pale tongue prevent me from performing certain kinds of treatments?
A pale tongue means there is not enough Qi to mount a purge, or to support a healing crisis. Heat may have consumed the Qi. If you were to try to release toxins, you would likely create a state of autointoxication where the toxins are released from their safe holding in latency, but are unable to move out through the exterior. Clear the Heat and nourish Fluids before trying to release other pathology.

My patient has Leaky Gut Syndrome and her tongue is very pale. I thought I would see Heat creating this damage.
A pale tongue can indicate that there is insufficient Stomach Yang to conduct the complete transformation of food and Fluids. Incompletely digested food irritates the gut wall.

My patient's tongue is very pale but very moist. I thought that after Qi was consumed, Fluids could not be generated or ascended.
You are likely seeing that the Spleen is losing its capacity to control Dampness and you are seeing evidence of the accumulation of Damp.

My patient can't digest anything and has explosive diarrhea. The pulses are very rapid in the Stomach, but the tongue is pale, swollen, and has a deep midline crack. So many Heat signs, but the tongue is so pale!

The Stomach and Spleen must be in balance. Ironically, digestion can be weak if there is too much Stomach Fire as the Heat damages Spleen Qi. The tongue has a deep midline crack showing a long history of Heat—or Heat from overthinking. It's pale because the Heat has consumed Qi. It's swollen because the Fire in the digestive tract has depleted Spleen Qi and damaged the mechanism of transformation.

What does it mean if the tongue is gray?

The Kidneys are trying hard to support the interior. Either the pathogen is so severe that Heat that has consumed Kidney Qi, or the Lungs and Spleen are so weak that Kidney Qi is valiantly trying to support them.

What does it mean if the tongue is black and shriveled?

Kidney Essence is severely depleted. Both Yin and Yang are decimated.

My patient's tongue is black but moist. What does this mean?

Heat has damaged the Kidneys causing Cold-Phlegm to accumulate.

My patient swears he doesn't eat anything on my list of things that exacerbate Stomach Fire, but his tongue has a deep midline crack and is quite red. He admits to reaching for sugar to keep going, though. He is the happy father of three teenagers. Where is the Heat coming from?

In modern urban settings, the cultivation of periods of seclusion and reflection is not valued. Constant mental stimulation takes a toll on the Middle Jiao. Heat accumulates as the Spleen struggles to process endless onslaught of stimuli, both meaningful and meaningless, important and unimportant. The Spleen and Stomach are constantly engaged in trying to keep up a supply of Qi for the conscious and unconscious maintenance and processing of these thoughts, with no prospect of respite. This creates Stomach Fire and Spleen depletion. The quest for more fuel for the incessantly-thinking brain creates sugar cravings. The sugar further depletes the Spleen-Pancreas and creates more Stomach Fire.

After a treatment to resolve Dampness, my patient's face and tongue became pale but the pulses stayed rapid. What did I do?

You might have forgotten to nourish Fluids as you cleared Dampness. And you probably also cleared Qi. If the face became pale and the pulse remained rapid, it's telling you that there is a deficit of Fluids—they should have been nourished prior to the clearing phase of the treatment. Don't worry; start with nourishing Fluids when you next see the patient.

My patient's tongue is very red all along the sides and particularly red at the tip but there is a thick white coat in the middle of the tongue. Why is the coat not yellow?
Heat affected the Liver which passed it up to the Heart. The Small Intestine syphoned some of the Heat off and brought the rest to the digestive tract, which then responded with Dampness. The Dampness suppressed or contained the Heat. Because the Dampness has not yet developed into stagnated Damp-Heat, it is still white in color.

My patient's tongue is dark red with no coat, but it's very swollen along the sides. Why hasn't the Heat consumed Fluids?
It probably has consumed Fluids; what you're seeing is compensation as the body tries to accumulate and hold on to Fluids pathologically. In this case, the body is likely holding onto Blood to conserve it. It could be holding Yin also, due to Dryness. You would be able to determine which Fluid is depleted by examining the width of the pulses in the Stomach, Liver, and Kidneys, respectively.

What might it mean if the tongue looks fairly regular but is purple?
The patient might be struggling to say what they really want to say. Treat the Heart Luo Channel by bleeding HT-5.

My patient's tongue is very red at the diaphragm area. Why is the redness isolated in this area?
There is diaphragmatic constraint. Vent the Heat through the Lung and Liver Channels, perhaps by reducing LU-6 and LR-6.

My patient's tongue is cracked and crimson all over but there is an unmistakably pale area in the center. Why might that be?
Fire has consumed Spleen Qi.

The tongue shows loss of Qi (it's pale) and is very dry and swollen. Where should I focus?
Begin with Fluids. Nourish Fluids so that you can move Qi.

My patient's tongue has a startlingly deep red body with a bright white coat. How can I make sense of this?
This presentation is often seen with Shen issues. Heat trapped particularly in the Upper Jiao becomes increasingly suppressed and moves into the interior, causing the Shen to become unsettled. The body responds with Dampness to control it. Antidepressants can make the coat white. Eventually, mania ensues as Heat moves more deeply, causing loss of memory and recognition problems.

My patient's tongue is simply dark. It's hard to label its color. It's muted.
When the tongue is dark all over, there may be fear in play. Treat the Kidneys and bleed GB-37.

What does it mean if the sublingual veins are very dark, almost black?
This can indicate deep trauma, which has affected the Kidneys. The Kidney Channel connects to the root of the tongue.

Questions About the Upper Jiao

My patient's very pointed tongue has red spots in the front third of the tongue. The area is precisely demarcated as though an invisible line were drawn across the tongue. What is happening?
It's likely you're seeing signs of a constrained diaphragm. Zong-Chest Qi is therefore constrained, pushing the tongue to form a sharp point. The body responds with Heat to move Qi to free the constraint, but the Heat has become trapped in the chest, showing as red papillae.

My patient's tongue tip is turned right under. What can this mean?
This can be a sign of deep disappointment. The Heart is not experiencing joy and is showing despair or dejection.

My patient's tongue is not particularly long, but the tip itself looks very stretched and pointy. Why?
The patient may be having a difficult time communicating. The Pericardium causes constriction in the blood vessels to protect the Heart.

My patient's tongue tip is stretched and constricted and there are tiny cracks behind the region of the Pericardium that appear to be caused by this constriction. What are the mechanisms in play?
The patient may have constraint in the Lungs as they try to convey the patient's conscience to the Heart for expression.

What does it mean when there is an elevation at the tip of the tongue covered in protrusions, with a tight band around the tip?
This can be an indication of latent Heat in the throat that might manifest as goiter, thyroid issues, constriction in the throat, or Plum Pit Qi.

I see a tight band right across the tip of the tongue. What does this mean?
This means there is Heat trapped somewhere above the Heart, perhaps the throat or the sensory orifices.

When my fertility patient shows her tongue, I don't see any indication of Blood or Fluid pathology. But there's a white patch on the Lung region. What am I missing?
The *Jia Yi Jing* reminds us that the Lungs command Qi to move Blood. The Lungs descend

Qi and Blood and disperse Wei-Defensive Qi. They instruct the Heart and Pericardium to move Blood. Hence Lung Qi is responsible not only for initiating bowel movements, but for beginning the period and for enabling conception as it descends the egg from the ovary to the fallopian tube. If the Lung region is white, the Lungs are depleted. Lung Qi has been consumed. The Lungs are the principle organ of fertility.

The tip of my patient's tongue is very elevated. What severe conditions might be present in such a tongue?

There may be rage, resentment, and seizures.

Questions About the Middle Jiao

My patient's tongue is huge, pale, and blocklike in the Middle and Upper Jiaos. The Lung pulse is weak. What is this scenario?

The Upper Jiao is responsible for moving Fluids. But here the Middle Jiao is not transforming the Fluids (and food) in the first place. Drain the Fluids (through the Lower Jiao), don't expel (through Upper Jiao). The Lungs are too weak for expulsion. If the tongue were not so pale, you might be able to strengthen the Lungs and expel concurrently.

My patient's tongue looks swollen from side to side right across the middle. What does this indicate?

When the middle third of the tongue is swollen all the way from one edge of the tongue to the other, it often means that grains are being poorly digested—usually wheat. The tongue shows accumulation of Dampness (the swelling) because the person is not keeping up with the task of processing, separating, moving, and eliminating what is incoming. Poor food combinations eventually cause problems. When digestion is slow, food ferments in the gut, causing autointoxication. Processed foods and refined sugars greatly aggravate this problem. Fermentation that originates in the gut eventually damages digestion, leading to accumulations and reactions even to foods that are easy to digest. The gut must be strengthened; start by tonifying the Spleen.

My patient's tongue is very red and has a swollen area right in the center. What could it mean?

It could mean that internal Heat is being smothered by Stomach Yin.

The sides of my patient's tongue are crimson and dry. What can this mean?

This can mean that Blood is being sacrificed to support Fluids. The Liver tries to stagnate the Blood. Heat responds to the stagnation. The pulses will clarify this for you.

What does it mean if the tongue is tiny and dry?

Jing-Essence is exhausted.

What could it mean if only the center portion of the sides of the tongue are scalloped and also covered in thorns?

The Liver or Gallbladder may be harboring fire toxins. The body is holding them in the Liver to prevent them reaching the Heart. As the Liver tries to contain them it stagnates its own Yin, causing the sides to swell and become scalloped.

What does it mean when the tongue is elevated all the way down the middle, like the opposite of a midline crack?

The sides are squeezing the tongue inward toward the center midline. The Liver and Gallbladder are constrained, creating weakness in the Spleen and Stomach.

I keep nourishing Fluids but my patient's tongue is stubbornly cracked right through the Middle Jiao. They are drinking water and eating fat, so why is nothing happening?

You don't mention the pulses. Perhaps the Lungs are weak and this is a distribution issue. The Lungs distribute and disperse Fluids. See if the Lungs are not diffusing in the pulses. LU-7 serves this purpose.

Questions About the Sides

How can I tell if my patient is eating too much protein?

The Liver and Gallbladder tongue regions will show swelling, stagnation, and Heat. Meat requires Stomach Heat (stomach acids) to digest. Since we can't directly use protein from food, we must digest it by breaking it up into amino acids. To protect the villi of the upper intestines as the steak and acid (acidic chyme) descend into the Small Intestine, bile (manufactured in the Liver) is excreted to neutralize the acid. Digestion of carbohydrates can then follow. The higher the protein consumption, the higher the volume of stomach acid, and therefore bile, required. The spent bile leaves behind bile salts, which are sent back to the Liver for processing and recycling. The amino acids proceed to the Small Intestine where they are separated. They're then transported to the Liver, where human proteins are synthesized from them. So the Liver is called upon not only to make sufficient bile, but to recycle the spent bile and to synthesize usable proteins at the end. When the Liver and Gallbladder are required to process too much protein, they become inflamed. Hence excess protein creates excess Heat. The sides of the tongue will be red.

The sides of my patient's tongue are a very purple and the middle of the tongue has a depression in the Spleen and Stomach region. What could be happening?

The patient might be eating too much protein. If the Gallbladder has been called upon too much, the sides of the tongue may be scalloped and have a purplish hue. These are signs that the

Gallbladder is constantly squeezing out bile. If the tongue is very purple, there may be gallstones due to stagnation of Qi. If the area around the mouth is yellow-greenish, the Gallbladder is overstimulated and the Spleen is weakening because its neighbor is overwhelming it. The eyes could be yellowed, too (jaundice).

The sides of my pregnant patient's tongue are a very deep purple. Why don't I feel slow pulses to indicate Cold?

In late pregnancy, some women crave very high protein foods that are very Yang, deep-fried greasy foods, pizza, and sugary foods such as cake and ice cream. These foods create constraint in the Gallbladder as it struggles to keep up with the demand for bile. They might also be worrying a lot, weakening the Spleen and causing a response in the Liver and Gallbladder. There may be a bitter taste in the mouth. The deep purple discoloration is often on the left, confirming the Gallbladder is constrained. Sour foods will neutralize the Heat: lemon, lime, artichokes, pickles. Sour berries also stimulate and move the Gallbladder.

My patient's tongue is purple on the sides but a normal color in the center. A deep midline crack is filled with a sticky deposit. What could this mean?

As emissary among Qi, Ying, and Blood, the Liver may be stagnating Qi to support Stomach Fluids, to help the body conserve them. The Middle is concurrently holding on to pathological Dampness to try to conserve Fluids.

The front of my patient's tongue is shaped as though it has been cut off. It's squared and retracted with a depression in the Lung region. The sides are crimped. The patient is unable to sleep without dreaming of flying.

This could be either a Liver deficiency or a Lung deficiency. Both areas are retracted due to deficiencies. They are unable to exercise their upward vectors (Lung Qi dispersing, Liver Qi ascending normally). The body then attempts to process and correct this, resulting in flying dreams.

What does it mean if the sides of the tongue are dry?

It means the Liver is depleted and constrained as it yields its Blood to support Kidney Yin.

My patient's tongue is scalloped all along the sides but the center of the tongue (the Spleen region) is not swollen at all. I thought scalloping is a sign of Spleen Qi deficiency!

Scalloping is only a sign of Spleen Qi deficiency if the center is swollen and that swelling extends to the edges. If the swelling is isolated on the edges, or mainly on the edges, or if it's clear that the swelling is not emanating from the center, the Liver is stagnating as it attempts to store more Blood. Spleen scalloping is a sign of deficiency; the Spleen is unable to control Damp. Liver scalloping is a sign of compensation; the Liver is unable to store sufficient Blood or there is insufficient Blood to store, or there is Liver Qi constraint preventing deep penetration of a pathogenic factor. The constrained Liver is unable to move Qi.

The sides of my patient's tongue are orange to smoky brown in color. What does this mean?
This can mean that the Gallbladder has been chronically overstimulated, usually by too much sugar, alcohol, or processed food. At the end of that spectrum, we see conditions like gallstones, hepatitis, fibrosis in the Liver, cirrhosis, even lymphoma. Sometimes even the coat can be orange.

If the tongue shoots forward, does it mean there is Stomach Fire?
It can, but the Heat has affected the Liver, causing the sides to lengthen and expand with the Heat. Heat is rampant.

My patient's tongue is very long and swollen. Is this a Spleen condition?
If the Spleen responds by retaining Dampness, the tongue swells, but is usually not long. Look for Liver constraint or Stomach Fire being controlled by Dampness.

In several of my patients I notice the color of the sides of the tongue differ markedly from the color of the rest of the tongue, especially the tip. Why?
This can mean that the Liver is active in trying to store Blood. You might see the tip red or pink at the same time the sides are pale or purple. The contrast is telling you the Liver is engaged in an action to compensate for too much expenditure of Blood.

The sides of my patient's tongue are severely cracked. How does this relate to her episodes of panic?
If the Liver is unable to astringe (store) Blood, it also cannot contain the emotions, since emotions reside in the Blood. As the Liver tightens to try to contain more Blood, the emotions stagnate further. (In her case the Blood may be affected at the Bladder Luo. Bleed BL-58.)

My patient's tongue is pale, but the sides are quite dark. His issues are emotional. Can a Blood deficiency cause this?
Yes. The Liver is trying to astringe Blood in response to a Blood deficiency and the Blood is stagnating and not moving enough. This is making the sides dark while the rest of the body is pale. There is enough Qi for the body to create this response. If there were not, you would see a dry, pale tongue all over, including the sides.

My patient has a tongue that is purple and extremely tight along the edges. The tip of the tongue is pushed to a sharp point that is not dark or red. Her pulses are wiry. What does this presentation indicate? And why is the tip not red or dark?
I imagine your patient is in a lot of pain with all that Liver constraint. The Liver is trying hard to astringe Blood, to store more Blood. This action of holding forces the tip forward. The tip of the tongue is paler than the sides because the Liver constraint is so severe, that the tip is

not filling up with Blood. There might be a shortage of Blood to the brain, causing memory loss, dizziness, and discomfort in the head. The Gallbladder is affected because it moves Blood in the Liver.

My patient is trying to get pregnant. Her pulses are wiry and the left side of her tongue is very swollen and scalloped. Why is this?

The Gallbladder manifests on the left side of the tongue. It might be trying to hold blood to nourish the Curious Organs, including the uterus. Don't interrupt that process but nourish Blood and adjust the diet. If all else is well, it will release on its own when replete.

The sides of my patient's tongue are quite orange and yet very wet. What does it mean?

There is likely Damp-Heat in the Gallbladder.

My patient has dementia and his tongue is very swollen on the left side. Why might the right side be paler and smaller than the left?

The Gallbladder connects to the Curious Organs. It may be working hard to move what little Blood there is in the Liver to the brain.

I'm trying to clear Dampness in the Spleen but my patient's tongue is stubbornly scalloped and swollen along the edges. I'm frustrated.

You don't mention the center of the tongue. Is the whole tongue swollen? If it is, then the Spleen may be Damp, but if the swelling is concentrated along the sides and the center is not so swollen, you're likely looking at Dampness accumulated in the Liver. Is the Liver pulse rapid? Maybe there is Heat in the Liver and you're trying to remove the intelligent response of the body—to quell the Heat. The body will resist your attempts to drain that if the body is strong enough. Or are the sides pale? Maybe there's a Blood deficiency. You might be trying to drain Damp when there isn't any. Have another look!

I often see swelling along the sides of tongue in women. Why?

The Liver is trying to conserve Blood. Modern culture doesn't treasure the Blood so much. People stay up late, stare at electronic screens, miss breakfast, don't eat much soup or stew, and don't take time to reflect and calm their emotions. As the body also becomes deficient in Qi, the sides stop swelling, turn pale, and have a crushed look about them.

Sometimes I see swelling on the sides while the sides are scalloped. Is this a Spleen sign?

No, this is still a Liver sign. If the Spleen were primary here, you'd see the entire middle section of the tongue swollen. If it's just the sides that are swollen and scalloped, the Liver is trying so hard to contain or conserve Blood that it's beginning to invade the Spleen. This is the classic scenario of Pre-Menstrual Stress Syndrome (PMS). Nourish Blood, and the Liver will relax and leave the Spleen alone.

The tongue body appears very dry, yet it is scalloped with a thick, greasy coat, especially in the middle. Looking at it from the sides, I can see that the tongue body is deep red. The pulses are very thin and only slightly slippery and slightly rapid. I would have expected a very slippery pulse given the dramatic thickness of the tongue. What am I missing?

Perhaps the thin pulses came first and there was tremendous Dryness which weakened the Spleen. If the Spleen is not moist, it cannot "steam" or "cook" food. Heat resulted from the Dryness. Then the body created Dampness both in response to the Dryness and to the Heat. The Dampness reduced the Heat as it combined with it, creating a thick, greasy coat, perhaps Hot-Phlegm. The Damp and the Heat will not clear unless you nourish Fluids as you go.

What does it mean if there are cracks on the sides of the tongue?

The Liver is dry. Dryness is affecting the peritoneum.

The sides of the tongue are very swollen, solid-looking, and appear cracked. What can this mean?

Swollen sides with cracks in the sides is a sign of food stagnation or constipation.

My patient is having trouble conceiving. Scalloping is far more prominent on the left side of her tongue than the right. Why is this?

When the left side is noticeably more swollen than the other side, there is more taxation on the Gallbladder than on the Liver. Remember, the Gallbladder is the link between the post-natal arena and the Curious Organs. In your case, the Gallbladder is likely trying to bring more and more Blood to the uterus in order to build its resources for a pregnancy.

My patient has dementia. I expected the tongue to look shrunken and depleted but it's very long with tight sides and a pale tip. I've been trying to relax the Liver but the condition is not improving. What is happening?

The Liver tries to astringe (hold onto) Blood by tightening up. (The prognosis is good in your case because the patient is able to create this response.) The tightening makes the sides of the tongue taut, pushing it forward and lengthening it. If it squeezes hard enough, Blood cannot reach the tip of the tongue (reflecting, in this case, the Upper Jiao, right up to the brain). The tip cannot fill up. There's insufficient Blood reaching the brain, causing the dementia. Nourish Blood to relax the Liver. If you release the Liver, you're telling the body to give up trying to nourish the brain.

The sides of my very frustrated and angry patient's tongue are like ground beef, they're so rough. The tip of the tongue is very pointed. Why does this happen?

As the Liver squeezes while trying valiantly to astringe Blood, the sides of the tongue are pushed toward the tip. The sides become rough because Qi is not moving smoothly. This leads to diaphragmatic constriction, and frustration with life. The tongue is pushed into a point, indicating constraint in the Heart. The patient feels they can't do everything they would like to do.

The sides of my patient's tongue are crimped like a pie crust.
When there is Liver Qi constraint, eventually the sides of the tongue may crimp. Irritability may become severe.

When the sides of the tongue look tight and there appears a demarcation on the sides of the tongue at the level of the diaphragm, are the Heart or Lungs necessarily constrained? What are the psychological differentiations between the two?
The Upper Jiao will eventually be affected by Liver Qi constraint (showing on the sides of the tongue). There will be rage, resentment, envy, or jealousy. If the Lungs are most affected, there may be resentment and envy. If the Heart is most affected, there may be jealousy. But these qualities can overlap. Stay focused on releasing the constraint.

Questions About the Lower Jiao

When my patient sticks her tongue out, I see that the tongue is very narrowed at the level of her lips, which would be about two thirds of the way back on the tongue. It's a sudden cinching. What does this mean?
This is showing you there is constraint in Dai Mai. Examine the pulses to see why. Are there bumps and deposits on the back of the tongue? Maybe it needs draining? Is there a thicker coat back there that otherwise looks okay? Maybe it needs consolidating? The pulses will enable you to make the right choice.

The rear of my patient's tongue is absolutely smooth and very dry. What does this mean?
The Bladder's function is to flush out the Lower Jiao. If these fluids are lacking, it won't be able to do this. Irrigate the Lower Jiao by treating perhaps the Large Intestine. You don't mention whether it's pale. Perhaps there is a Blood or Qi deficiency there. The pulses will clarify this for you.

What does it mean if sides of the rear of my patient's tongue are dry and the tongue looks very narrow at the rear?
The Large Intestine is unable to manage Fluids. It cannot control Jin-Thin Fluids. Perhaps these Fluids are not available.

The rear of my patient's tongue is dry and has thorns all over it. The Small Intestine pulse is very thin and is the most rapid pulse. Are these connected?
Yes, the Small Intestine is responsible for internalizing pathology that cannot be let go due to the systemic lack of mediumship or Qi with which to transport it. If there are thorns on the rear of the tongue and the left moderate cun pulse is thin and rapid, the Small Intestine is unable to

maintain or find latency for pathology. The pathology is then released into the system and can reach the organs. Clear Heat and nourish Jin-Thin and Ye-Thick Fluids.

What does it mean if the rear of the tongue is very moist and healthy-looking?
The Bladder can easily move Fluids and Jing-Essence is bountiful.

What does it mean if the coat on the back of the tongue looks as though you could easily scrape it off?
It depends on the area of the tongue. On the middle and front of the tongue, a coat that can be scraped is not a problem. But if the rear of the tongue has a coat that is not rooted, it means that the constitution has been damaged. The body is unable to consolidate Jing-Essence.

My patient's tongue has a thick, cheesy deposit precisely in the middle of the very rear of the tongue. What does this mean?
The center of the very rear of the tongue reflects the Kidneys. They might be struggling to store Yin and the body may be compensating by accumulating Dampness, but it's so long-term that the Damp has developed into or has become Phlegm or otherwise turbid. This can indicate prostatitis, cysts, and masses. Don't clear the Damp at first; nourish Yin so the body can let the pathological Damp go. Once Yin has been nourished, clear the Damp that remains.

The rear of my patient's tongue is very Damp and has little rough patches on it, but the pulses are not slippery. Why is this? Her period is very delayed.
The Liver might be trying to hold onto Yin to help nourish the Kidney Yin. This would explain the delayed period and the rough spots on the back of the tongue. Or the Lungs may be trying to move Yin to the Kidneys and are distracted from moving Wei Qi to the uterus.

The back of my patient's tongue is very dark. Why?
The body may be trying to contain Blood in the Lower Jiao. Perhaps there is a Blood deficiency and the body has formed fibroids in response.

What might be the pathological mechanism present when the tongue is noticeably dry (particularly at the rear) in a patient who has difficulty speaking?
It could mean the Kidneys are unable to diffuse Qi at the root of the tongue.

My patient has a very thick yellow coat at the rear of the tongue and I can't seem to clear it. The sides of his tongue are very bumpy and irregular. He's angry, has hypertension, and is very attached to his pizza, fried chicken, peanuts, and fries. Sigh.
He's holding onto Yin as much as he can and it must be for good reason. A hormonally deficient person will likely accumulate Damp in the Lower Jiao. This can develop into prostate or reproductive issues. The patient will crave fatty foods so that they have adequate cholesterol to create hormones. Remember, cholesterol is the precursor of all hormones and is essential in

the diet. The choice of low-quality fat here is difficult for the Liver to process, as you can see by the roughness of the tongue sides. He'd be better off eating a lot of seeds throughout the day and very small amounts of animal fat including butter. Too much will strain his Liver further. Alter the diet, then relax the Liver to bring the blood pressure down. Once these changes are enacted, the body will accumulate Yin and release the Damp. Clear Dampness when the Kidney Yin pulse is wide and well-defined.

The back of my patient's tongue is completely dry, narrow, and has no coat.
This is rare and means the constitution is very depleted. The Kidneys and Intestines are dry, Yin is depleted. This is what you might see before protrusions begin to appear, as the Intestines thin and release into the bloodstream toxins that are no longer buffered by Yin. Heat has consumed Qi and Yin. Clear Heat before you nourish Yin.

My five year-old patient has a crack at the rear of the tongue. The rest of the tongue is unremarkable.
This would indicate constitutional Heat. The child might have contracted the Heat in utero. Perhaps medications, drugs, or alcohol were in play during gestation. The Jing may be affected by vaccines. Seaweed would be an important addition in this case.

What does it mean if the rear of the tongue is swollen but there are no cracks or protrusions?
The body may be trying to conserve Jing.

What does it mean if my patient has cracks on the side of the tongue and large protrusions at the back of the tongue? Tests for cancer are negative.
Large protrusions at the rear, along with cracks in the side of the tongue, can mean fecal matter is stuck in the Large Intestine. There may be intestinal polyps.

What is the difference between large and tiny thorns on the back of the tongue?
Tiny thorns may indicate inflammation of the mucus membranes of the uterus, bladder, or large intestine. Large thorns indicate large deposits of toxins. Toxins play an integral part in the development of masses.

Why is my Parkinson's patient's tongue smooth in the front two thirds and then abruptly strewn with cracks and dramatic roughness in the rear third?
Roughness and cracks can accumulate in the Lower Jiao due to Liver constraint as it pushes its Yin to control latency of Heat, Damp, or Wind. There will be headaches, abdominal symptoms and Wind signs.

Why are some tongues concave in the rear?
This means there is weakness in the Kidneys. Kidney Yin is insufficient to fill out the tongue and there is insufficient Yang to uphold it. There could be Qi collapsing, hernias, prolapses, sinking Spleen Qi, since Kidneys are unable to support the Spleen.

My patient eats pizza and drinks diet soda despite my suggestions, but I see no Dampness in the Middle Jiao on the tongue. Why is there a thick coat only at the rear?
The Stomach is moving Dampness to the Bladder for disinhibition.

The rear of the tongue is brown with protrusions.
The bowels are severely affected with Damp-Heat.

If the coat is thick at the rear, should I disinhibit Dampness?

Usually, yes, since the Dampness is in the Lower Jiao. But if the Kidney pulses are rapid at the deep level, the Dampness might be holding that Heat in check, in which case, leave it there and clear Heat first.

Why might my patient's tongue be very wet at the back?
The patient may be retaining water. They might do well with a barley soup or porridge to help drain it.

What does it mean when the rear of the tongue is sunken?
Wherever the tongue is sunken, there is a Qi deficiency reflected. If the rear is sunken, there may be a Kidney Qi deficiency.

Questions About the Chong Mai Tongue

My patient has discernible raised bars immediately on either side of the midline of the tongue. What does this mean?
Sometimes you'll see a tongue that has two raised beams or rails either side of the midline, usually in the Middle Jiao region. Called the hidden beams, they show that rectus abdominis is being unconsciously held tightly as armor. This occurs if basic physiological and psychological needs were or are not met, if there has been inadequate soothing, if touch has been missing in childhood, if in childhood the patient felt unprotected. Culture and nature have been at odds. The sense of not having been accepted elicits a posture of rejection; allergies may arise, Qi begins to stagnate. The corresponding tongue has the same two hidden beams.

What does it mean if the tongue has pronounced Chong rails on the rear of the tongue?
This means Jing is being lost as it is broken down to support Blood.

Does the Chong tongue always mean there is stagnation of Qi?
Yes. Chong Mai harmonizes Stomach and Spleen, which have downward and upward vectors respectively. If not harmonized, the distribution of Blood and Fluids cannot happen. When

Chong Mai stagnates, its distribution of Fluids to the Lungs and Kidneys, and Blood to the Heart and uterus, is stymied; there is stagnation all through the torso. Nutrients are not in flow, perhaps leading to wasting (prediabetes). The fifth trajectory of Chong Mai includes transportation points (ST-30, ST-36, ST-37, ST-39) to reinstate its distributive function.

Questions About Cracks

I saw a lot of sticky, gluey stuff in the cracks of my patient's tongue so I cleared Damp and the next day my patient had a severe toothache. Is this a coincidence?

It's likely that the two are connected. You cleared the Dampness that was responding to the Heat and then the unchecked Heat rose upward as it will do, and vented through the teeth. Or, the draining treatment depleted Jing in a way that allowed the teeth to reveal their toxins. (Remember the teeth are key sites of latency.) If there was barely enough dampness to restrain the expression of the pathology, a strong Damp clearing treatment may be enough to allow the Heat to become rampant. Clear Heat and nourish Fluids. (I would bleed the Large Intestine Luo. It clears Heat from the teeth beautifully.)

What does it mean when a midline crack deviates at the diaphragm area?

It means the Heat is looking for venting options in the Middle Jiao. Perhaps excess Stomach Fire is moving to the Liver or the Spleen.

What does it mean when a midline crack splits into two as it reaches the Upper Jiao?

It means that Heat is being syphoned up to the Upper Jiao, perhaps to the Lungs or the Pericardium.

My patient is three years old, has frequent seizures, and was born with a deep midline crack. Is there a connection?

The deep Dryness is likely of constitutional (prenatal) origin. Treat with Chong Mai before moving to Yang Qiao Mai. Briefly reduce TH-4 and ST-42. (Vibrate a needle, lift to the superficial level, intend the Heat to vent from the constitution, then push the needle back down to protect the Yuan-Source level.)

All the cracks on my patient's tongue are transverse (horizontal). What does this mean?

There is Dryness. Moisten dryness and nourish Yin to generate Fluids.

My patient's tongue is covered with cracks and yet is very swollen. Why is this happening?

The body is accumulating pathological Dampness in an attempt to hydrate itself. Moisten so that the body doesn't need to resort to Dampness.

My patient has a deep midline crack that further deepens as it reaches the rear third of the tongue. What might this indicate?
The Heat has reached the constitution. Work with Chong Mai or consolidate Yin.

My patient has a crack right through the tip of the tongue. What could this mean?
This could indicate stenosis in the Heart, arising due to anxiety. Or perhaps there has been a life of disappointment.

The cracks in my patient's tongue fan out before they get to the Heart region. They don't actually reach the Heart. What is happening?
When cracks approach the Heart region, but don't actually make it in, the Pericardium has intercepted the Heat, or buffered it. Often the Heat that approaches the Heart is coming from a constrained Liver. Were it to reach the Heart, there would be anxiety and uncontrolled emotions and potentially arrhythmia. The Pericardium buffers and cools the Heart.

My patient has a crack that goes all the way from the Heart to the rear of the tongue. When it gets to the rear, it forks. What could this mean?
It could mean that Heat in the Upper Jiao was affecting the Heart and Lungs and the Pericardium buffered that Heat. (Heart and Lungs meet via the Pericardium.) To protect Heart, the Pericardium used its connection to the Kidneys to move the Heat downward away from the Heart, but now it's consuming the resources of the Kidneys. This would be a picture of Steaming Bone Syndrome or autoimmune diseases.

A patient I hadn't seen in years returned and the cracks in her tongue had migrated further across the tongue. What does this mean?
Wind is present.

My patient has both transverse cracks and a midline crack.
Dryness manifests in transverse (horizontal) cracks and consumption of fluids, and Heat manifests in vertical ones. Both can be present. But a deep midline crack is usually present in people who are constantly engaged in thinking.

The side of the tongue in the left rear is missing, completely eroded. What does this mean?
The left side is Yang, so consider the Small Intestine and the Large Intestine. Small Intestine is more focused on the left, so it's more likely that the issue is the Small Intestine. Missing flesh reflects a severe deficiency of Yin, perhaps damage to the mucosa and villi. Nourish Thick-Ye Fluids.

How does a geographic tongue relate to Fluids?
The Spleen and Stomach may be engendering fluids but if the tongue is geographic, the Fluids are not being distributed.

What in the diet is most likely to cause deep cracks in the middle of the tongue?
Hot spices, garlic, and onion. (The body is not handling these foods.)

What in the diet is most likely to cause deep cracks in the sides of the tongue?
Alcohol and excess protein. (The body is not handling these foods.)

What in the diet is most likely to cause cracks in the front of the tongue?
Coffee, chocolate, and tobacco. (The body is not handling these items.) Note: All these can create cracks anywhere in the tongue.

I'm treating a child with a very deep midline crack that was not present at birth. What does this mean?
Deep cracks in children that were not present at birth show trauma to the constitution that probably occurred before the age of three. That trauma could relate to emotions, shock, medications, vaccines, antibiotics, etc. Some children are born with a deep crack, indicating inherited trauma to the constitution. Chong Mai treatments will treat these issues (and, perhaps surprisingly, will ameliorate such cracks).

Questions About Spots and Protrusions

My patient has fine white spots all over the tongue. There are patches of thick coat on the tongue. She has various cancer metastases.
These spots are signs of fire toxins. The patches of coat show that Dampness is responding to the Heat. It's important not to drain it. Draining would not only remove what's left of the body's buffering mechanism (Damp restrains the fire toxins, preventing further metastasis), but would damage Fluids, since the Heat would be free to consume more of them. The Heat has been latent a long time, hence the appearance of fire toxins. Don't attempt to clear this unless you have plenty of Fluids, Blood, and Yin; otherwise you'll create further autointoxication. When there are enough Fluids, the body will attempt to sweat or defecate some of the toxins out. Until then, use the Divergent Channels to prevent disease progression.

In many of my patients, I see red spots in the area between the Liver and the Spleen regions. What does it mean and why is it so common?
This is a sign of disharmony between Spleen and Liver. It's generally caused by poor dietary habits, which are endemic in our culture. Sometimes the spots are pale, sometimes red. Sometimes there are no dots in these regions, but elevated bands. The body is trying to work out how to deal with Dampness or Heat. Dietary change is essential in these cases.

My patient's tongue is covered in patches of purplish spots. What might this mean?
There may be emotional trauma resulting in or caused by long-term Blood stagnation.

What does it mean when there are black spots at the posterior underside of the tongue?
Pathology is likely at the Yuan level.

I see many fine white dots at the front of my patient's tongue. They are confined to a very small area near the tip. What does this mean?
This is a sign of fire toxins in the Upper Jiao. Check the pulses of the Upper Jiao—the left and right cun positions—and look for rapid pulses at the deep level. If there is insufficient mediumship to move toxins, put them into latency using the Divergent Channels.

Why is my patient's entire tongue rough, like ground beef, covered in protrusions and cracks?
Extreme and unresolved Heat is drying the tongue body. Clear Heat.

My patient's tongue is entirely covered in thorns. The tongue is pale and shiny. The edges are as dry as cardboard. What does this mean?
This type of tongue has a difficult prognosis. Heat has consumed Qi, Blood, and Yin, leaving the tongue shiny, pale, and dry respectively. The body has lost the resources it would need to hold toxins latent or move them out if it chose to do so. The toxins are rampant systemically. If you're interested in the Complement Channels, check the Triple Heater pulse and consider starting with Triple Heater Divergent Channel, deep-superficial-deep insertion.

If I see a cluster of thorns in a certain area, does it mean that the fire toxins are located there?
Yes, but likely not only there. Remember that the body will move fire toxins until it can find an exit or latency (hiding) for them. The tongue might only be showing you the location of the exit or place of deposit being explored by the body. The pulse will give you the original location. Look for the location of deep and rapid pulses. Clear Heat from these areas also.

My patient has a cluster of red petechiae at the tip of the tongue and nowhere else.
This will occurs when Qi has gathered in the chest and is unable to move.

My patient was given intravenous barbiturates for persistent migraines and then presented with fine white thorns all over the tongue.
Intravenous drugs become systemic immediately. The thorns can emerge overnight, since the body is unable to contain the toxicity.

The back of my patient's tongue is covered in thorns. They are large and dark, like cut-off cones. Is his "no carb" diet a factor in the tongue presentation?
Probably. This kind of presentation is contraindicated to a high protein diet. Thorns at the back of the tongue indicate that latency of fire toxins has been lost. The fire toxins have become systemic and burned the lining of the intestines. Excess Yang from the overconsumption of protein will spread the disease (toxins).

Questions About Froth and Wind

The tongue is undulating, moving like a rolling sea.
This is a sign of systemic Wind. Build the medium that is deficient before treating the Wind.

I see a tongue with normal appearance so why it is noticeably shaking?
There may be a strong external pathogenic factor that is lingering after antibiotics were taken. The antibiotics suppressed the body's response to the pathogenic factor, sending its escort, Wind, deeper into the body.

My patient's tongue is deep red all over and shaking very finely.
Heat originating anywhere can cause shaking. Exuberant Heat results in Wind due to consumption of fluids.

My patient's tongue is pale and shaking. He cannot hold it still and yet he is exhausted. The sides of the tongue are dry, slightly purple, and pinched tightly. The Kidney pulses are both found up in the Wei level.
The Kidney Primary Channel connects to the tongue and so the behavior of the tongue can reflect Kidney pathology. If Kidney Yin is insufficient to ground Kidney Yang and bring it to a state of rest, Kidney Yang will escape, causing instability. The Yin deficiency leads to congestion of Liver Qi as it tries to stagnate Yin to conserve it. This causes the sides of the tongue to crimp. As Yin is not able to move efficiently, the body's efforts to move it create more instability, resulting in Wind. The tongue then shakes.

Why might the froth on my patient's tongue be concentrated at the back?
There may be a crisis resulting in a Kidney Yin deficiency. Lung Yin and Liver Blood are trying to support the Kidneys and these commodities are moving to the Lower Jiao with urgency.

Why is there froth concentrated near the tip of the tongue?
Lung Yin has been insulted by the Liver. Regulate the Liver.

Why are the sides of my patient's tongue very tight, red, and stretched out, with frothy lines on it?
The Liver may be struggling to move Qi. It's constrained and the stagnation has caused Heat to accumulate. As the Liver tries to create movement, it stirs Yin, producing froth. Clear Heat and relax the Liver. Consider bleeding some Luo points to release the Heat.

Why is my epileptic patient's tongue covered in froth, mainly along the edges but also in lines halfway between the edge and the midline?
Usually this pattern has an emotional etiology. There's a persistent emotion that the patient cannot resolve or shift. The Heat created as a result of that emotion stirs and depletes Yin, creating Wind,

which rises to the sensory orifices, causing tics, tremors or seizures, and sometimes epilepsy, as in the Wind-Phlegm presentation of your patient. The patient is somatizing their protest, demanding resolution and change but not knowing how to achieve it, the body engaging in violent outbursts. The Mind must be treated. In cases like this, I often bleed the points and varicosities I find along the Yang Qiao Mai trajectory and then complete a course in needling Yang Qiao Mai.

I was clearing Damp and suddenly Wind emerged even though there was no froth on the tongue at all.

The Dampness that was controlling the Wind was suddenly cleared, leaving Heat unchecked. The Heat stirred up Wind that had been held in latency. Be careful not to clear Dampness when it is generated as a buffer for the true pathology.

APPENDIX I

The Invitation to Show the Tongue

The way the practitioner asks a patient to show their tongue greatly affects the way the patient presents the tongue. If unprepared, new patients can find the request plainly bizarre. Children can find it hilarious. Others may find it embarrassing for a number of reasons. Perhaps they just ate something and they know there's food stuck on it, or perhaps they think it's rude. Or perhaps they think their tongue is ugly. Some apologize for not having scraped it that day. Some may find it an imposition, or feel exposed.

The way around all this can be to give a mini-lesson, since patients mostly want to understand what you're doing. After scrawling a very quick map of the tongue, I explain that although the pulses are the main source of information for diagnosis, the tongue can be quite useful in seeing where the inflammation or dehydration has been referred. Then, leaning back a little, and without expectation, I say, "If it's okay, I'd like to take a quick look at your tongue in case it's offering some more information." That keeps the patient in charge (they can refuse) and keeps the patient from feeling pressured (I'm not saying I have to see it).

Sometimes the patient will ask how to show it: "Should I just stick it out?" to which I lightly answer, "When the mouth is opened they tend to show themselves, no worries." This enables the patient to release the task to the tongue itself.

Most often the patient will open their mouth and allow the tongue to emerge. Some will try to be extra helpful and stick it out as far as they can. In some, the tongue will dart out quickly and appear quite rigid, in others it will flop, doglike. Some patients will open their mouths but not allow the tongue to move beyond the teeth. In some of these cases, Qi is retracting the tongue, in others, the tongue is simply short. All these possibilities are in themselves clues to diagnosis. Occasionally a patient will stick out their tongue but clamp around it very firmly as if to say, "I don't like this, and I feel intruded upon." In these cases, as soon as you can, indicate you've seen enough and thank them—honor their tacit request for privacy.

(See Tongue Posture, page 30)

The Examination of the Tongue

If you've been taking pulses and are next to the patient, be sure to move away a little before asking to see the tongue. Tongue diagnosis must happen fairly quickly because the act of holding the tongue in an unnatural position causes changes in color, posture, moisture. Nonetheless, it does take a little time at least. While the tongue is out, run commentary to buy time while you look quickly and efficiently. For example, "Perfect, thank you. Okay, I see some redness, a little swelling in the middle, a little thickening of the coat at the back. Thank you." The patient will focus on what you're saying instead of their tongue sticking out. Some patients might allow you to take a photograph of their tongue if you reassure them that you will only photograph the tongue. It's important to ask permission, of course. Be careful not to photograph the entire face so that when they see the photo they're not distracted or worried that such a photo exists. If they appear a little reluctant to allow it, they might be more amenable to the photo being taken on their phone. And if you get the feeling they really don't want any of it, it's not a good idea; the tension will adversely affect the treatment to follow. The advantage of having a photo is that you can leisurely take them on a diagnostic tour of their tongue and they can see what you're speaking about. This can be empowering to the patient, and can also raise their confidence in the wonderful treatment they are about to receive.

APPENDIX II

The Passage of a Pathogenic Factor

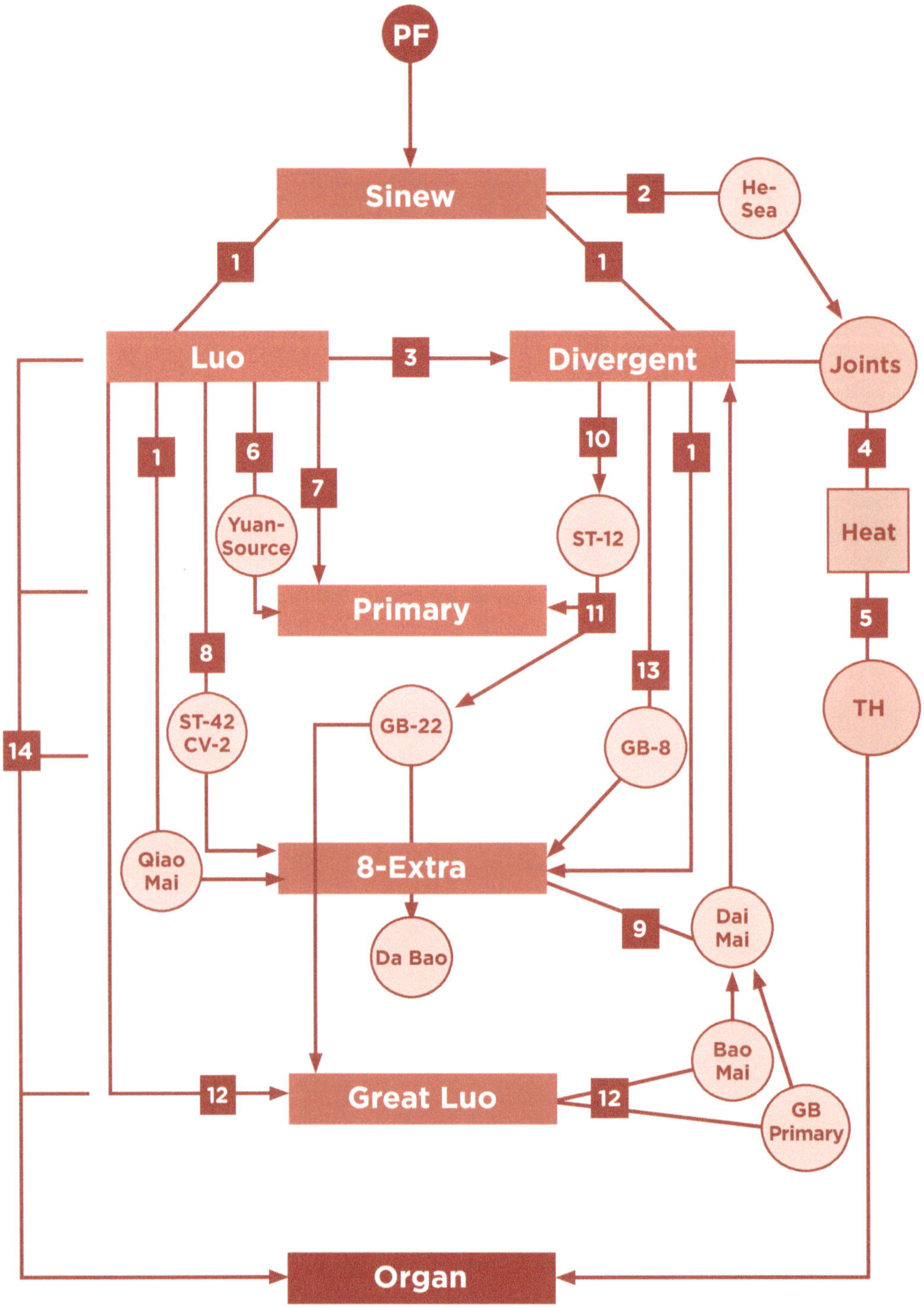

The complete acupuncture system comprises the Primary Channels—the channels responsible for the moment-to-moment functioning of the organs—and the Complement Channels (the Sinew, Luo, Divergent and Eight Extraordinary Channels). The function of the Complement Channels is to steer pathogenic factors away from the viscera, ensuring uninterrupted function of the Primary Channels. The diagram on the facing page shows the brilliant design of the entire network, the connections and interactions between the channels as they act to preserve life.

1. If the Sinews fail, the pathogen moves either to the Divergent or to the Luo Channels. When those avenues are exhausted, the Eight Extra Channels can absorb the pathology. When a pathogen is being held latent in the Luos, Divergents or Eight Extras, there are no signs or symptoms.

2. If the Tai Yang Sinew—the very first line of defense for an external pathogenic factor—fails and the Luo Channels do not absorb the pathogen, the pathogen can enter the He-Sea point of the Bladder Primary Channel. The body diverts the pathogen from the Bladder organ (to which the He-Sea has access) to the joints. The pathogen has entered the Divergent Channel sequence at that point.

3. If the Luo Channels are taxed due to Ying (Blood or Fluid) deficiency, the pathogen can go to the Divergent Channels.

4. If the Sinews fail due to insufficient Yang, the pathogen can go to the joints. As Jing declines, latency is lost (symptoms emerge as the pathogen becomes unhidden in the joints) and arthritis ensues.

5. If Ying is taxed by heat, the Jing may step in and use its cold to hold the pathogen. When latency is lost from the Jing, heat along with the pathology is released, causing the Triple Heater pulse to float as it tries to clear the Jing of pathology. The pathogen then has access to the organs. Therefore the body will try at all costs to find an alternative reservoir of latency.

6. The Luo Channels can empty into the Yuan-Source level if they overflow with pathology and fail to find a neighboring Luo to occupy.

7. The Luos can empty into their related Primary Channel or a neighboring Luo.

8. Pathology in the Luos can find its way to the Eight Extra Channels. The last Yang Luo (the Gallbladder Luo) can empty its pathology to ST-42 which connects to Chong Mai, and the last Yin Luo (the Liver Luo) can empty into the Ren Mai at the end of its trajectory, CV-2, giving entry to the Constitution.

9. The Constitution can pass the pathology to its main reservoir, Dai Mai. When Dai Mai fills, it should drain, but if it cannot, it uses Kidney Divergent Channel to extend its field of latency.

10. Once in a Divergent Channel, the pathogen can then move through the Divergent Channel sequence until it reaches the last confluence, the Large Intestine and Lung Divergent Channels.

11. At the end of the Divergent Channel sequence, the pathogen can enter the Primary Channels at ST-12, but the body may try to push the pathology to the Da Bao at GB-22 which is another point on the Lung Divergent Channel trajectory. GB-22 is also the Great Luo of the Spleen and the pathogen can find latency in the Luo arena there, also.

12. When the Great Luo of the Spleen fills, the pathology can spill down via either the GB Primary Channel or Bao Mai to Dai Mai, a major holding site.

13. At the end of the Divergent Channel sequence, the pathogen can go to Du Mai at GB-8.

14. When the capacity to hold the pathogen in latency is exhausted, the pathogen moves to the organs and the disease becomes terminal.

With knowledge of all the channels of acupuncture, a full set of classical techniques, and a clear diagnosis, the opportunities for healing are limitless, and the results of treatment can be astonishing. While there is life and while there is breath, all possibilities are open.

Acknowledgments

Thank you to the extraordinary team that helped put this book together.

Thank you to **Cody Dodo**, my great friend, and such a blessing, for making yet another beautiful, clear book, and for so many unique and precise diagrams. These books couldn't happen without you.

Thank you **Mark Phillips**, my right hand, friend, and manager of our Press, website, and outreach, whose steady and expert steering of this ship on its many and varied journeys is treasured beyond measure.

Thank you again, **Dr Linda Puckette** for your perennial encouragement, your expertise, invaluable feedback, and friendship.

Thanks to the quality control team of giant hearts: **Andrew Sterman**, **Gabrielle Zlotnik**, **Melpi Magliveras**, **Miriam Sterman**, and **Kathleen Furlong** for their eagle eyes, and for their dedication to the re-deepening of the practice of acupuncture. Thank you **Rosie O'Shea**, **Tanya Reydel**, **Misha Reydel**, **Susan Plourde**, **Pamela Gregg Flax**, **Min Sun Chung**, **Karen Hershman**, and **Chelsea Horenstein** for your steady support of this book. Thanks to **Lois Greenfield** for your professional advice and wise counsel. Thank you **Armin Madani-Nejad** for your invaluable help with this book, and for your dedication to the medicine.
Thanks to all the countless colleagues who sent photographs, and to their patients who generously allowed photos of their tongues to be published.
Thanks to the **Ripples** and **Chat communities** for your support, and for your love of the medicine.
Thank you **Ivan Zavala** for expertly translating references, especially those of Chao Yuan Fang.
Thank you, again, **Martha Oatis** for your poignant poem.
Thank you **Dr Hung Tran**, for your friendship and deep encouragement.
Thank you **Monica Martin** for your friendship and deep support.
Thank you **Dorian Hastings** for your expert proof-reading and polishing of the manuscript.
Thank you **Doug McGill** for always seeing the clear, heart-centered way, for holding open space for me, and for your friendship.
Thank you **Neil Bender** and **Marika Bender** for your wise counsel, friendship and deep kindness.

Thank you again, **Andrew Sterman**, my partner in thought and love.

And in the center of my heart, again I thank my teacher, **Dr. Jeffrey Yuen**, for his vast teachings and for urging me to make the medicine my own. I am forever grateful and inspired.

Further Reading

Dr. Jeffrey Yuen, oral transmission. A primary source of oral transmission of Classical Chinese Medicine at an international level is Jeffrey Yuen, the 88th generation of his Taoist lineage: Yu Ching Huang Lao Pai, (Jade Purity School, Yellow Emperor/Lao Tzu sect); 26th generation of Chuan Chen Lung Men Pai (Complete Reality School, Dragon Gate Sect).

Wu Jing-Nuan, translator, *Ling Shu* or *The Spiritual Pivot* (Honolulu: University of Hawaii Press, 1993).

Zhongjing Zhang, Feng Ye, Nigel Wiseman, Craig Mitchell, and Ye Feng, *Shang Han Lun*, *On Cold Damage* (Brookline: Paradigm, 1999).

Bing Wang with Nelson Liansheng Wu, Andrew Qi Wu, translators, *Yellow Emperor's Canon Internal Medicine* (Beijing: China Science and Technology Press, 1999).

Maoshing Ni, *The Yellow Emperor's Classic of Medicine* (Boston: Shambhala, 1995).

Paul Unschuld, general editor and translator, Hermann Tessenow, translator, *Huang Di Nei Jing Su Wen: An Annotated Translation of Huang Di's Inner Classic* (Berkeley: University of California Press, 2011).

Huang-Fu Mi, *The Systematic Classic of Acupuncture and Moxibustion* (Boulder: Blue Poppy Press, 1993).

Paul Unschuld, translator, *Nan Ching, Classic of Difficult Issues* (Berkeley: University of California Press, 1986).

Andrew Sterman, *Welcoming Food, Diet as Medicine for the Home Cook and Other Healers*, 2 volumes (New York: Classical Wellness Press, 2020).

Ioannis Solos, *Gold Mirrors and Tongue Reflections: The Cornerstone Classics of Chinese Medicine Tongue Diagnosis - The Ao Shi Shang Han Jin Jing Lu, and the Shang Han She Jian* (Vancouver, Canada: Singing Dragon Press, 2012). This book translates the first textbook of tongue diagnosis, Scholar Ao's *Gold Mirror Records*, first published in 1341; and a second book, *Tongue Reflections in Cold Damage*, first published in 1668, featuring the tongue color analysis.

Nancy Holroyde-Downing, *Tongues on Fire: On the Origins and Transmission of a System of Tongue Diagnosis*, PhD dissertation, University College London, 2017.

About the Author

Ann Cecil-Sterman, MS, LAc, is the author of the widely acclaimed books, *The Art of Pulse Diagnosis*, *Illustrations of the Complete Acupuncture System*, and *Advanced Acupuncture: A Clinic Manual*, a required text in many acupuncture schools in the United States. She travels all over the world, to Spain, England, Mexico, Italy, Australia, Canada, Poland, and all over the United States, to teach the application and methodology of the Complement Channels, the art of pulse diagnosis, and with her husband, Andrew Sterman, the use of food as medicine. For many years she taught Advanced Clinical Observation and was a senior clinic supervisor at the school of acupuncture founded by Dr. Jeffrey Yuen in 1997 in New York City. She is a long-time student of Dr. Yuen, having extensively studied acupuncture, diet, Chinese medical history, herbs, Qigong, essential oils, stones, and philosophy with him across North America. Ann was director of the Classical Wellness Center in Manhattan where for many years she practiced and taught classes on advanced diagnosis and the theory and application of Classical Chinese Medicine. Currently, her patients—children and adults of all ages—come from all over the world, working through illnesses, or on personal cultivation. Ann's practice features the Complement Channels of acupuncture—the Sinew, Luo, Divergent, and Eight Extraordinary Channels—and is augmented with Classical Chinese dietary therapeutic guidance. Ann also paints large-scale abstract works depicting physiological function, especially pulses. As a musician, one of her three CDs was nominated for an ARIA (Australian Grammy). She occasionally tours with the Philip Glass Ensemble, having toured with them in Europe, Australia and the United States. She lives in Chelsea, Manhattan, with her husband and two children. www.anncecilsterman.com

About the Designer

Cody Dodo, MS, LAc, studied acupuncture under Dr. Jeffrey Yuen at the Swedish Institute in New York and later completed advanced studies with Dr. Yuen in acupuncture and Chinese dietary therapy. Prior to his pursuit of acupuncture, Cody had a long career as a graphic designer in the publishing industry. Cody has a private acupuncture practice in Manhattan, and teaches Classical Acupuncture internationally, and at Pacific College of Health and Science. He also designed the author's other books, *Advanced Acupuncture: A Clinic Manual* (2012, 2018), *Illustrations of the Complete Acupuncture System* (2014), and *The Art of Pulse Diagnosis* (2015).

INDEX

E

F

G

H

I

J

K

L

M

N

O

P

T

U

V

W

X

Y

Z

www.ingramcontent.com/pod-product-compliance
Ingram Content Group UK Ltd.
Pitfield, Milton Keynes, MK11 3LW, UK
UKHW061413111026
15625UKWH00050B/587
* 9 7 8 0 9 8 3 7 7 2 0 2 6 *